Practices in Children's Nursing

For Churchill Livingstone:

Publishing Manager, Health Professions: Ellen Green/Inta Ozols
Head of Project Management: Ewan Halley
Project Development Manager: Valerie Dearing
Designers: Judith Wright/George Ajayi
Page Make-up: Gerard Heyburn

Practices in Children's Nursing

Guidelines for Hospital and Community

Edited by

Sally Huband BA RGN RSCN SCM RNT
Formerly Senior Lecturer, Paediatrics, Sussex and Kent Institute, Brighton, UK

Ethel Trigg MBA RN RSCN DMS FETC
Head of Clinical Practice, Worthing and Southlands Hospitals NHS Trust, West Sussex, UK

Foreword by

Dame Yvonne Moores
Chief Nursing Officer/Director of Nursing, Department of Health, London, UK

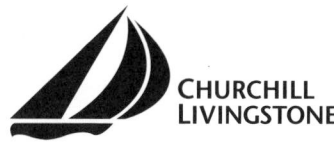

CHURCHILL
LIVINGSTONE

EDINBURGH   LONDON   NEW YORK   PHILADELPHIA   ST LOUIS   SYDNEY   TORONTO 2000

CHURCHILL LIVINGSTONE
An imprint of Harcourt Publishers Limited

First published 2000

ISBN 0 443 05875 X

British Library Cataloguing in Publication Data
A catalogue record for this book is available from the British
Library.

Library of Congress Cataloging in Publication Data
A catalog record for this book is available from the Library of
Congress.

Note
Medical knowledge is constantly changing. As new information becomes available, changes in treatment, procedures,
equipment and the use of drugs become necessary.
The editors, contributors and the publishers have, as far as it
is possible, taken care to ensure that the information given in
this text is accurate and up to date. However, readers are
strongly advised to confirm that the information, especially
with regard to drug usage, complies with current legislation
and standards of practice.

Printed in China

Contents

Clinical and Community Coordinators

CLINICAL COORDINATORS

SHEFFIELD
Allison Butler RGN RSCN EN(G) MHS (cert)
Senior Nurse, Sheffield Children's Hospital NHS Trust, Sheffield, UK

Practices 5, 8, 23, 25, 27, 28, 31, 38, 39

BIRMINGHAM
Julia Fearon RGN RSCN EB 934, 998, 870 C & G 730
Clinical Coordinator, Birmingham Children's Hospital NHS Trust, Birmingham, UK

Practices 3, 4, 12, 19, 20, 22, 26, 32

BRISTOL
Jenny Kay MBA BA (Hons) RGN RSCN ENB 415 998
Formerly Clinical Manager, Paediatrics, Southmead Health Services NHS Trust, Bristol, UK
Presently Nursing Officer, Communications, Department of Health, London, UK

Practices 1, 9, 10, 11, 14, 16, 29, 36

Jenny Kay wrote the above practices whilst working at Bristol. The practices therefore do not necessarily reflect government policy.

GREAT ORMOND STREET
Susan MacQueen MSC RGN RSCN
Clinical Nurse Specialist Infection Control, Great Ormond Street Hospital for Children NHS Trust, Great Ormond Street, London, UK
Control of infection; Practices 2, 6, 18, 21, 30, 33, 34, 35, 42

GLASGOW
Toby A Mohammed MN (Specialty in Educ) RGN RSCN PGCE
Lecturer in Children's Nursing, Glasgow Caledonian University, Glasgow. UK

Practices 7, 13, 15, 17, 23, 24, 37, 40, 41

COMMUNITY COORDINATORS

Pam Masini RGN RSCN ENB 931 (Continuing Care of the Dying Patient and Family), 998, N51 (Principles of Managing Children's Pain)
Paediatric Community Office, Stoke Mandeville Hospital NHS Trust, Aylesbury, UK with advice and support from:
Julia O'Dwyer BMedSci (Hons) Specialist and Community Health Care Practice RGN RSCN R52 (Paediatric Oncology Course)
Community Children's Nurse, Rotherham Priority Health NHS Trust, Rotherham, UK

Introduction to Community

Contributors

Anni Black RGN RSCN DPSN
Sister, Sheffield Children's Hospital NHS Trust, Sheffield, UK

Practice 39

Janice Colson MA RSCN RGN Dip of Nursing
Education RNT
Principal Lecturer Child Health, Faculty of Health Care & Social Sciences, University of Luton, Stoke Mandeville Hospital, Aylesbury, UK

Concepts

Jacqueline Denyer RGN RSCN RHV
Clinical Nurse Specialist Epidermolysis Bullosa, Department of Dermatology, Great Ormond Street Hospital for Children NHS Trust, London, UK

Practice 33

Barbara Doyle BSci (Hons) RGN RSCN CertOnc
Senior Sister, Sheffield Children's Hospital NHS Trust, Sheffield, UK

Practice 8

Tricia Deeley RGN RSCN
Senior Nurse Sedationist, Great Ormond Street Hospital for Children NHS Trust, Great Ormond Street, London, UK

Practice 30

Susan M Fisher RSCN
Clinical Nurse Specialist Pain Relief, Pain Relief Service, Yorkhill NHS Trust, Glasgow, UK

Practice 23

Faith Gibson MSc (Cancer Nursing) RGN RSCN
OncCert CertEd
Senior Lecturer Nurse Researcher, South Bank University, London, UK and Great Ormond Street Hospital for Children NHS Trust, London, UK

Practices 21, 42

Jane Hutchins RGN RSCN DPSN
Sister, Sheffield Children's Hospital NHS Trust, Sheffield, UK

Practice 38

Helen Johnson BSc (Hons) RGN RSCN ENB 216
Clinical Nurse Specialist, Stoma Care, Great Ormond Street Hospital for Children NHS Trust, London, UK

Practice 35

Julie Knowles RGN RSCN
Paediatric Diabetes Nurse, Community Health Sheffield/Sheffield Children's Hospital NHS Trust, Sheffield, UK

Practice 5

Fiona Lynch RGN RSCN
Staff Nurse, Sheffield Children's Hospital NHS Trust, Sheffield, UK

Practice 31

Harriet Martin GradDipPhys MRCP
Senior Physiotherapist, Birmingham Children's

Hospital NHS Trust, Birmingham,UK

Practice 26

Becky McClelland RGN RSCN
Staff Nurse, Sheffield Children's Hospital NHS
Trust, Sheffield, UK

Practice 27

Wendy Nelson NZRN DipNurs RSCN BSc (Hons)
Nursing Studies
Nursing Practice Educator, Great Ormond Street
Hospital for Children NHS Trust, London, UK

Practice 21

Sue Pickup MMedSci (Clinical Nursing) RGN RSCN
CNS Pain Management, Sheffield Children's
NHS Trust, Sheffield, UK

Practice 23

Gill Rennie RGN RSCN SCM ENB 405
SCBU Liaison Nurse, Stoke Mandeville Hospital
NHS Trust, Aylesbury, UK

Practice 22

Stephen Rowley RGN RSCN BSc (Hons)
Charge Nurse, Ward PPW3, University College
London Hospitals, London, UK

Practice 2

Anita Ryan BSc (Hons) Child Health RGN RM RSCN
AdDipChild Development
Ward Sister, Dermatology Unit, Great Ormond
Street Hospital for Children NHS Trust, London, UK

Practice 42

Helen Shipton NNEB HPSEB AEB Counselling 7307
Teaching Certificate
Formerly Community Play Specialist, Stoke
Mandeville NHS Trust, Aylesbury, UK

Appendix: Play

Sue Spurling MA RGN RSCN RCNT RHV (Dip) ENB
405 RCST TIDHA MRQA
Senior Lecturer, Paediatrics, Faculty of Health
Care & Social Sciences, University of Luton,
High Wycombe, UK

Appendix: Complementary Therapies

Rosemary Turnbull RSCN BSc (Hons) Child Health
ENB N25 998
Formerly Paediatric Dermatology Nurse, Great
Ormond Street Hospital for Children NHS Trust,
London, UK

Practice 33

Alison Warren RGN RSCN ENB 415 998
Sister, Paediatric Intensive Care Unit,
Birmingham Children's Hospital NHS Trust,
Birmingham, UK

Aileen Wilson DCR
Superintendent of Cross Sectional Imaging,
Worthing and Southlands NHS Trust, UK

Practice 30

Frances Wood RGN RSCN DPSN BA (Hons) HCP
Sister, Sheffield Children's Hospital NHS Trust,
Sheffield, UK

Practice 25

Preface

This book aims to provide nursing students and qualified staff with a manual of common practices in children's nursing.

Why is this book needed?

Children's nursing textbooks generally do not aim to give details of the actual practices that students and qualified nurses are called upon to undertake. Some hospitals have their own 'procedure book' but in district general hospitals this is likely to be adult oriented.

We hope this book will be a useful reference for those working with children in hospital and in the community. It is not intended to cover neonatal and children's intensive care areas, as the editors felt that if these were included the practices would become too cumbersome.

About the book

The clinical nursing staff of five well-known children's centres (Glasgow, Sheffield, Birmingham, Bristol and Great Ormond Street) have been involved in researching and writing the practices. All practices were then reviewed by another centre, to avoid the book becoming parochial. In spite of this, we are aware that some centres will disagree with some of the content. The practices have also been read by community children's nurses and additions made, where necessary, to enable nurses caring for children in the community to utilise the book.

To avoid repetition in the book, some issues are addressed in the introductory part, and we would strongly recommend that those chapters, which underpin all clinical practice, are read first. Children's nursing is family centred and although not every practice refers to parents, carers and siblings, the editors would like to stress that it is a fundamental principle that they should be included wherever possible.

There are two appendixes: the use of play as a distraction when nursing children is well known and the brief appendix on play in intended to reinforce this; there is also an appendix on complementary therapies, as these are becoming more commonly used and many families may be using one or more, as well as more traditional medicine.

It was decided not to follow a nursing model for the practices as there are many different ones in use and most units have developed their own, so we felt that using a model would cause unnecessary confusion. For ease of use and reference, most practices are discussed under the following headings:

- Introduction
- Rationale
- Factors to note
- Guidelines
- Equipment
- Method
- Special observations and complications
- Dos and Do Nots
- References and Further Reading

The practices are supported by illustrations as appropriate.

We would like to think that this practice manual would become a well-thumbed book in a variety of clinical settings. We hope that it will be useful and will help nurses reflect on their practice and assist them in seeing that the children in their care receive the highest standard of nursing that is possible.

Sally Huband
Ethel Trigg

Sussex 1999

Acknowledgements

Allison Butler would like to thank Nichola Butler and Ruth White, Respiratory Nurses, and Pat Wilson, Practice Development Nurse, who assisted in the review process, Hussein Khatib, Chief Nurse Executive, for his support, and all staff who assisted the authors in the writing of the guidelines. Julia Fearon would like to thank The Procedure Group, Birmingham Children's Hospital NHS Trust: Elaine Berry RN (Child) DipNurs; Julie Clissett RGN RSCN; Pauline Dewick RGN RSCN ENB 415, The Bereavement Trust and The Nutritional Care Team and Birmingham Children's Hospital NHS Trust. Jenny Kay would like to thank Linda Prime, Pam Carpenter, Jenny Lewis, Maureen Betts, Gill Rothwell, David Murray, the entire Paediatric team and the library staff at Southmead Health Services NHS Trust, Bristol, Helen Langton and Lin Law, at the University of the West of England, William Booth at the Bristol Children's Hospital, and Cathy Cairns at Frenchay Healthcare NHS Trust. Toby A. Mohammed would like to thank Maureen Lilley (Nurse Practitioner), Morag Liddell (Ward Manager), Liz Johnston (former Midwifery Sister), Susan Maxwell (ITU Sister), Alma Matheson (Renal Unit Sister), Diane King (Home Care Renal Sister), all from Yorkhill Hospitals NHS Trust in Glasgow, for reviewing completed drafts. Also thanks to Cath McColl, Clinical Director/Service Manager for support and encouragement.

Foreword

I am delighted to write the Foreword to this excellent book. I know that children's nurses everywhere will welcome this textbook, which discusses the clinical nursing care of children and their families as a unique area of expertise. It does not just apply standard nursing techniques to children as though they were small adults. It addresses the special needs and problems of children at all stages of their development, from baby to young adult. The family contribution to care is seen as central to the well being of the child. I am also pleased to see the emphasis on care at home.

The authors have given a wealth of information, tips and ideas. They share their own breadth of experience in practice, which has come from across all regions in the UK. All practice is evidence based and it is balanced with the sometimes difficult art of nursing children and their families in hospital and at home. The authors have achieved the complex task of effectively combining theory and practice, as well as the art and science of nursing.

In 'Making a Difference', the recently published strategy for nursing, midwifery and health visiting in England, the Government sets out the relevance of their quality framework, outlined in a 'First Class Service' for nurses. These plans are built around setting standards, delivering them at a local level and monitoring standards through benchmarking and clinical audit. This book provides a practical example of just that - it sets high, evidence based standards of practice, and suggests ways of delivering these at local level. I am sure that nurses across the country will also see the potential to use these standards as benchmarks against which their own practice can be audited.

Congratulations to all the chapter authors, Sally Huband and Ethel Trigg, the editors, and Harcourt Publishers. They have created a textbook that will, I am sure, be a standard reference for nursing students, as well as qualified nurses in practice, management and education for many years to come.

Concepts

Introduction

In the latter part of the 20th century members of western society are generally better educated, more informed about their rights, and thus have greater expectations of health care provision (Atherton 1994). These circumstances have inevitably created more demands on the nursing profession. In response, nursing has had to move away from the traditional image in which nurses were seen as handmaidens to the doctor.

The handmaiden image is being replaced by that of a professional practitioner, with an ever extending repertoire of skills, who is educated to practise from a sound, research-based knowledge. Today's practitioners in children's nursing sometimes feel that they do not have the opportunity to provide much 'hands-on care'. This is because the philosophy of family-centred care has been almost nationally embraced. Therefore, whilst parents and other family members are doing what were previously considered 'nursing duties', nurses are having to be responsible for teaching families, providing support and helping families to make decisions in the best interests of their sick child. These activities may often present nurses with situations in which they have to make some difficult decisions. Such circumstances, therefore, suggest that nurses have to feel competent about the delivery of their practical skills in addition to thinking in a clear and rational manner about the emotional and social care they provide.

The aim of this text is to provide nurses with a guide to the many and varied practical skills which they may be required to undertake when caring for sick children. Before commencing any practice there are a number of issues with which all nurses should be familiar. These issues include the nurse's own accountability for her actions, her role as an advocate for children and parents, the provision of information to children and parents, enabling them to consent from an informed basis, and finally an awareness of the elements of risk management.

This chapter will provide an overview of the issues identified above and aims to place them in context for nurses caring for sick children in a variety of care environments. Whilst each concept will be discussed under a separate heading within the text, they are interrelated and, when appropriate, cross-references will be made.

Accountability

Accountability may be defined as 'the taking of responsibility for one's own behaviour' (Curtin & Flaherty 1982, p. 72).

The definition provides evidence of an abstract concept which nurses should explore further since it is a term frequently used by and about nurses. Student nurses often ask questions such as: 'If we give a wrong drug, who is accountable?' or 'Supposing a child injures himself whilst he is playing with me in the playroom, am I accountable?' Students have every right to pose such questions and they should be exploring the issues whilst they are still students. Although it is impossible to explore every conceivable situation, students should be provided with guiding principles which will help in their decision-making.

Students are not the only ones to have unanswered questions about accountability. Qualified nurses also have unanswered questions about their ever extending scope of professional practice. They are, on the whole, very aware of the implications of ever expanding boundaries of practice and thus realise that there is not room for complacency. So just what does it mean for a nurse to be accountable? Pyne (1988) suggests that the UKCC *Code of Professional Conduct* (1992a) is an extended definition of professional accountability. However, it may be argued that this code provides guidelines for the professions and, like all guidelines, it is open to interpretation by individuals.

Nurses should avoid individual interpretations of their professional accountability since in so doing they may bring their careers into jeopardy, together with the reputations of their employing institutions and the profession. Heywood Jones (1990) stresses the importance of every practitioner conforming to the code. Therefore, in an attempt to demystify the existing ambiguity, it would seem appropriate to explore what accountability means to the nurse. Howard (1997) states that practice with accountability is a key concept in the effective delivery of health care in modern nursing. This suggests that nurses have not always been willing or able to be accountable for their practice. Nursing has changed and is still changing. These changes include extending the boundaries of practice, for example administering intravenous drugs, taking blood samples via venous access and in some very specialist roles, such as the neonatal nurse practitioner, attending deliveries of infants in place of a doctor. The majority of nurses undertaking these specialist skills are now educated to diploma and degree level, with an increasing number achieving higher academic accolades. This chapter is about practice and the aim is to explore how this educational status might inform practice.

Practice for the children's nurse may involve undertaking all aspects of care for a child who, for example, is highly dependent on nursing care. Conversely, it may entail teaching parents how to carry out care such as administering nutritional needs via a nasogastric tube or more commonly, where the child has a long-term need, via a gastrostomy (Dearmun et al 1995).

Whatever the practice, the nurse is accountable for her decisions and actions. This fact is emphasised in *The Scope of Professional Practice* (UKCC 1992b). The document also emphasises the practitioner's need to maintain and develop knowledge and competence. Examples of maintaining and developing knowledge in the field of children's nursing may range from the technical knowledge of how to prime and maintain the latest syringe driver for the delivery of intravenous postoperative analgesia to the application of wet wrap bandages for the treatment of a child suffering with eczema (Donaldson 1997). In both of these situations the responsibility to practise intelligently is with the individual nurse.

In the course of their learning student nurses frequently rotate to new areas of practice, where they may encounter different, unfamiliar practices and new equipment. In such circumstances they must indicate their knowledge deficit and request appropriate orientation. It is the responsibility of all nurses to question when unsure. Curtin & Flaherty (1982) emphasise the importance of nurses constantly striving to add to their personal knowledge and to perfect their professional skills. Nurses must recognise that they can learn from each other and, in addition, be proactive in seeking out appropriate study days and courses to attend. By undertaking these activities they uphold a commitment to education and sound practice.

However, in some instances the development of practice has been in advance of educational provision. Perhaps one of the most significant of these is the increasing trend towards caring for sick children in their own homes (Whiting 1997). This activity may be seen as responding to and upholding recommendations made repeatedly since the Platt Report was published in 1958.

The introduction to the section on nursing practices in the community addresses the role of the community children's nurse. These nurses are often isolated from colleagues for long periods during their working day, making it difficult to discuss issues when uncertainty arises. They should not feel obligated to undertake practices for which they do not have appropriate skills. However, they are responsible for their own knowledge base and effective decision-making, since their level of accountability is no more or less than that of any other nurse.

Care for a sick child at home is mainly provided by the parents, but when the community nurse visits she will be expected to provide support, guidance and some care. Parents need to see evidence of a competent and confident practitioner. Such situations provide the ultimate opportunity for nurses to exercise their professional judgement. Carter & Campbell (1997) identify professional judgement as a complex concept and state that 'no single decision will be the same as another individual decision' (p. 5).

The administration of intravenous drugs is one area where nurses are constantly expanding the boundaries of their practice. Nurses who are willing and able to be accountable for the administration of often extremely potent cocktails of intravenous drugs can enable the maintenance of care for very sick children at home and in hospital. This type of work does not come within the remit of all nurses. Nurses who undertake such work will have completed specialist courses beyond registration, thus ensuring that they have the requisite knowledge and skills. However, it is each individual's responsibility to ensure that she maintains the knowledge through regular updating and the skills by practising when the opportunity arises.

Finally in accounting for her actions, the nurse must ensure that those actions are:

- explainable
- defendable
- based on knowledge rather than on tradition or myth.

These points link back to the current education and training of nurses. There is no need for nurses to base their actions on tradition or myth any longer because there is now an existing body of knowledge from which to draw in support of all actions.

Informed consent

Consent may be defined as 'giving permission, to acquiesce or accept something which is done or planned by someone else'. To be informed is 'to have information, to be conversant with' (Hanks 1987). When these two words are combined they indicate that a person understands the nature of what he or she is giving permission for someone else to do to him or her.

Traditionally it has been accepted that consent is being given for medical and nursing treatments by virtue of the child being in hospital. Formal consent, by the signing of a form, was only requested and given prior to surgery. These circumstances meant that parents returning to their child after a brief spell of absence might find some change in the treatment regime. A further test may have been carried out or a new intravenous line inserted; the list is endless. Such situations clearly did not provide opportunities for information to be exchanged and consent given.

When children require medical and nursing care, consent should be obtained before any treatment is given. The question of who provides that consent is a frequently debated issue within medical and nursing circles. The debate on informed consent was once confined to the involvement of children within the research process. Richardson & Webber (1995) and Coyne (1998) write about the involvement of children in the research process at some length and other writers cite the Nuremberg Code as the first attempt to provide a code of practice for any researchers using human subjects in their experiments (Brykczyńska 1989). This section is about informed consent to the more routine practices of nursing care.

Recipients of today's health service are generally more aware of their rights to appropriate information on which to base consent to, or refusal of, treatment and care. Since the introduction of the Children Act in 1989, many aspects of issues relating to children's rights have been highlighted. Dickenson (1994) states that statute law has endowed children with more rights whilst case law has decreased their choices regarding their own treatment. In brief, this means that young people under the age of 18 years may give consent to treatment, but they have no right to refuse treatment.

In a text which is primarily about practices that may be undertaken in the delivery of care to children, it would seem most appropriate to provide some exploration of what is required of nurses before they administer any care to a child. Additionally, the rights of the child and family regarding consent to and participation in the procedure are central issues for consideration. It is not possible to look at every practice within this text; rather, a general discussion will be provided with a selection of examples from practice.

Consent is now a more everyday, practical issue. The age of the child and the level of cognitive development in relation to competence are factors central to the debate (Coyne 1998, Orr 1999). The concept of informed consent, therefore, should be considered in the context of specific situations. However, a basic understanding of the concept and relevant supporting criteria is necessary first.

The following section will aim to explore the concept as it relates to children in a variety of health and illness situations.

From the definition of consent, it is easy to see how, in naiveté, an individual may be harmed if he is neither informed of nor conversant with the appropriate detail of what is planned by another person. This particular issue is discussed below. Because of their age and stage of development, children are a particularly vulnerable group who, even when provided with information about an aspect of care, may not comprehend the implications.

There are a number of general principles relating to consent as identified by Dimond (1996). These include:

- Competent adults have a right to give or refuse consent to treatment.
- Without consent or other justification, any touching of the person would constitute in law a trespass on the person. For example, an operation carried out without a consent form being signed prior to administration of the premedication could constitute a trespass.
- Where there has been a trespass on the person then the victim can claim compensation through a court action without proof of harm.
- To claim that the action was undertaken for the benefit of the patient would not be a valid defence if there were not consent or other justification recognised in law.

Charles-Edwards (1995) also stresses the importance of consent before any bodily touching takes place. Without consent, touching another person, be they patient or not, could be held as an assault. Frequently, consent is implied informally rather than stated in a formal manner, as for example when a form is signed prior to surgery.

It is essential that informed consent is obtained before any treatment or care is given to a patient. Nicholson (1986) emphasises the importance of this by stating that voluntary and informed consent is mandatory to turn what would otherwise be a trespass or assault into a legally sanctioned act. Trespass or assault may result in civil or criminal proceedings. Additionally, for the consent to be legally valid, the following essential elements should be included:

- sufficient information
- the capacity to understand the information
- consent is given voluntarily without coercion (Charles-Edwards 1995).

These essential elements provide a useful framework on which to base further exploration.

Sufficient information

The information given should include a full explanation of the proposed treatment and any incidental procedures which may be involved. This should apply to nursing practices as well as to surgical and medical procedures. The information should be provided in a manner intelligible to the child and parents. Jargon should be avoided. This is particularly important for children who readily misinterpret statements like 'being put to sleep' as what happened to their pet they never saw again. 'Coming back from theatre with a plaster on' has a different meaning when the operation is to be an osteotomy from when a band aid is applied for a grazed knee or cut finger. The child is likely to be more familiar with the latter and the difference needs to be made clear with the use of toys and diagrams, according to the child's age and cognitive level. Furthermore, it should not be assumed that parents will always understand the information they are offered. Perhaps this experience of hospital is the first for the parents as well as the child.

Issues such as risks, benefits and alternatives to the proposed treatment may be particularly difficult for some parents to come to terms with, making their responsibility to provide informed consent on behalf of their child particularly hard. Parents probably find it easier to provide consent for themselves than on behalf of their child (Alderson 1990). The risks and benefits of all options should be explained in clear, logical terms, avoiding misinformation or omission.

Doctors have a duty to inform the child and parents about medical procedures. Parents may assume that the doctors know best, which in fact places a heavy burden on their shoulders when, for example, all treatment options carry equally high risks. Doctors may use their medical knowledge and terminology to avoid questions from parents. Such situations provide evidence of poor communication and may leave parents to make decisions on consent in ignorance.

Nurses have a particular role in preparing children for procedures, be they medical or nursing. Often this has to be done in stages. An overview may be given initially, but this may be insufficient for the young child. At this point it would seem appropriate to cite the example of Bobbie, who was being nursed in a hip spica plaster. Following his operation he would not eat. Several days of coaxing made little difference to his non-existent appetite. Explanations about the importance of food for getting better had no effect, but suddenly the 4-year-old started to cry and all was revealed. He did not want to eat because he thought the plaster cast was covering his anus and so preventing him from having his bowels open. Therefore, if he did not eat he would not need to defecate.

This scenario illustrates the importance of the provision of ongoing information. The resolution of Bobbie's problem was achieved through the simple play activity of applying a similar plaster to a doll and providing the necessary explanation. Many situations are less complex. For example, when a nurse is performing a dressing, she may have told the child what she is going to do, but it is nonetheless important to explain each step of the procedure as well. This is particularly relevant if the child cannot or does not wish to look at what is happening.

The capacity to understand the information

In the case of children and young people, the capacity to understand the information is probably the most controversial aspect of obtaining informed consent. Two major issues arise out of this. They are the child's ability to be rational according to his level of cognitive development and the recognition by others of the child's autonomy.

The child's chronological age and competence will naturally influence his ability to participate in the decision-making process. Therefore, in the early years of life such decisions are usually made by the child's parents (Charles-Edwards 1995). However, children do have views and these can provide a rich source of information on how they feel in any given situation (Coyne 1998).

Parents, by virtue of that title, have a responsibility for the health and well-being of their children. When a child is ill, parents may be faced with some very difficult decisions about the best possible treatment options for their child. They may spend considerable time in discussion with medical and nursing staff about the course of the treatment and potential outcomes.

Parents who consent on behalf of their child are consenting by proxy. Informed proxy consent requires the exchange and evaluation of information to enable the best possible or least harmful decision to be made for the child. Whenever possible the child should be involved in the process (Alderson 1990). Proxy consent may be seen as a contentious issue with arguments that children do not authorise the proxy. If they were competent to do that they could make the decision for themselves. Doctors sometimes feel that they should act as the proxy, rather than the parents.

Proxy consent cannot provide complete protection, but it should allow for questioning and examination of decisions and increase the potential for children to receive the best possible care.

As children develop they have a right to information about their care and this should be provided in an age-appropriate and child-friendly way (Purssell 1995). Donaldson (1987) writes in support of the ability of preschool children to understand the feelings of other people when they are provided in social terms familiar to the child in everyday life. This suggests that preschool children may well be capable of contributing to aspects of decisions about their care. The preschool child will be able to have choice, for example in which hand or arm an intravenous infusion will be sited, or whether he would prefer to remove the tape holding the dressing in place. These may seem simple activities, but they allow the child to retain some degree of control over his well-being, and in giving choice the nurse demonstrates respect for the child's increasing autonomy. The doctrine of informed consent is a reminder to all members of the health care team that they should respect the patient's rights.

Studies undertaken in the United States found that 5-year-olds with terminal cancer were able to make decisions about future therapy versus supportive care regardless of parental involvement (Nitschke et al 1982). There is no substantial evidence of replication of such studies. They were undertaken with groups of particular children in circumstances where they had more experience of health care than many other children. Nonetheless, providers of health care should be cognisant of such work and be prepared to involve

children in the decision-making process. Alderson (1990) states that consent is more than being passively informed. Citing the revised Declaration of Helsinki in 1983 she emphasises that when minor children are able to give consent then that consent should be obtained together with the consent of the minor's legal guardian. A further recommendation is that from the age of 7 a child's assent should be sought, and from the age of 14 the child's consent. Assent is agreement, consent is informed and voluntary commitment (Alderson 1990).

With a child's increasing age the issues relating to informed consent become more complex. Weithorn & Campbell (1982) identified that the majority of 14-year-olds have the same ability as adults to make decisions about their health care.

More recently, Orr (1999) supports earlier writers in stating that children at the concrete operational stage of development are competent to give informed consent if they have had concrete experience of the planned treatment. In discussing this issue Orr cites that case of Jaymee Bowen (child B) who had two courses of chemotherapy and a bone marrow transplant in her fight against leukaemia in 1995. It is argued that because of these experiences Jaymee was in a position to understand the meaning and implications of further proposed treatment.

However, English common law is vague about the age of consent to medical treatment (Alderson 1990). Under the Family Law Reform Act of 1969 a child aged 16 or 17 years is able to provide valid consent to treatment (Dimond 1996). There are limitations to this in as much as it does not give young persons in this age group the right to consent to organ or blood donation. This may be permissible under common law providing the young person has the competence to make the decision (Dimond 1996). Parents or legal guardians are, therefore, expected to sign a consent for anyone under 16 years of age, particularly within the hospital setting.

However, in other situations young persons under the age of 16 have been allowed to make decisions about their health care without parental involvement. These circumstances were brought about following the Gillick case in 1983–1984 (Gillick 1985) which helped to establish a standard of competence known as 'Gillick Competence' (Dimond 1996). A Gillick competent child is one who is deemed to have sufficient maturity to understand the nature of the treatment being offered and to make a decision about that in his or her own right (Richardson & Webber 1995). The judge also held that parents' interest in their child's welfare did not amount to a right, but should more accurately be described as a responsibility (Dimond 1996). This particular issue has now been more strongly emphasised in the Children Act 1989.

Consent is given voluntarily without coercion

When communicating information, coercion must be avoided since consent is nullified by coercion. Coercion is most likely to occur when parents and child (if his cognitive ability allows) adopt the attitude that the doctor knows best. This may well be the situation when the procedure is complex and it is the doctor who is obtaining consent.

Alderson (1990) identifies three types of coercive power:

- obvious coercion, which is the provision or withholding of treatment in the knowledge that the course of action is not what the child or parents want
- the provision of treatment which the patient or parent is unlikely to want combined with the blocking of questions from parents about possible alternatives
- preventing patients from making a choice because they do not realise that there are alternatives available.

These particular powers seem harsh, but in reality they do happen and she provides examples from experiences with children and parents in a cardiothoracic unit. Parents and children who are deemed competent should not feel coerced into agreeing to a course of treatment.

Parents may find it difficult to refuse treatment on behalf of their children for a variety of reasons. Primarily, it is accepted that parents want the best for their child and if this means pursuing lengthy courses of drug therapy or extensive surgical intervention they probably feel the prospect of a positive outcome is worth the endurance of a harsh intervening period. However, adults make decisions for children from an adult perspective (Richardson & Webber 1995). Although well intentioned, this may not be what the child wants. Additionally, it may stifle the child's developing autonomy.

As discussed above, children are capable of making some choices about their health care and treatment from an early age. With increasing age they can become more involved, and it is perhaps between the older age group and parents that conflicts about treatment choices are likely to arise. Where the question arises over whether treatment should be continued or cease in the case of a young person with cancer, parents may, want the treatment. The young person who is having to suffer the consequences may, with the confidence of youth, be more able to say that enough is enough and further treatment should be withdrawn. In these or similar circumstances the child's viewpoint may be ignored.

Many nurses using this text may not be involved in major life and death issues. They are more likely to have to deal frequently with children and young people who may not wish to undergo some of the treatments described in the clinical skills sections of this book. In such circumstances the Children Act 1989 serves as a reminder that children in our society can exercise more autonomy and, where possible, the views of the child should be taken into account'.

In this section, the issues which surround informed consent have been explored and have included the essential elements of consent and the conflicts which may arise when child and parents are in dispute over the best course of action. Alderson (1990) states that if consent is not reasonably informed, signing a consent can be worse than an empty gesture. It amounts to making a decision which may later cause remorse.

Advocacy

Advocacy has been defined by the United Kingdom Central Council for Nursing, Midwifery and Health Visiting as being 'concerned with promoting and safeguarding the well being and interests of patients and clients' (UKCC 1989, p. 12).

Rushton and colleagues (1996) state that advocacy on behalf of patients and their families is central to the practice of nursing, and they provide a very similar definition to the one offered by the UKCC. Gates (1995) reminds readers of the origins of the word advocate, from the Latin *advocatus*, meaning one who is summoned to give evidence. Woodrow (1997) states that the concept of advocacy comes from legal practice, thus producing visions of courtroom scenes with lawyers pleading the case of their client. This concept and the Latin origins of the word advocate would appear to have some significance for nurses since much of the literature on advocacy is concerned with patients' complaints (Mallik 1997). In such circumstances nurses may well be called to give evidence about the care they have provided. Whether the evidence is verbal or in the form of written statements, there are important implications for the nurse. If a patient or a member of the patient's family complains about the care he has received, nurses may be held accountable. Nurses are expected to uphold their *Code of Professional Conduct* (UKCC 1992a). Circumstances such as these provide nurses with ethical dilemmas and difficult decisions. In circumstances where nurses are working in partnership with parents and the child, trust is an essential element. The nurse is allowed into a privileged position and it is, therefore, important that she is aware of her own values and principles in any given situation.

Children's nurses often struggle when attempting to define their advocacy role (Rushton et al 1996). Anecdotal evidence would suggest that they do not view it in the terms described above. Rather, they interpret it within their daily activities of caring for children, speaking out and acting on behalf of the child. Examples of good practice from nurses' reflections on their role as advocate are provided below. A student nurse recalled how she had prevented a doctor from inserting an intravenous cannula into Jack's arm because he had not had EMLA cream applied for the prescribed time. In a similar situation, Stephanie was hysterical at the thought of yet another blood test. Initially, her parents and the nurse could do nothing to calm her. The doctor was anxious to get the blood samples and requested that she should be held tightly to gain cooperation (Collier & Robinson 1997). The nurse, sensing the tensions, asked the doctor to wait whilst she got the bubble tubes. These brightly coloured objects provided perfect distraction and the test went ahead without further problems. Nurses frequently feel uncomfortable about restraining children for procedures when alternative methods may be as effective (RCN 1999). Furthermore, in a survey by Collier & Robinson (1997), the majority of nurses felt that restraint rather than pain was the most likely cause of distress. The scenarios provide evidence of nurses acting in the child's best interests based on knowledge supported by research.

These scenarios also highlight the probable imbalance of power between health care professionals and patients, particularly between doctors and children. They indicate the vulnerability of sick children and their need for support when confronted by paternalistic medical professionals (Chambers 1992). Whilst it would be unjust to label all doctors as paternalistic, there has been a tradition within medicine that the doctor knows best and therefore patients and nurses will do as they are told.

In fairness to medical colleagues, nurses are also sometimes eager to exert power over children and parents in their care. Making judgemental statements about parental skills, displaying negative attitudes and failing to provide opportunities for parents to participate in their child's care are just some examples of how nurses might demonstrate that they think they know best.

Phillips (1994) states that it takes less time to tell a child what to do than to consult with him about his wishes. Ondrusek, Abramovitch et al (1998) suggest that children will say yes because it is seen as what they should do. Although this refers to the involvement of children in a research study it may readily be translated into a variety of other situations including treatments. Such behaviour may enable the busy nurse, working within a punishing timescale, to complete the dressing, administer the intravenous drugs or apply the skin care. Children may comply with this type of behaviour, but it does not reflect the spirit of advocacy and raises questions about whose best interests are being served.

There are times when nurses may think that they are acting in a child's best interests. For example, in another situation, a staff nurse returned from the operating theatre to the children's ward with a child before her operation, because the anaesthetist was not ready to receive her into the anaesthetic room. The staff nurse had decided that it was in the child's best interests to wait in the less stressful ward environment rather than in the busy corridor by the operating theatre.

This decision was made by the staff nurse in what she considered the child's best interests. There is no evidence to suggest that she had consulted with the child. Furthermore, the child may have been told that by the time she returned to the ward her operation would be over. Also, the nurse may have caused the child's parents to be unnecessarily alarmed by her action of returning to the ward. In this scenario the nurse may have created more tension. It would seem that, if she had not consulted with the child or explained her actions, she had confused her role of advocate with that of exerting power.

In almost every situation when a child is sick, parents and immediate family are faced with uncertainty and ambiguity about the treatment and outcomes of the illness. Additionally, in accepting that the child is ill, parents have to accept that the child needs to be cared for by health professionals and thus as parents they may have to relinquish some of their former parenting roles (Altschuler 1997). It would seem that there is a strong argument for not asking parents to relinquish their parenting role, but rather enabling them to adapt. Adaptation would involve re-establishing the parenting role from being parents of a well child to being parents of a sick child (Rennick 1986).

When introducing the concept of re-establishing the parenting role, Rennick (1986) was discussing parents of children admitted to a children's intensive care unit. However, the strategies are readily transferable to the majority of paediatric care situations. Indeed, such strategies provide ideal opportunities for nurses to act in the child's best interests. This may be done through negotiating what care parents wish to participate in and that which they prefer to hand over to nurses. The idea of nurses being told by parents what they may do for their child could be difficult for some nurses to accept, particularly if they have to embrace the concepts of family-centred care and partnership. However, if the nurse views advocacy as a dimension of her role, then it would seem essential that the other aspects have to be incorporated into the nursing strategy. This very factor may in turn cause nurses to ask themselves some pertinent and leading questions.

It would, therefore, seem relevant to return to further consideration of the application of advocacy within the role of the children's nurse.

Within the concept of family-centred care, the child is seen as part of the family; therefore, when advocating for the child the nurse should also be an advocate for the family – or should she? This raises questions of how nurses view their advocacy role, particularly when confronted with situations where there may be conflicts of interest.

When they occur, conflicts of interest can place the nurse in a very difficult position. Conflicts of interest may arise out of a variety of situations. For example, when children express their views about care regimes (as discussed in the section on informed consent), those views may be negative. Simon, aged 13, has been started on another course of painful intravenous antibiotic therapy. He is still very ill and cannot see an end or even improvement in this illness. He expresses his unhappiness to his nurse and asks that the drugs are stopped. Purssell (1995) suggests that children need a powerful advocate and parents or guardians are in an ideal position for the role. In Simon's case this is not so. Mary, the nurse, knows that Simon's prognosis is poor and feels that she should raise the issue at the forthcoming multi-disciplinary team meeting. She is also aware that Simon's parents and the team members will oppose any suggestions to review the care regime; they want everything possible to be done.

Issues of power and control are raised from this scenario. Mary thinks she will be acting in Simon's best interests. She is the nurse who has most interactions with him; she knows how ill he feels, but that he tries to be cheerful for his parents. Mary also feels that colleagues will experience a sense of failure if they change the care regime. Therefore, they will exert power over Simon and her to continue the treatment.

A further example of where nurses feel that conflicts of interest arise concerns video surveillance of parents when they are suspected of child abuse. Nurses are expected to assume a partnership with parents, whilst at the same time they know that parents are being subjected to covert video surveillance when left alone to care for their child. In situations such as these, nurses and other providers of care for children have to justify carefully what is essentially an invasion of privacy when they take steps to override parental prerogatives (Kohrman et al 1995).

Whilst the above situation arises infrequently and usually in units specially designed for monitoring work with parents who are suspected of abuse, it may be an issue for nurses in other care environments.

Another dimension of the nurse's advocacy role may be seen in working with parents to gain their child's cooperation in a treatment regime, for example teaching the child newly diagnosed as having diabetes about his diet and administration of insulin. Similarly, an older child with cystic fibrosis may find the frequent drugs and physiotherapy tedious. Negotiation with child and parents can enable a more positive approach with everyone acting in the child's best interests.

Finally, when nurses claim to be advocates for children, they should be fighting for appropriate standards of care for all children (Casey 1997). This includes the environment in which children are cared for and the qualifications of those who care for them.

Risk management

'Risk is the potential for an unexpected or unwanted outcome' (Russell 1995, p. 607).

The complex and diverse nature of health care creates a forum for risk activities. Bowden (1996) argues that doctors and nurses should not be prevented from taking risks in the development of treatments and care regimes for patients, providing that the risks are as a result of decisions based on sound knowledge and an understanding of what might be the possible consequences.

Symons (1995) states that risk management is an important feature of current health care systems and should be given a high profile within all organisations. Bowden (1996) urges managers to be proactive in risk management and he identifies three aspects. First, *risk assess-*

ment allows for systems which identify potential litigious events to be put into place. Time should be spent with staff identifying areas in which they feel vulnerable to risks. A breach in the nurse's duty of care as perceived by a patient is cited by Russell (1995) as one example. Secondly, a nurse or student may be asked to undertake a procedure which is beyond her competence. *Risk reduction and control* is the second aspect of risk management. The employment of risk managers may be one effective method of initiating and coordinating the risk-management programme. However, clinical and other line managers should accept risk as to high priority within their responsibility (Bowden 1996). Issues such as the lack of available equipment, perceived staffing shortages and ineffective communications are highlighted by Dineen (1995) as other relevant factors. Finally, *risk transference* is about institutions being covered through insurance for claims that may be brought against them. Tingle (1995) cites the failure of communications as being a central feature in an analysis of complaints about the National Health Service written to *The Times* between 1993 and 1994. Such complaints have escalated since the launch of government reforms in the early 1990s.

At a time when patients and parents are even more aware of their personal rights, legislation and government initiatives such as The Patients Charter Services for Children and Young People (1996), they are invited to complain and of course they do. However, according to Symons (1995), for all the letters of criticism there are approximately 10 times more of commendation received by hospitals. This is an encouraging fact and nurses should be eager to record all comments so that good practice can be extended and poor practices changed.

Health professionals who are aware of the consequences of risk-taking will enter into situations from an informed position and they will be accountable for their actions. Conversely, many risks occur by accident or mistake. The source of such risks may arise from one or more of the following (Bowden 1996):

- a lack of clear policies
- deficient working practices
- poorly defined responsibilities
- inadequate communications
- staff working beyond their level of competence.

The list above combined with the opening quotation from Russell (1995) emphasises the negative connotations of risk. Every health care worker has good reason to be aware of the negative elements of risk since a failure to do so may result in litigation. Solon (1995) cites

litigation as a 'fact of life', with all health care workers being in the potential firing line.

There would appear to be three categories of risk. They might be identified as follows:

- the risks for the child and parents
- the risks for the nurse
- the risks arising from research, which include both the patient and nurse.

Within the context of this book the aim is to facilitate nurses in minimising risk both to the child and parents and to themselves through effective risk management. Risks arising from research may be read about elsewhere (Charles-Edwards 1995 Coyne 1998). However, all nurses should be cognisant of the ethical issues of being involved and involving patients in the research process.

Risks for the child and parents relate to the care and treatment they are being offered. When consenting to treatment and care, children who have the cognitive ability and all parents will judge the information they receive in the light of their own values and circumstances (Charles-Edwards 1995). Decisions will be made after balancing the risks versus the benefits (see Informed consent, above).

With reference to treatment and care, risks are associated with benefits and considered in categories of high risk low benefit and low risk high benefit. An example of high risk low benefit might be the child who is being offered a second heart–lung transplant following rejection of the first one. Conversely, the measles, mumps and rubella (MMR) vaccination may be considered as a low risk high benefit treatment (Richardson & Webber 1995). Family-centred care is a concept central to philosophies in the majority of areas where children are nursed. Nurses should be aware of the risks involved when they do not define clearly what they mean by family-centred care. They should be able to provide evidence of negotiation which has taken place to establish exactly who will undertake which elements of care for the child. There is rather too much evidence which suggests that parents may feel unsupported and neglected in the care of their sick child (Darbyshire 1994).

Aspects of family-centred care provide many additional examples of risks for children, parents and nurses. Feeding, or the provision of food for the child to feed himself, is usually considered to be a normal 'parenting skill'. However, when that food is to be administered via a nasogastric tube or gastrostomy, questions may arise over who should give the feeds. If the parents wish to give the feeds, then nurses must ensure a low risk high benefit situation by teaching the parents this 'new skill' and monitoring their ability until all parties feel equally confident that the parents can carry out the practice. The risk is in handing over to parents what has previously been conceived as nursing care; the benefit is that parents and child can share the closeness of a meal time together. Principles from this scenario can be transferred to many other practices which may involve parents, student nurses or nurses previously unfamiliar with a particular practice.

Risks for nurses may originate from two sources. First some risks arise from complaints by parents as a result of the nurse failing in her duty of care. Examples of the nurse failing in her duty of care might include inadequate securing of a nasogastric tube, resulting in the infant removing the tube and necessitating the passage of another, causing him further distress. In caring for a child who is receiving fluids via a peripheral venous line, the nurse may fail to notice the swelling on the child's arm. When the electronic pump continues to alarm, a second nurse discovers the child's arm is oedematous and hard, indicating the severity of the extravasion.

A lack of written instructions may also give rise to failure in duty of care. For example, at the change-over of shifts, Nurse Small tells Nurse Knight that Joe is having 20 ml of milk 2-hourly and that his bottles are ready in the refrigerator. When the day staff have left, Nurse Knight checks the care plan only to realise that Nurse Small has not completed this for her shift.

The nurse completing the shift has not provided details of the care given; the new nurse has only the verbal report to rely on. This may lead to inappropriate care, with both nurses implicated for failing in their duty of care. Accurate, well-written care plans provide clinical evidence for determining the delivery of care and minimise risk.

Secondly, there are risks which the nurse accepts in exercising her duty of care, for example looking after an infectious patient (Chadwick & Tadd 1992), dealing with an aggressive person in the accident and emergency department, or teaching children and parents in the administration of drugs. Chadwick & Tadd (1992) emphasise that members of the nursing and medical professions are expected to assume a certain level of personal risk as part of their professional obligation.

In order to avoid litigation, management strategies which aim to reduce the incidence of sub-optimal events must be adopted (Dineen 1995). Bowden (1996) argues that a lot of everyday risk management is undertaken on an ad hoc basis in an uncoordinated way. This then raises the question of what strategies should be adopted in order to achieve positive, organised risk management. The remainder of this section will aim to suggest strategies for risk management which may be applicable to the care of children.

The management of risks must become everybody's business. All nurses should be aware of the potential risks each time they enter into a situation with a child and/or his parents. There may be a need for changes in the value system of the organisation which will lead to openness and honesty, enabling individuals to admit to potential or actual mistakes. Only when such incidents are recorded and discussed can action be taken to avoid recurrence. Tingle (1995) suggests that clinical supervision has great potential as a tool to reduce litigation and complaint levels. Many complaints arise from poor communication and records which lack clarity. The potential for this in children's nursing is possibly greater, owing to the tripartite relationship between child, parents and nurse. Where a system such as individualised nursing or named nursing does not exist and everyone contributes, channels of communication may become blurred and there may be no evidence of which nurse did what procedure for which child. The implementation of a clinical supervision programme which facilitates improvements in communication with children and parents and the inclusion of more detail in records could go some way towards effective risk management.

The risk-assessment process should enable the creation of a risk profile and action plan which highlights issues for the most urgent attention. Risk reduction and control is the next stage. Bowden (1996) suggests the employment of risk managers, but theirs would be an advisory and supportive role. The day-to-day organisation relating to the number, types, location and management of claims, complaints and adverse incidents would be undertaken by line managers (Symons 1995, Bowden 1996). The importance of record-keeping is highlighted by Solon (1995) who stresses that records should be used as a tool for more accurate and professional work. Keeping records of all interactions with children and parents should be given equal parity with 'getting the job done' (UKCC 1998).

The third stage in the process is risk transference in which Bowden discusses insurance by trusts to cover claims on their behalf. Although this may seem beyond the domain of the majority of readers, the fact that there are funds to cover claims should not be a cause for complacency.

In conclusion, risk management is about the prevention or minimisation of risks within the process of providing care. Benefits of a risk-management programme are improvements in the quality of patient care, reductions in damage and injury to patients, increases in patient activity and a better environment for staff. Strategies identified to achieve this include improved communications and record-keeping which involve the child and family as active participants. The child and family should be encouraged to voice their opinions of the care received through systematic channels. Finally, clinical supervision may enable a more open and honest approach to the delivery of care both in hospital and the community. Utilising these strategies may enable a positive and proactive approach to risk management in the future.

Summary

This chapter has explored a number of key concepts which should be considered as the cornerstones of practice for the professional nurse. Although each concept has been discussed as a separate entity, in practice they are interrelated. The nurse has to understand the elements of risk within any situation in order to act as a responsible professional who is accountable to patients, employers and the profession. When providing information to children and parents, the nurse should be aware of her own values and opinions, so that she gives an unbiased, rational explanation. Practitioners who are able to do this are true advocates for their patients. Advocacy also requires that the practitioner is cognisant of the risks for the patient. Therefore, sound research-based knowledge should underpin the key concepts of this chapter.

The confines of this chapter have only permitted a relatively superficial exploration of the concepts of accountability, informed consent, advocacy and risk management. It is suggested that readers use the references for further reading.

Finally, many of the issues raised give nurses cause for concern. They are everyday incidents in practice, and nurses should be encouraged to discuss their practice with colleagues. This might happen at the changeover of shifts, during clinical supervision or in the more formal setting of a seminar. Whatever the chosen setting, the importance of dialogue cannot be overestimated. Each nurse should accept responsibility for encouraging colleagues to speak out about their practice, keep themselves updated and share knowledge and skills.

As they approach the new millennium nurses now have more opportunity than ever before to develop their knowledge and skills to enhance practice. Nurses should be proud of this practice and be prepared to share what they do well, as the many practices provided in this text prove.

References

Alderson P 1990 Choosing for children: parents consent to surgery. Oxford University Press, Oxford

Altschuler J 1997 Family relationships during serious illness. Nursing Times 93(7): 48–49

Atherton T M 1994 The rights of the child in health care. In: Lindsay B (ed) The child and family: contemporary issues in child health and care. Baillière Tindall, London

Bowden D 1996 Calculate the risk. Nursing Management 3(4): 10–11

Brykczyńska G M 1989 Ethics in paediatric nursing. Chapman Hall, London

Carter B, Campbell S 1997 Children's nurses as critical thinkers. Journal of Child Health Care 1(1): 5

Casey A 1997 So much to do. Paediatric Nursing 9(9): 3

Chadwick R, Tadd W 1992 Ethics and nursing practice. Macmillan Education, London

Chambers M A 1992 Who speaks for the children? Journal of Clinical Nursing 1(2): 73–76

Charles-Edwards I 1995 Moral ethical and legal perspectives. In: Carter B, Dearmun A (eds) Child health care nursing – concepts, theory and practice. Blackwell Science, Oxford

Collier J, Robinson S 1997 Holding children still for procedures. Paediatric Nursing 9(9): 12–14

Coyne IT 1998 Researching children: some methodological and ethical considerations. Journal of Clinical Nursing 7(5): 409–416

Curtin L, Flaherty M J 1982 Nursing ethics: theories and pragmatics. Prentice/Hall International, Englewood Cliffs

Darbyshire P 1994 Living with a sick child in hospital: the experiences of parents and nurses. Chapman & Hall, London

Dearmun A K, Campbell S, Ballow J 1995 Meeting the needs of the child and family with altered gastro-intestinal function. In: Carter B, Dearmun A K (eds) Child health care nursing – concepts, theory and practice. Blackwell Science, Oxford

Department of Health 1996 The Patients Charter Services for Children and Yourng People. London, HMSO

Dickenson D 1994 Children's informed consent to treatment: is the law an ass? Journal of Medical Ethics 20: 205–206

Dimond B 1996 The legal aspects of child health care. Blackwell Science, Oxford

Dineen M 1995 Clinical risk management – a pragmatic approach. British Journal of Health Care Management 1(14): 724–727

Donaldson M 1987 Children's minds. Fontana Press, London

Donaldson S 1997 Atopic eczema: management and control. Paediatric Nursing 9(8): 29–34

Gates B 1995 Whose best interests? Nursing Times 91(4): 31–32

Gillick V 1985 Dear Mrs Gillick. Marshall, Basingstoke

Great Britain Parliament 1969 Family Law Reform Act, HMSO, London

Hanks P 1987 The new Collins concise dictionary of the English language. Guild Publishing, London

Heywood Jones I 1990 The nurse's code. Macmillan Press, London

HMSO 1989 Children Act. HMSO, London

Howard R 1997 Grasping the opportunities within evolving nursing boundaries. Journal of Child Health Care 1(2): 81–83

Kohrman A, Clayton E W, Frader J E et al 1995 Informed consent, parental permission and assent in pediatric practice. Pediatrics 95(2): 314–317

Mallik M 1997 Patient representatives: a new role in advocacy. British Journal of Nursing 6(2): 108–113

Nicholson R (ed) 1986 Medical research with children: ethics, law and practice. Oxford University Press, Oxford

Nitschke R, Humphrey B, Sexauer C, Catron B, Wunder S, Jay S 1982 Therapeutic choices made by patients with end stage cancer. Journal of Pediatrics 101(3): 471–476

Ondrusek N, Abramovitch R Pencharz P, Koren G 1998 Empirical examination of the ability of children to consent to clinical research. Journal of Medical Ethics 24(3): 158–165

Orr FE 1999 The role of the paediatric nurse in promoting paediatric right to consent. Journal of Clinical Nursing 8(1): 291–298

Phillips T 1994 Children and power. In: Lindsay B (ed) The child and family: contemporary nursing issues in child health and care. Baillière Tindall, London

Purssell E 1995 Listening to children: medical treatment and consent. Journal of Advanced Nursing 21(4): 623–624

Pyne R 1988 On being accountable. Health Visitor 61: 173–175

RCN 1999 Restraining, holding still and containing Children. Guidance for good practice. RCN, London

Rennick J 1986 Re-establishing the parental role in a pediatric intensive care unit. Journal of Pediatric Nursing 1(1): 40–44

Richardson J, Webber I 1995 Ethical issues in child health care. Mosby, London

Rushton C H, Armstrong L, McEnhill M 1996 Establishing therapeutic boundaries as patients' advocates. Pediatric Nursing 22(3): 185–189

Russell S 1995 Risk management. British Journal of Nursing 4(10): 607

Solon M 1995 How not to go to court – keep the record straight. British Journal of Health Care Management 1(14): 719

Symons J 1995 Making staff aware of risks. Health Manpower Management 21(4): 15–19

Tingle J 1995 Clinical supervision is an effective risk management tool. British Journal of Nursing 4(14): 794

United Kingdom Central Council for Nursing, Midwifery and Health Visiting (UKCC) 1989 Exercising accountability. UKCC, London

United Kingdom Central Council for Nursing, Midwifery and Health Visiting (UKCC) 1992a Code of professional conduct, 3rd edn. UKCC, London

United Kingdom Central Council for Nursing, Midwifery and Health Visiting (UKCC) 1992b The scope of professional practice. UKCC, London

United Kingdom Central Council for Nursing, Midwifery and Health Visiting (UKCC) 1998 Guidelines for record and record keeping. UKCC, London

Weithorn L A, Campbell S B 1982 The competency in children and adolescents to make informed treatment decisions. Child Development 53: 1589–1598

Whiting M 1997 Community children's nursing: a bright future? Paediatric Nursing 9(4): 6–8

Woodrow P 1997 Nurse advocacy: is it in the patient's best interests? British Journal of Nursing 6(4): 225–229

Control of Infection

Introduction

Many practical procedures carried out by a nurse can be a source of infection. The nurse has both a legal and a professional duty of care towards patients, staff and visitors and must ensure that procedures are performed safely. Families and staff are more likely to complain or take legal action if they think that there has been negligence from either an individual or the health authority.

Infection control is an important part of risk management and there is a legal obligation to take appropriate precautions (Public Health (Infectious Disease) Regulations (HMSO 1988)). The Health and Safety at Work Act (HMSO 1974) and various European regulations (see Box 1) stipulate that there must be formal risk assessment written management procedures in place and with audit trials where there may be hazards from infection towards patients, visitors or staff in the workplace. This includes care in the community. Guidelines clarifying responsibilities for infection control arrangements are described in the Hospital Infection Working Group report (Cooke Report) DoH/PHLS 1995 and in RCN guidelines (RCN 1994).

Prevalence surveys of hospitalised patients indicate that approximately 10% suffer a hospital-acquired infection (HAI) – nosocomial infection (Emmerson et al 1996).

Box 1	Health and safety at work regulations

1. The Control of Substances Hazardous to Health Regulations (HSE 1988) (COSHH) which include hazards from microorganisms, chemicals including drugs, and dust.
2. Personal Protective Equipment at Work Regulations (HSE 1992a)
3. Provision and Use of Work Equipment Regulations (HSE 1992b)
4. Food Safety (General Food Hygiene) Regulations (HMSO 1995)

This is increased in high-risk patients such as those in special care baby units, intensive care or who are immunosuppressed (Drews et al 1995, Rogers & Barnes 1988). It is estimated that approximately 30% of these HAI infections are avoidable if health care workers (HCW) adhere to evidence-based practice (Haley et al 1985a,b). The cost of these infections is high (Mehtar et al 1989). The estimated cost of HAI in England was £115 million in 1987 and it was suggested that £36 million could be saved (Currie & Maynard 1989).

The Communicable Disease Surveillance Centre and Public Health Laboratory Service coordinate nation-wide epidemiological studies in both hospital-acquired infection (HAI) and community-acquired infection (CAI). The Nosocomial Infection National Surveillance Scheme (NINSS) allows hospitals to join the scheme voluntarily.

Medical and nursing cultural influences may play a part in non-compliance with evidence-based infection control practice. Ethnographic studies (Macqueen 1995) have indicated that nurses wash their hands more frequently before aseptic procedures than after 'dirty' tasks, and that they perceive babies as being 'less dirty' than older children. Ongoing education, training and support for all staff must therefore be an integral part of an infection control programme.

The chain of infection

The chain of infection consists of the microorganism, a source, a susceptible host and a means of transmission.

The microorganism

Most nosocomial infections are caused by bacteria and viruses but problems with fungi are increasingly being identified, especially in immunosuppressed patients.

The most important characteristics of the organism are:

- pathogenicity – ability to produce disease
- infectivity – ability to spread from person to person

- invasiveness – ability to spread within the host
- virulence – the severity of the illness
- properties of adherence to synthetic materials such as implanted devices, e.g. *Staphylococcus epidermidis* adheres well to some synthetic material.

When foreign material is inserted into the body, the material interacts with the host's natural defence mechanism and the risk of infection increases. The surface of the foreign body (e.g. a plastic catheter) is covered with host-derived proteins such as albumin, fibrinogen, fibronectin, collagen, laminin, vitronectin and immunoglobulins. Some of these components (e.g. albumin) may serve to retard microbial adherence, whilst others such as fibronectin may serve as receptors for bacteria. This complex of host and bacterial constituents is known as a biofilm (Bisno 1995). It is important that nurses are aware of different catheter materials in order that the most appropriate for the procedure may be selected to reduce the risk of infection. Considerations of availability, cost, site and length of time of insertion, and chemicals with which the material may come in contact, such as drugs or intravenous solutions, must be taken into account.

The antigenic make-up of an organism may also change through the use of antibiotics and disinfectants. Outbreaks of multiply antibiotic-resistant Gram-negative bacteria such as *Klebsiella*, *Escherichia coli* and *Pseudomonas* and Gram-positive bacteria such as methicillin-resistant *Staphylococcus aureus* (MRSA) are becoming more common in both the hospital and the community setting (Kelly & Chivers 1996, O'Brien 1997).

The source of infection

The infection may be endogenous, arising from the child's own flora, or exogenous, arising from the environment. The source may be children, parents, staff or visitors or, more rarely, animals. It may include:

- those with acute disease
- persons in the incubation period of a disease
- persons who are colonised with an infectious agent but who do not have the disease (asymptomatic carriers)
- those who are chronic carriers of an infectious agent.

Environmental transmission of the organism may be increased through air movement and dust.

The following have all been cited as environmental sources of hospital-acquired infections:

- lack of adherence by health care workers to basic infection control guidelines

- overcrowding of patient beds (Haley & Bregman 1982)
- a badly maintained environment, e.g. torn chairs or mattresses, soiled curtains, cracked tiles
- inadequate decontamination and maintenance of equipment
- inadequate disposal of clinical and household waste
- lack of pest control, e.g. the sighting of cockroaches, mice or rats
- inadequate food hygiene practice
- improper air flow
- lack of isolation facilities.

Mode of transmission

Microorganisms are carried on inanimate or animate objects from a reservoir to a source. The reservoir is the place where the organism maintains its presence, metabolises and replicates. The source is the place from which the infectious agent passes to the host either by direct or indirect contact through a vehicle as the means of transmission.

Transmission may occur by one or more of five different routes.

Contact:

- Direct contact as in person-to-person spread when nursing or turning a child or between two children physically playing together.
- Indirect contact such as in inadequate decontamination of equipment.

Droplet.   Droplets are generated by the source person during sneezing, coughing or talking and during procedures such as suctioning or bronchoscopy. Transmission occurs when droplets containing organisms are propelled a short distance through the air and deposited on the host's conjunctivae, nasal mucosa or mouth. Droplets do not remain suspended in the air and therefore this should not be confused with airborne transmission.

Airborne.   Dissemination via this route is of either airborne droplet nuclei (small particle residue of evaporated droplets 5 nm or less in size that remain suspended in the air for long periods of time) or dust particles containing the infective organism. Organisms can be widely dispersed by air currents and inhaled by susceptible hosts either in the same room or over a further distance therefore special air-handling and ventilation may be required to prevent airborne transmission. Varicella (chickenpox), measles virus and *Mycobacterium tuberculosis* are examples of organisms transmitted by the airborne route.

Common vehicle. This applies to organisms transmitted by contaminated items such as food, water, medications, devices and equipment.

Vector-borne. Organisms may be carried by vectors such as flies, cockroaches, mice, rats and other vermin.

The host

Host factors that influence the development of infections are the site of deposition of the organism and the host's defence mechanism. See Table 1.

Table 1 **Common risk factors for infection**

Risk factors	Reasons
Gestational age: < 32 weeks	The stratum corneum is very scant and permeable to bacteria. The skin is an effective barrier by 37 weeks gestation Humoral defence mechanism–complement activation is only 20–40% of adult values (full-term newborn is 50–80% of adult value) Maternal IgG begins passing transplacentally at approximately 15 weeks' gestation but does not reach the optimum until about 33 weeks. The fetus begins to synthesise IgM at about 30 weeks gestation
Low birth weight	Risk of infection is increased in babies weighing < 1000 g and less in babies > 2500 g
Method of nutrition	Infection occurs less in breastfed babies because of protection from maternal antibody transference Infection occurs more in bottle-fed babies because of lack of hygiene in equipment, preparation and storage
Umbilical cord stump	Associated with infection especially after placement of umbilical vein catheters
Congenital abnormalities	Such as abnormal immune function (severe combined immune deficiency, DiGeorge syndrome, Down syndrome), congenital infection (rubella, cytomegalovirus, hepatitis) or congenital cardiac or renal disease
Acquired disease processes	Other infections or chronic disease processes
Invasive devices	External devices such as intravascular, urinary, endotracheal tubes, nasogastric, gastrostomy, drainage systems. Internal devices such as ventricular atrial/peritoneal shunts, heart valves and artificial patches
Surgery	Type and length of surgery
Chemotherapy	Antibiotic therapy has been associated with *Clostridium difficile* and necrotising enterocolitis. Certain drugs such as steroids alter immunity
Length of stay in hospital	Increases the risk of colonisation/invasion with pathogenic organisms
Increased handling by hospital staff	Hands of staff have been associated with cross-infection of pathogenic organisms in hospitalised patients
Equipment	Equipment includes suction apparatus, respiratory equipment, humidifiers, feeding utensils, thermometers, pedal bins, incubators, scalp electrodes, stethoscopes, laryngoscopes, surgical instruments, communal ointments

Precautions to be taken

The application of source isolation or protective precautions (barrier nursing) was revised by the Communicable Disease Center in Atlanta, USA, in 1996 and the terms 'standard' precautions and 'transmission' precautions are now felt to be more appropriate (Garner 1996). This encompasses the need to control the increasing emergence of multiple antibiotic-resistant organisms, common outbreaks of viral diarrhoeal illnesses and the recognition of blood-borne viruses. Although local practices may vary, the principles of infection control remain the same.

Standard precautions

These precautions are designed to reduce the risk of transmission of microorganisms from both recognised and unrecognised sources of infection. They should be practised in both hospital and the community when care may involve coming into contact with:

- blood
- all body secretions and excretions regardless of whether they contain blood
- non-intact skin
- mucous membrane.

The key principles include:

- handwashing before and after patient contact
- wearing protective clothing to avoid contamination of the skin or mucosal surfaces – gloves, aprons, face protection as appropriate
- safe handling and disposal of sharp instruments and needles
- safe disposal of clinical waste
- safe disposal of foul and infected linen
- safe handling and transportation of specimens
- maintaining a clean environment
- regular maintenance and appropriate cleaning, disinfection or sterilisation of equipment.

Transmission-based precautions

These precautions are designed for:

1. children known or suspected to be infected or colonised with pathogens for which additional precautions are required to interrupt transmission; this may include one or more of airborne, droplet or contact transmission
2. children who are immunosuppressed and require an environment with special air filtration (high-efficiency particulate air – HEPA) to prevent the risk of acquiring airborne fungal infections such as *Aspergillus*.

Depending on the causative organism, the route of transmission, the need for a special environment and resources available, the child may need to be:

- nursed in an individual cubicle preferably with handwashing and toilet facilities
- cohorted (placed with other children) in a separate area on the ward with others who are infected/colonised with the same pathogen
- nursed in a room with negative pressure with at least six exchanges of air per hour. There is usually an air-lock and the door must be kept closed.
- nursed in a room with high-efficiency filtered positive air pressure. There is usually an air-lock and the door must be kept closed. This is usually reserved for severely immunosuppressed children such as those undergoing transplantation.
- nursed at home away from susceptible people if the risk factor of infection to others is felt to be high, such as small babies or those with significant immunosuppression.

Hand hygiene

Hand hygiene is the single most cost-effective method of reducing cross-infection (APIC 1995). The purpose of handwashing is to remove dirt, organic material and transient microorganisms (Gould 1991). Transient hand carriage, especially of Gram-negative organisms, has been reported in 20–30% of hospital staff and may persist for several weeks. One study (Sneddon 1990) demonstrated that Gram-negative organisms were isolated from 44% of nurses' hands before washing and from 12% after washing; 40% of hands sampled after dirty activity and 25% after clean activity were contaminated. Only 52% of the handwashes were considered good.

Cuts and abrasions of any exposed areas of skin must be covered with a dressing that is semipermeable and an effective bacterial and viral barrier. Health care workers with exfoliating skin lesions must report to an occupational health department

Requirements:
- A hand basin with running warm water.
- An appropriate liquid soap, antiseptic detergent and/or alcohol hand-rub.
- Disposable towels. A variety of methods of hand drying are available. There is no conclusive microbiological evidence to distinguish between the efficacy of hot air hand dryers and paper towels.

A clean, laundered non-disposable towel can be used in the home setting.

- Where the above is not possible, an alcohol rub will suffice where hands are not heavily contaminated.

Handwashing method.   The correct method of handwashing is shown in Figure 1. Table 2 lists methods of hand hygiene practice – the method used will depend on the type of practice to be undertaken.

Risk factors for infection:

- Skin lesions, e.g. eczema, paronychia, cuts and abrasions.
- Nail polish, artificial nails or long nails.

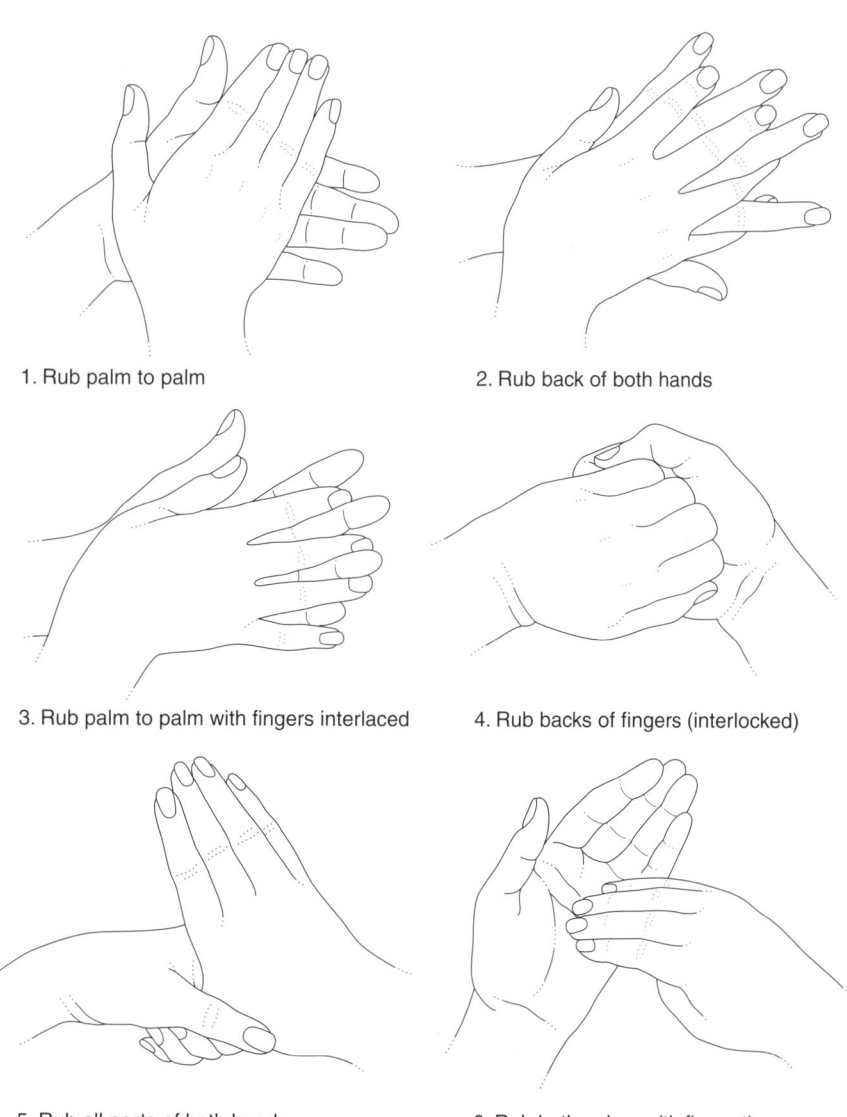

Wet hands, apply soap and use the following procedure

1. Rub palm to palm

2. Rub back of both hands

3. Rub palm to palm with fingers interlaced

4. Rub backs of fingers (interlocked)

5. Rub all parts of both hands

6. Rub both palms with finger tips

7. Rinse hands under running water and dry thoroughly on a clean towel

Figure 1
How to wash hands correctly and reduce infection.

Table 2   **Methods of hand hygiene practice**

Description	Purpose	Method
Social hand-wash	To remove soil and transient microorganisms	Liquid soap or detergent for at least 10–15 seconds
Hand antisepsis	To remove or destroy transient microorganisms	Antimicrobial soap or detergent or alcohol-based hand rub for at least 10–15 seconds
Surgical hand-scrub	To remove or destroy transient microorganisms and reduce resident flora	Antimicrobial soap or detergent preparation with brush (sterile) to achieve friction for at least 120 seconds or alcohol-based preparation for at least 20 seconds

- Jewellery, e.g. rings, watches, bracelets. These may harbour pathogenic organisms.
- Non-compliance – handwashing occurs in approximately half of the instances in which it is indicated.
- Communal hand lotion.
- Cloth hand towels in an institutional setting.
- Large reusable containers and 'topping up' antiseptics and liquid soap.
- Communal bar soap.
- Alcohol hand-rub is not as effective in the presence of physical dirt.
- Moisturising agents and surfactants may interfere with the residual activity of chlorhexidine.
- Lack of sufficient handwashing facilities.
- Waste pedal bins with broken lids which have to be opened with the hand.

Protective clothing

A risk assessment of the task to be performed must be made (Fig. 2) and protective clothing must always be available. The assessment may differ between parents and health care workers who are more exposed to a variety of pathogens during their duties. However, risk factors in association with blood-borne viruses such as HIV, hepatitis B or C, for example, may be the same. The increasing recognition of latex allergy in both patients and health care workers must be taken into consideration (Johnson 1997, Markey 1994). Any blood or body secretions/excretions may contain microbial pathogens and must be handled as potentially infectious. In young children, especially in the nappy-wearing age, the bowel flora is commonly distributed over the skin and in the upper respiratory tract.

Disposable gloves
- Gloves provide added protection when the risk of microbial contamination is increased such as during nappy changing when a child has diarrhoea.
- Non-sterile gloves must be worn for direct contact with blood or body fluids, non-intact skin and mucous membrane.

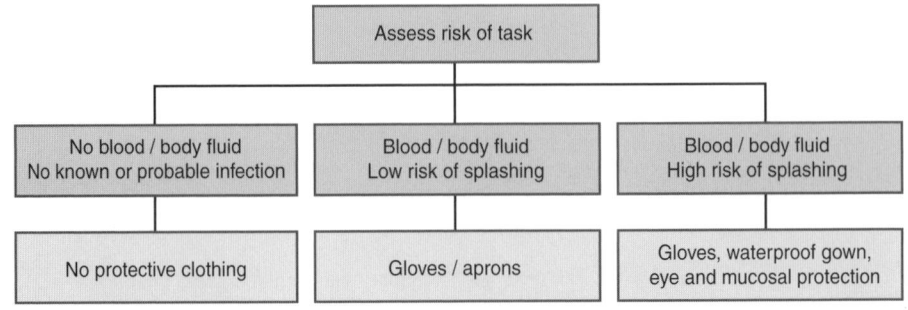

Figure 2
Risk assessment.

- Wear gloves for all care if intact skin is a source of contamination, such as when the child is colonised with multiply antibiotic-resistant organisms. Certain pathogens such as klebsiellae have increased adherence properties to the skin and may be found on the hands after social handwashing (Casewell & Phillips 1977).
- Gloves should be disposable and discarded between patients or contaminated body sites.
- Hands have become contaminated even when wearing gloves and therefore a soap and water hand-wash or alcohol hand-rub is recommended after removal of gloves.

Risks factors for infection:
- Quality of gloves – leakage has been reported in 4–63% of vinyl gloves and 3–52% of latex gloves (Korniewicz et al 1989).
- Petroleum-based or oil emollients may affect the integrity of latex.
- Dermatitis due to allergy to latex or glove powder.

Plastic aprons
Cotton gowns offer minimal microbial protection (Donowitz 1986) and therefore should be replaced with single-use disposable plastic aprons. Hands must be washed after removal of the apron.

Aprons should be changed between clean and dirty tasks and should be worn for:

- all patient care
- aseptic techniques
- serving meals and feeding patients
- performing dirty tasks
- bedmaking.

Facial protection
This may include masks, visors or goggles and is worn to protect both the patient and the health care worker.

Surgical masks are worn in theatre to protect the patient against large particle droplets from the surgical team immediately over the operation site (Belkin 1997). More research is required as to the risk of infection to the patient from members of the circulating theatre team or during minor surgery.

Facial protection should be worn when performing procedures which may generate splashes or sprays of blood or body fluid, secretions or excretions and where there is a risk of contaminating the mucosal surfaces of the eyes, nose or mouth.

Factors to consider:
- Compliance with wearing the protective device correctly.

- Type of filter in mask.
- Procedures which generate aerosols, e.g. bronchoscopy or suctioning.
- Risk of splattering of blood or other body fluids.
- Open pulmonary tuberculosis and multiply antibiotic-resistant tuberculosis (MRTB).
- Risk to and from the child and health care worker.

Protective gowns and headwear
These should not only be made of appropriate material to minimise 'strike through' or leakage of blood and body fluids, or but also be comfortable to the wearer. Hair should be covered by the hood/hat. They should be available where the risk of contamination with blood and body fluids is increased such as in the operating theatre, intensive care or accident and emergency units

Foot protection
Contamination of the feet with blood/body fluids will be minimised if boots/theatre shoes are worn in high-risk areas such as the operating theatre, intensive care or accident and emergency units. Theatre footwear should not be worn outside the theatre complex. It maybe washed in a heat disinfector and dried after each use. Overshoes have not been shown to reduce infection and may indeed increase the risk by contaminating hands on application or removal.

Waste disposal

All contaminated waste must be placed into yellow clinical sacks. It must be secured and the source area identified, i.e. the responsible local health authority (check local policy for hospitals and the community), before it is removed from the premises for incineration (Health and Safety Executive 1992, 1995a).

Sharps.   Needles, blades and other sharp instruments must be placed in a rigid, puncture-proof sharps container immediately after use. Discard needles and syringe as one unit into the sharps box. Do not resheath contaminated needles as this increases the risk of injury (Jagger et al 1990). Never fill the container more than two-thirds full and ensure that it is securely closed and labelled before disposal and incineration (BMA 1990).

Uncontaminated paper and other household waste should be placed in a black bag, secured ready for collection and landfill.

Risk factors for infection:
- Resheathing needles.

- Breaking the hub of the needle to take blood from neonates.
- Leaving sharps lying around and not disposing of them immediately into a sharps bin.
- Overfilling sharps bins or clinical waste bags.
- Handing sharp instruments to another person instead of laying them down safely so that they can be picked up, especially in the operating theatre where the risk of injury maybe increased.

Disposal of infected linen

Local policies for the handling of laundry must be followed (Health and Safety Executive 1995a). Foul and infected linen should be segregated and placed in a red water-soluble bag contained in an outer bag and labelled 'danger of infection'.

Soiled linen may also be contaminated with pathogenic microorganisms and should be placed directly into appropriate laundry containers. Baby clothes, blankets etc. should be laundered centrally in an institution. If performed at local level, a separate room with adequately maintained washing and drying facilities must be available.

Risk factors for infection:

- Washing baby clothes in the kitchen or dirty utility room in an institution.
- Not maintaining adequate washing temperatures for disinfection (70–71°C for at least 3 minutes).
- Inadequate maintenance of washing/drying machines.
- Transporting dirty linen on the same trolley as that used for transporting and serving food.
- Storing clean linen in unhygienic conditions.

Eating utensils such as dishes, cups, glasses, baby bottles

Eating utensils carry a risk of transmitting infection.

Factors to note:

- All feeding utensils should be washed in a well-maintained dishwasher. They should be placed in the dishwasher immediately after use and not left lying around.
- Where dishwashers are not available, feeding utensils should be thoroughly washed in hot water and detergent, rinsed in hot water and dried.
- Baby feeding bottles and equipment should be washed in a well-maintained dishwasher or a commercial Steam Sterilizer. It is not necessary to sterilise them in an autoclave in hospital.
- Feeding utensils for severely immunosuppressed children, such as those undergoing transplantation,

should be washed in a dishwasher, thoroughly dried and stored separately. Sterilisation by autoclave is not considered necessary.
- Where a heat process is not available, baby bottles and feeding equipment should be thoroughly cleaned before immersion in a chemical sterilant such as hypochlorite or dichloroisocyanurate for the recommended time and stored in a clean container afterwards.
- Equipment for expressing breast milk should be sterile and single use, and breast pumps should be decontaminated and maintained regularly.
- Although disposable utensils may be used for infected patients, it is not considered necessary if the above facilities are available.

Risk factors for infection.   Candida infection has been associated with inadequate decontamination of teats and dummies.

The environment and the use of disinfectants

The following definitions (Ayliffe et al 1993) are used to standardise different methods of decontamination.

Sterilisation.   A process used to render an object free from all living organisms.

Disinfection.   A process used to reduce the number of microorganisms but not usually of bacterial spores. The process does not necessarily kill or remove all microorganisms but reduces the number to a level which is not harmful to health.

Cleaning.   A process that removes contaminants including dust, soil, large numbers of microorganisms and the organic matter (e.g. faeces, blood) that protects the organisms. Cleaning is always necessary before sterilisation or the use of disinfectants.

The risks to patients from the environment and equipment maybe classified as follows:

1. High risk – items in close contact with a break in the skin or mucous membrane or introduced into a normally sterile body area should be *sterile*.
2. Intermediate risk – items in contact with mucous membrane or other items contaminated with particularly virulent or readily transmissible organisms, or items to be used on highly susceptible patients should be *disinfected*.
3. Low risk – items in contact with normal and intact skin should be *cleaned* and dried.

Advice on the use of disinfectants should be followed (Ayliffe et al 1993, Rutala 1990) and local policies adhered to. The use of disinfectants in the paediatric setting should be kept to a minimum to ensure safety. Care must be taken to keep them locked away out of reach of children.

Hot water and detergent with thorough drying is considered adequate for most environmental cleaning. The environment must be kept clean and a high standard of housekeeping maintained. However, studies have shown that viruses causing diarrhoea such as rotavirus can remain viable on inanimate surfaces for several days (Satter et al 1994). Touching contaminated surfaces can transfer infectious virus to the hands and aid spread. Ethyl alcohol (ethanol) wipes are an effective disinfectant against these viruses.

Factors to note:
- Equipment must be cleaned with hot water and detergent before sterilisation or disinfection. Always follow manufacturers' instructions regarding decontamination. Chemicals may react adversely on some materials, for example alcohol will produce opaqueness on Perspex material or hypochlorites may rust metals.
- Always use moist heat sterilisation and heat disinfection where possible. Some materials are heat labile and chemical sterilisation or disinfection may need to be used, such as with endoscopic equipment.
- A risk assessment to the child and health care worker must be made with any chemical used in accordance with the Control of Substances Hazardous to Health (COSHH) Regulations.
- The use of phenolic disinfectants has been associated with neonatal hyperbilirubinaemia (Wysowski 1978).
- Hypochlorite disinfectant is used for:
  – 1.0% (10 000 ppm available chlorine) – disinfection of heavy spillages of blood and body fluids
  – 0.1% (1000 ppm available chlorine) – general cleaning when disinfection is required
  – 0.025% (250 ppm available chlorine) – disinfecting babies' bottles, teats, dummies.
- Walls should be cleaned if visibly dirty.
- After cleaning a room which has housed a child with an infection, it is unnecessary to leave it to air for a set period of time.

Risk factors for infection:
- Not cleaning equipment before using chemical disinfection. Many disinfectants are inactivated in the presence of organic matter such as blood, dirt or grease.
- 'Topping up' bottles of disinfectant or antiseptics.
- Not making up fresh solutions or using the correct dilution.

- Hypochlorite solutions are unstable and must be renewed every 24 hours.
- Mixing incompatible chemicals.
- A poorly maintained environment encourages infestation and inhibits adequate cleaning.

Equipment

It is preferable that all equipment is cleaned and maintained in a central unit where documentation and quality control can be monitored. Manufacturing guidelines must be followed according to the type of equipment and level of decontamination required, e.g. sterilisation, disinfection or cleaning (Fuller 1992).

Factors to note:
- Equipment must be decontaminated before service or repair; see HSG(93)26 (DoH 1993).
- Single-use items must not be reused unless the health authority have in place an adequate quality assurance programme and accept liability (MDA 1995).
- Equipment such as wooden spatulas have been used as splints for intravenous cannulation sites, for which they were not designed, and consequentially caused serious fungal infection (Holzel et al 1998).

Risk factors for infection:
- Torn mattresses, pillow covers and chairs causing difficulty in cleaning.
- Poorly maintained equipment such as suction apparatus, breast pumps or blood gas machines.
- Inadequately cleaned equipment such as urine- or stool-testing equipment, thermometers, laryngoscopes, incubators and respiratory ventilators/humidifiers.

Occupational health

All health care workers should have access to an occupational health department and should report:

- For a pre-employment health review and to be advised on immunisations and relevant immunity status such as after vaccination against hepatitis B. A small percentage of people do not produce antibodies to some immunisations and therefore remain susceptible to the disease (Salisbury & Begg 1996).
- If on immunosuppressive therapy or pregnant, when appropriate advice to reduce the risk of infection can be given (Advisory Committee on Dangerous Pathogens 1997).
- If they have suffered from an infectious disease and have been at work or wish to return to work.

- If they feel that they are likely to be or are infected with a blood-borne virus such as human immunodeficiency virus, hepatitis B or C and are performing exposure-prone procedures during their work (HSG(93)40 (NHSME 1993) and Addendum (DoH 1996), RCN 1997).
- For all accidents, including those involving:
  – sharps injuries or contamination of mucosal surfaces of the eyes, nose or mouth with blood or body fluids
  – blood or body fluids on non-intact skin.
- When allergic reactions occur such as with latex or chemicals.

Risk factors for infection:
- Not adhering to handwashing procedures.
- Not wearing recommended protective clothing.
- Working with exfoliating skin lesions or uncovered broken skin.
- Working with children who have certain infectious diseases such as chickenpox and not being immune.
- Not being protected from infectious diseases where immunisation is available.
- Travelling abroad and not taking health care advice.

Surveillance of infection and auditing practice

Surveillance of infection and ongoing audit of hospital-acquired infection should be seen as a collaborative multidisciplinary undertaking between the infection control team, clinical staff and managers.

Documentation of increased-risk factors, such as insertion and removal of devices including intravascular and urinary catheters, respiratory intubation or any invasive procedure, must be maintained. Surveillance methods vary (Glenister et al 1993, Millward et al 1993) and should be discussed with the local infection control team.

The role of the nurse as a health educator can be of particular importance to the child and family when explaining about infectious diseases. The nurse must feel confident in her knowledge and be able to individualise care safely and explain basic hygiene precautions. Children and their families should have a right to expect that their health will be protected as well as promoted when receiving health care services.

References

Advisory Committee on Dangerous Pathogens 1997 Infection risks to new and expectant mothers in the workplace. HSE, London

Association for Professionals in Infection Control and Epidemiology (APIC) 1995 APIC guideline for handwashing and antisepsis in health care settings. American Journal of Infection Control 23: 251–269

Ayliffe G A J, Coates D, Hoffman P N 1993 Chemical disinfection in hospitals, 2nd edn. Public Health Laboratory Service, London

Belkin N L 1997 The evolution of the surgical mask: filtering efficiency versus effectiveness. Infection Control and Hospital Epidemiology 18: 49–57

Bisno A L 1995 Molecular aspects of bacterial colonization. Infection Control and Hospital Epidemiology 16: 648–657

British Medical Association (BMA) 1990 A code of practice for the safe use and disposal of sharps. BMA, London

Casewell M, Phillips I 1977 Hands as a route of transmission for *Klebsiella* species. British Medical Journal 2(6098): 1315–1317

Currie E, Maynard A 1989 The economics of hospital acquired infection. Discussion paper 65. University of York, York

Department of Health (DoH) 1993 Decontamination of equipment prior to inspection, service or repair. HSG(93)26. HMSO, London

Department of Health (DoH) 1996 Addendum to HSG(93)40: protecting health care workers and patients from hepatitis B. DoH, Wetherby

DoH/PHLS Hospital Infection Working Group 1995 Hospital infection control: guidance on the control of infection in hospitals (Cooke Report). DoH/PHLS, London

Donowitz L G 1986 Failure of the overgown to prevent nosocomial infection in a paediatric intensive care unit. Pediatrics 77: 35–38

Drews M B, Ludwig A C, Leititis J U, Daschner F D 1995 Low birthweight and nosocomial infection of neonates in a neonatal intensive care unit. Journal of Hospital Infection 30: 65–72

Emmerson A M, Enstone J E, Griffin M, Kelsey M C, Smyth E T M 1996 The second national prevalence survey of infection in hospitals – overview of the results. Journal of Hospital Infection 32: 157–190

Fuller A 1992 Sterilising instruments. Journal of Infection Control Nursing, Nursing Times 88(50): 64–65

Garner J S 1996 Guidelines for isolation precautions in hospitals. American Journal of Infection Control 24: 24–52

Glenister H M, Taylor L J, Bartlett C L R, Cooke E M, Sedgwick J A, Mackintosh C A 1993 An evaluation of surveillance methods for detecting infections in hospital inpatients. Journal of Hospital Infection 23: 229–242

Gould D 1991 Nurses' hands as vectors of hospital-acquired infection: a review. Journal of Advanced Nursing 16: 1216–1225

Haley R W, Bregman D A 1982 The role of understaffing and overcrowding in recurrent outbreaks of staphylococcal infection in a neonatal special-care unit. Journal of Infectious Diseases 145: 875–885

Haley R W, Culver D H, White J W 1985a The efficacy of infection surveillance and control programs in preventing nosocomial infections in university hospitals. (SENIC study) American Journal of Epidemiology 121: 182–205

Haley R W, Morgan W M, Culver D H, White J W, Emori T G, Mosser J, Hughes J M 1985b Update from the SENIC project: hospital infection control: recent progress and opportunities under prospective payment. American Journal of Infection Control 13(3): 97–108

Health and Safety Executive (HSE) 1988 Control of substances hazardous to health regulations. HMSO, London

Health and Safety Executive (HSE) 1992 Personal protective equipment at work regulations. HMSO, London

Health and Safety Executive (HSE) 1992 Provision and use of work equipment regulations. HMSO, London

Health and Safety Executive (HSE) 1995 Hospital laundry arrangements for used and infected linen. HSG (95)18. HMSO, London

Health and Safety Executive Health Guidance Note 1995 Safe disposal of clinical waste whole hospital policy guidance. HMSO, London

Health and Safety Executive, Health Services Advisory Committee 1992 Safe disposal of clinical waste. HMSO, London

HMSO 1994 Health and Safety at Work Act. HMSO, London

HMSO 1988 Public Health (Infectious Disease) Regulations. (SI 1988: 1546) HMSO, London

HMSO 1995 Food safety (general food hygiene) regulations. HMSO, London

Holzel H H, Macqueen S, MacDonald A et al 1998 *Rhizopus microsporus*: a major threat or minor inconvenience. Journal of Hospital Infection 38: 113–118

Jagger J, Hunt E H, Pearson R D 1990 Sharp object injuries in the hospital: causes and strategies for prevention. American Journal of Infection Control 18: 227–231

Johnson G 1997 Time to take the gloves off. Occupational Health 25–28

Kelly J, Chivers G 1996 Built-in resistance. Journal of Infection Control Nursing, Nursing Times 92(2): 50–54

Korniewicz D M, Laughton B E, Butz A, Larson E 1989 Integrity of vinyl and latex procedure gloves. Nursing Research 38(3): 144–146

Macqueen S 1995 Anthropology and germ theory. Journal of Hospital Infection 30(suppl): 116–126

Markey J 1994 Latex allergy: implications for healthcare personnel and infusion therapy patients. Journal of Intravenous Nursing 17(1): 35–39

Medical Devices Agency (MDA) 1995 Reuse of medical devices supplied for single use only. Device Bulletin MDA DB 9501. MDA, London

Mehtar S, Drabu Y J, Mayet F 1989 Expenses incurred during a 5-week epidemic methicillin-resistant *Staphylococcus aureus* outbreak. Journal of Hospital Infection 13: 199–220

Millward S, Barnett J, Thomlinson D A 1993 A clinical infection control audit programme: evaluation of an audit tool used by infection control nurses to monitor standards and assess effective staff training. Journal of Hospital Infection 24: 219–232

National Health Service Management Executive (NHSME) 1992 Management of food services and food hygiene in the National Health Service. DoH, London

National Health Service Management Executive (NHSME) 1993 Protecting health care workers and patients from hepatitis B. HSG(93)40. DoH, London

O'Brien T F 1997 The global epidemic nature of antimicrobial resistance and the need to monitor and manage it locally. Clinical Infectious Diseases 24(suppl 1): S2–S8

Rogers T R, Barnes R A 1988 Prevention of airborne fungal infection in immunocompromised patients. Journal of Hospital Infection 11(suppl A): 15–20

Royal College of Nursing (RCN) 1994 Guidelines on infection control for nurses in general practice. RCN, London

Royal College of Nursing (RCN) 1997 Hepatitis guidelines. RCN, London

Rutala W A 1990 APIC guidelines for selection and use of disinfectants. American Journal of Infection Control 18: 99–117

Salisbury D M, Begg N 1996 Immunisation against infectious diseases. HMSO, London

Satter S Y, Jacobson H, Rahman H, Cusack T M, Rubino J R 1994 Interruption of rotavirus spread through chemical disinfection. Infection Control and Hospital Epidemiology 15: 751–756

Sneddon J G 1990 A preventable course of infection: carriage of Gram-negative bacilli on hands. Professional Nurse 6(2): 98–104

Wysowski D M et al 1978 Epidemic neonatal hyperbilirubinaemia and the use of phenolic disinfection. Paediatrics 16(2): 165–170

Further reading

Advisory committee on dangerous pathogens 1998 Transmissible spongiform encephalopathy agents: Safe working and the prevention of infection. HMSO, London

Begg N T 1992 Update – control of meningococcal disease. Communicable Disease Report 2: R65

Boucher I Third report of group of experts 1998 Cryptospiridium in water supply. HMSO, London

Bowell B 1992 A risk to others. Nursing Times 88(4): 38–40

Claxton R, Harrison T 1991 Caring for children with HIV and AIDS. Edward Arnold, London

Department of Health (DoH) 1989 High security infectious disease units (HSIDU): transport arrangements. EL(89)P/133. HMSO, London

Department of Health (DoH) 1989 HIV infection, breast feeding and milk banking in UK. PL/CMO(89)4, PL/CNO(89)3. HMSO, London

Department of Health (DoH) 1991 Decontamination of equipment, linen or other surface contaminated with hepatitis B and/or human immunodeficiency virus. HC(91)33. HMSO, London

Evans R 1992 Child's play. Journal of Infection Control Nursing, Nursing Times 88(24): 63–64, 66–67

Expert advisory group on AIDs and the advisory group on hepatitis 1998 Guidance for clinical health care workers: protection against infection with blood – borne viruses. HMSO, London

HMSO 1989 Guide to good manufacturing practice for National Health Service sterile services departments. HMSO, London

HMSO 1990 Further evaluation of transportable steam sterilizers for unwrapped instruments and utensils. HMSO, London

Horton R 1993 Introducing high quality infection control in a hospital setting. British Journal of Nursing 2(15): 746–754

Hunter P R 1991 Application of hazard analysis critical control point (HACCP) to the handling of expressed breast milk on a neonatal unit. Journal of Hospital Infection 17: 139–146

Infection control nurses association 1997 Guidelines for hand hygiene (obtained from ICNA Tel: 01506 811077)

Inter departmental working group on tuberculosis 1998 The prevention and control of tuberculosis in the United Kingdom. HMSO, London

London Ambulance Service 1991 Categories for the conveyance of patients with infectious diseases.

Macqueen S 1996 Think globally, act locally: germ invasion and risk analysis. Journal of Neonatal Nursing 2(1): 20–25

Madge P, Paton J Y, McColl J H, Mackie P L K 1992 Prospective controlled study of four infection control procedures to prevent nosocomial infection with respiratory syncitial virus. Lancet 340: 1079–1083

Medical Devices Agency (MDA) 1996 Decontamination of endoscopes. MDA DB 9607. MDA, London

National Health Service Management Executive (NHSME) 1992 Management of food services and food hygiene in the National Health Service. DoH, London

PHLS Hepatitis Subcommittee 1992 Exposure to hepatitis B virus: guidelines on post-exposure prophylaxis. Communicable Disease Report 2: R97–101

PHLS Meningococcal Infections Working Party 1989 The epidemiology and control of meningococcal disease. Communicable Disease Report 89/08: 3–5

PHLS Salmonella Sub-committee 1990 Notes on the control of human sources of gastrointestinal infections, infestations and bacterial intoxications in the United Kingdom. Communicable Disease Report (suppl 1): 1–13

Public Health Medicine Environmental Group 1996 Guidelines on the control of infection in residential and nursing homes. DoH, London

Purssell E 1996 Preventing nosocomial infection in paediatric wards. Journal of Clinical Nursing 5: 313–318

RCN 1995 Guidance on infection control in hospitals. RCN, London

Report of a Combined Working Party of the Hospital Infection Society and the British Society for Antimicrobial Chemotherapy 1990 Revised guidelines for the control of epidemic methicillin-resistant *Staphylococcus aureus*. Journal of Hospital Infection 16: 351–377

Royal College of Obstetricians and Gynaecologists (RCOG) 1990 HIV infection in maternity care and gynaecology. Revised report of the RCOG sub-committee on problems associated with AIDS in relation to obstetrics and gynaecology. RCOG, London

Teare E L, Peacock A 1996 The development of an infection control link-nurse programme in a district general hospital. Journal of Hospital Infection 34: 267–278

UK Health Department 1997 Guidelines on post-exposure prophylaxis for health care workers exposed to HIV. DoH, London

Webster O, Bowell E 1986 Thinking prevention. Nursing Times 82(23): 68–74

Wilson J 1995 Infection control in clinical practice. Baillière Tindall, London

Introduction to Community

Over the past decade increasing numbers of sick children have been nursed in their own homes, although the concept is not new. In 1949, the first paediatric domiciliary service was set up in Rotherham in an attempt to reduce the high rate of infant mortality thought to be caused by cross-infection in hospital (Winter & Teare 1997). 10 years later the Ministry of Health gave recognition to the fact that children's psychological needs were best met at home, and they should only be admitted to hospital when they were too sick to be nursed at home (MoH 1959). The increase in numbers of sick children requiring nursing at home has been due partly to the increased survival rates of children with life-threatening conditions and infants of short gestational age who still need care on discharge from hospital (Langlands & McDonagh 1995), the increase in day surgery for children and also the reduction in the length of time that a child admitted to hospital is likely to stay as an inpatient.

Whereas the right of sick adults to be cared for at home by appropriately trained nurses has long been recognised, the right of sick children to have a similar service has only recently been acknowledged. Parents will always be the main carers in the home but should have access to community children's nurses (CCNs) (Roe 1997). Thornes (1991) states that once a child has returned home following day surgery, nursing support should be provided by nurses trained in the care of sick children. Although there has been a significant increase in the number of children's community nurses over the past decade, with 52 general teams and 124 specialist teams in 1993 (Woodroffe et al 1993), there are still areas of the country with no service available. Roe (1997) states that 50% of children in England have access to a CCN but only 10% to a 24-hour service. Children and their parents are therefore being deprived of their right to an early discharge from hospital or may be discharged into the care of competent but not children's trained community nurses. Fradd (1990) writes of children being nursed at home with more technical support than ever before and that these changing patterns of care necessitate the involvement of children's nurses who will be appropriately equipped to give support.

The aims of community care for sick children are:

- to provide skilled nursing care, which involves planning and implementing family-centred care for both short- and long-term situations
- to be aware of and able to manage available resources
- to work in partnership with the family, thus promoting consumer choice
- to evaluate and monitor standards of care (Gastrell 1993).

Recent analysis of models of CCN services identified that both generalist and specialist teams may operate from either acute or community bases (RCN 1994). Generalist teams usually cover the catchment area in which they are based and the range of their work is great, varying from postoperative visits to children following day surgery through a whole range of childhood conditions which may include caring for a child with home ventilation or a child requiring terminal care. The specialist nurse's expertise is in fields such as oncology, cystic fibrosis and neonatology (Kelly et al 1995) and as such she can act as a resource for the generalist nurses. CCN teams may be based either within primary health care teams, for example in a health centre, or as an extension of a hospital paediatric department.

One of the aims of Project 2000 Child Branch courses was that students would be prepared to become practitioners capable of working in institutional and non-institutional settings. However, there is proving to be a wide diversity in the experience that these students gain during their training (Cash et al 1994). In a study conducted in the Thames region in 1995, it was found that the average length of student placement with a CCN was 8.7 days (Whiting 1997). There may be opportunities for diplomates to work within the community, but it would need to be in a clearly defined role, working alongside experienced staff. Prior to working as a CCN, they are likely to need further education on one of the newly developed community pathways.

Currently, most CCNs are 'very experienced hospital children's nurses who decide to extend their practice into the community' (Cash et al 1994). Initially District Nursing courses were structured to meet the needs of adult nursing. As the demand for CCNs increased, paediatric strands to these courses were developed, but these did not always meet the needs of the practitioners (Whiting 1994). 1995 saw the graduation of the first two paediatric nurses to undertake a community health care course which encompassed specialist strands focusing on individual learning needs (Langlands & McDonagh 1995, Muir 1995). The increasing demand has led to the development of undergraduate programmes leading to a professional qualification in community children's nursing (Parker & Colson 1995).

In spite of the increasing opportunities for children's nurses to pursue their careers in the community with more appropriate educational back up, there may still be difficulties with regard to getting secondment for the courses and funding for setting up new teams. In times of economic difficulties, trusts may not see this as a priority.

Implementing a successful transition of care from hospital to home needs careful planning. The aim of this planning is to ensure that the child's care is continuous and the parents receive the support and education that enables them to provide safe care without undue stress. For children with complex problems, this planning may be initiated some weeks before the child leaves hospital. Ideally the CCN will visit the family in hospital so that relationships can be initiated and practical details discussed. The CCN can familiarise herself with the care that the child is currently receiving and identify the resources that will be required in the home. Education programmes can be initiated for the parents, who should be encouraged to discuss any concerns that they may have so that they are able to give informed consent to the care that they are being asked to undertake.

Charles-Edwards & Casey (1992) pose ethical issues for children's nurses about parental involvement and voluntary consent. They discuss the need for the benefits of home care being weighed against any potential risks which might occur if the family felt under pressure to take on the nursing role, or were not competent to undertake the care, or were given insufficient information. The hospital (or general practitioner if he accepts medical responsibility) 'retains the duty of care in the laws of negligence for the safety of the child' (Dimond 1996). It is therefore the responsibility of the individual practitioner to ensure that she has 'followed the reasonable standard of the responsible nurse working in those circumstances with those particular patients' (Dimond 1996). Documentation should record what has been shown to parents. This should also demonstrate that the instruction has been understood and that the parents are capable of undertaking the procedure competently, being aware of all the problems that might occur and what action to take.

Communication between the hospital and the primary health care team is essential. The CCN is often ideally placed to act as a liaison and may be able to involve the general practitioner and the health visitor at an early stage in the planning. Health visitors have a unique position in that they have access to families of the under-fives in health and should be able to identify when family relationships are suffering after a child has been to hospital (Muller et al 1986). Families should always be given the option of handing back control if they feel that they can no longer cope.

The choice of how to document nursing interventions and assessment of care is determined locally. Some teams share parent-held record books which give good lines of communication to health visitors, but might be insufficient for complex cases who require more detailed care plans. Some parents may wish to contribute to this documentation; others will not. Their choice should be respected. The recommendation of the British Paediatric Association is that the use of parent-held records contributes to high-quality child health care (Dimond 1996). The CCN may decide to use the parent-held records, with the team holding a duplicate set.

It may seem obvious that when visiting families in their own homes, the nurse is the visitor. However, it is only when this reversal of roles is experienced that the nurse appreciates the difference. Usually she will be welcomed into the home and will feel comfortable in the environment. However, it must be borne in mind that on the first visit the nurse will have no idea what she will encounter, be it blaring television or exuberant pets determined to undermine every principle of aseptic technique. The facilities for handwashing may be limited and there may be a lack of working surfaces. The CCN has to be flexible in her approach, whilst maintaining a high standard of care.

Initially, it may seem an abdication of responsibility to look on whilst the parent undertakes the nursing care that might have seemed the remit of the nursing staff in a hospital setting. The role of the CCN is to give positive reinforcement to the nursing care given by the families, rather than taking over the 'hands-on care' for the short period of the visit. Sometimes it is appropriate for the CCN to perform hands-on care, or to assist in care if necessary. She has to assess the situation, and the care being given, ensuring that she does not undermine the parent's confidence but acts as a support and reinforcer. The parents often become expert in caring for their sick children, and in the use of sophisticated technology. The CCN may need to accept that the parent is more familiar with the equipment than she is herself. The CCN will have a wider view of care and can therefore implement new strategies as appropriate. She may need to obtain specialised equipment or extra help for the family, whether this be physical or emotional support.

The personal safety of the CCN has to be considered. It is important that someone at base is aware of her visiting schedules and should endeavour to contact her if concerned that she has not returned to base within a certain time. Should a nurse feel threatened in a home, either by the family members or friends, she should leave as soon as possible and on subsequent visits take another member of staff with her. Mobile phones are an additional safety measure and in some areas are an essential part of the nurse's equipment. Nurse's cars contain syringes and needles and may therefore be targeted by drug users. In some areas, nurses undertaking night visits go in pairs and inform police of their whereabouts.

It may be difficult for families to have time for themselves when caring for a sick child at home. Going shopping or going out for social reasons may become a logistical nightmare and participating in family events an impossibility. There are some areas where respite services have been organised to meet this need (Argles & Tomsett 1995) and trained children's nurses or especially trained carers are available to allow families some life apart from caring for a sick child. It cannot be emphasised enough that the expectations that professionals may have of carers, and that carers have of themselves, may in time place an overwhelming burden on families. It is vital that the named nurse should be constantly watching for signs of stress amongst family members. The care of a sick child at home can be physically and emotionally exhausting and the support of the CCN or other professionals can empower the families to continue caring at home. The CCN is also in a position to ensure that the families are not swamped by too much professional input when different professionals are involved.

Finally, a thought for the nurses. Empowering families to look after their sick child at home is a challenging and fulfilling role. However, it can also be a lonely one. The CCN can become burdened with the problems facing the family, which may not be directly related to the sick child but affect the ability of the family to cope. The relationships developed during the care of a very sick or dying child are likely to be very intense and call for a great deal of emotional input from nurses. To survive these challenges and to remain objective and effec-

tive, it is essential to have readily accessible support networks, be these peer support or a more formal type of supervision. Whyte (1996) states that when working with families, some supervision should always be available. To watch a terminally ill child lying peacefully at home amongst the hubbub of family life reinforces the view that it is the right of the child to remain at home with his family, with support from an appropriately trained sick children's nurse. However, the emotional effect that this may have on the individual nurse should be acknowledged.

References

Argles J, Tomsett A 1995 Giving help where it is needed. Child Health 2(6): 221–223

Cash K, Compston H, Grant J, Livesley J, McAndrew P, Williams G 1994 The preparation of sick children's nurses to work in the community (P2000 evaluation). ENB, London, p 154

Charles-Edwards I, Casey A 1992 Parental involvement and voluntary consent. Paediatric Nursing 4(1): 16–18

Dimond B 1996 The legal aspects of child health care. Mosby, London, ch 8, p 82

Fradd E 1990 Setting up a paediatric community nursing service. Senior Nurse 10(7): 4–7

Gastrell P 1993 Diploma courses for paediatric district nurses. Paediatric Nursing 5(10): 13–14

Kelly P J, Taylor C, Tatman M A 1995 Hospital outreach or community nursing? Child Health 2(4): 160–163

Langlands T, McDonagh L 1995 The pathways to specialism. Paediatric Nursing 7(8): 6–7

Ministry of Health (MoH) 1959 The welfare of children in hospital. Report of Central Health Services Council (Platt Report). HMSO, London

Muir J 1995 Community. The student perspective. Paediatric Nursing 7(8): 25–27

Muller D, Harris P, Wattley L, Taylor J 1986 Nursing children: psychology, research and practice, 2nd edn. Chapman & Hall, London, ch 10, p 155

Parker E, Colson J 1995 Equity or discrimination? Paediatric Nursing 7(1): 10–12

Roe M 1997 Health services for children. Paediatric Nursing 9(3): 6–7

Royal College of Nursing (RCN) 1994 Directory of paediatric community nursing services, 11th edn. RCN, London

Thornes R 1991 Caring for children in the health services – just for the day. NAWCH, London

Whiting M 1994 Meeting needs: RSCN's in the community. Paediatric Nursing 6(1): 9–11

Whiting M 1997 Community children's nursing: a bright future? Paediatric Nursing 9(4): 6–8

Whyte D 1996 Expanding the boundaries of care. Paediatric Nursing 8(4): 20–23

Winter A, Teare J 1997 Construction and application of paediatric community nursing services. Journal of Child Health Care 1(1): 24–29

Woodroffe C, Glickman M, Barker M, Power C 1993 Children, teenagers and health. The key data. Open University Press, Birmingham

1

Administration of Medicines

Introduction and rationale

Of all nursing practices, the responsibility for safe administration of medication probably causes the most anxiety amongst learner nurses. Anxiety is healthy; complacency is dangerous. Complacency can lead to errors, the consequences of which can damage a child's health, and also possibly the nurse's career. However, nurses should be reassured that if they follow the simple measures described here, which should be part of every nurse's routine, each time they check medication, the medication will be given correctly.

Administering medication to children is doubly difficult; not only do the dosages vary according to the child's weight, but gaining a child's cooperation can be an enormous challenge. The variety of routes by which medication can be administered also adds confusion. A paediatric nurse must be familiar with the most common routes and be skilled in the different techniques required.

Learning outcomes

After reading this section the nurse should understand:

- the principles by which medications can be administered safely
- techniques for gaining a child's cooperation
- routes of administration, and suitable techniques for each route.

Factors to note

The recent Health Select Committee report (1997) highlighted concern over the licensing of drugs for children. Many of the most common preparations used for children are in fact only licensed for adults, owing to ethical and practical difficulties in conducting clinical trials in children.

While many of these drugs are clearly documented in well-known paediatric formularies (Alder Hey, Guy's), and have been prescribed and administered without problem for years, nurses must ensure that they are con-fident of local policy regarding the nurse's role in administering unlicensed drugs. Some new drugs will initially be licensed on a named-patient basis only, or as part of clinical trials. Local policy will often dictate that approval for new drugs be sought through the Trust Drugs and Therapeutics Committee, or via the Trust Formulary.

Many parents administer drugs to their children, such as the occasional antibiotic, dose of paracetamol, or complex drug regimes that may be given to children with chronic illness at home. The nurse forms a vital part of the team, which also includes doctors and pharmacists, that teaches and prepares parents for this role. Parents will often develop routines and techniques that are peculiar to the family but work well, and these should be respected.

Confusion can occur if the task of drug administration is shared between nurse and parent on the ward. While in many trusts parents are allowed, and in fact encouraged, to administer medication to their children, this forms part of the partnership of trust and understanding between parent and nurse which must exist within the framework of an established policy. Communication and accountability must be clearly defined in this partnership. Issues such as storage, communication and cost must be considered, as well as the willingness of parents to participate; they may indeed welcome and need a break from such responsibility (Fradd 1990, Sutherland et al 1995).

Single nurse administration is now well established on adult wards. One argument for single nurse checking is that it crystallises accountability. Where two nurses check drugs they can abdicate responsibility to the point where neither nurse checks properly; if just one nurse checks drugs she is more likely to take care to get it right. Paediatric areas have been slower to initiate single nurse checking, because of anxieties over the complexity of drug administration and dose calculation in children. Single nurse checking has, however, been introduced successfully in some paediatric wards.

Guidelines

The UKCC booklet *Standards for the Administration of Medicines* (1992), along with local trust policies, gives nurses ample guidance on safe administration of medicines. The UKCC expects the nurse not just to administer medications in a technically safe manner, but to make a much broader clinical and professional contribution to the process. The nurse must have sufficient understanding of pharmacology, including normal doses and side-effects, as well as an understanding of the environment and of clinical and psychological considerations, in order to contribute positively with the other members of the clinical team.

To administer medication safely the nurse must ensure:

- That the *correct patient* receives the medication. The identity of the patient must be checked. Name bands are routinely used to confirm identity, but parental confirmation of identity is also valuable. Williams (1996) mentions the use of photographs on drug charts to confirm identity. Be particularly careful if there are children with similar names on the ward, if children have siblings (particularly twins) visiting, or if the child is in a large group of children, for example in the playroom.
- That the child receives the *correct drug*. Many hand-written prescriptions can be difficult to decipher, or poorly written. It is very easy to confuse drug names which have the same root (e.g. ceftazidime, cefotaxime). The nurse must *not* make assumptions about what the doctor has written, but must ask the doctor to rewrite the prescription clearly and legibly, using block capitals (Dillner 1992).
- That the child receives the *correct dose*. A serious error in paediatrics is to administer 10 times the correct dose, either because the prescribing doctor has made a mistake and the nurse has failed to identify it, or because the nurse has calculated the amount incorrectly. Calculating paediatric dosages requires a reasonable level of numeracy, and the nurse must be confident of her arithmetical ability. Relying on a calculator and a formula is not sufficient; the numbers themselves must make sense (Bayne & Bindler 1988). The nurse must be familiar with the correct range of doses for each drug and, if she is not familiar with the correct dosage, should check in the formulary. Confusion is possible between milligrams, micrograms and nanograms, especially if abbreviations are used.
- That the dose is administered by the *correct route*. If the route is incorrect, the consequences may range from the minor (sub-therapeutic drug plasma levels) to the major (intravenous embolism if oral substances are given intravenously).
- That the dose is administered at the *correct time*. If it is impossible to administer the medication at the correct time, record why, and when it was administered and inform medical staff. Administration of medications should be a priority in the organisation of patient care, and if drugs are often being given late, attention should be given to whether ward routines need to be adjusted. Happily, many wards have abandoned the formal drug round, and instead rely on nurses to take responsibility for administering medication to their own named patients, at times that suit the child's routine and medication schedule. If staffing pressures are contributing towards any significant delay, the senior manager must be informed.
- That *expiry dates* are checked for each drug, every time.

The ward culture is crucial in creating an environment in which administration of medications is safe. The following guidance may be helpful to ward managers and their staff:

- Do not allow anyone to interrupt a nurse who is checking medications.
- On children's wards safe storage of all medications is a *must*. Cupboards and drug trolleys must be locked at all times, and must never be left unattended if open. To allow accidental poisoning because of sloppy practice is unacceptable. Remember, even seemingly innocuous substances may kill a child (e.g. iron tablets, paracetamol, cleaning substances). The storage of hazardous substances, which would include medications in children's areas, is covered within recent COSHH (Control of Substances Hazardous to Health) legislation.
- Efficient ordering and stock control systems will eliminate overstocking, reduce the number of scarcely used medicines on the ward, and reduce risk.
- Ensure that the nurse who is caring for the child, and that nurse only, takes responsibility for the child's medication.
- Ensure that all nurses are skilled and confident in necessary techniques, e.g. intravenous infusion, so that continuity of patient care is not interrupted.
- Drugs should not be prepared before they can be given, for example left sitting on children's lockers, or in the treatment room.
- Ensure that safety of drug administration has a high profile, that if mistakes occur they are declared

openly, and that lessons are learned and communicated.

■ Drug administration should be the focus of a 'zero defect' attitude to quality care. The tendency of humans to make mistakes should be minimised by tight procedures.

■ Encourage a culture where it is acceptable to challenge and question even the most senior members of the team.

Developmental considerations

As soon as the child reaches an age of even basic comprehension, informed consent to treatment becomes possible (McCall-Smith 1992). Most parents and nurses will have experienced the rebelliousness of the 2-year-old, the playfulness of the 5-year-old, and the downright subversion of the 13-year-old. Most nurses (and parents) will have at some stage in their careers held a child extremely firmly and 'forced' him to swallow medicines against his wishes, but this should be avoided if at all possible.

Helping the child understand why he must have the medication, and what will happen if he does not, can be achieved at a remarkably early age (Holdsworth, unpublished work, 1995). The parents may well have developed strategies at home that will help in hospital. Children enjoy routines, and if medicine is to be taken long term, making medicine time fun and building it into fun daily routines, such as bathtime and toothbrushing, can be helpful. Rewarding cooperative behaviour with praise, hugs and cuddles, as well as the occasional treat, while not overreacting to difficult behaviour, will teach most children that cooperation is the better option.

Mary Poppins knew what she was talking about when she sang 'a spoonful of sugar helps the medicine go down'. This age-old technique softens the bitter taste of medicine, provides a reward for good behaviour, and uses the traditional, and very useful tool of bribery. Over-sweet medicines, however, should be used with care, as dental caries can occur in long-term use of high-sugar medicines (Manley et al 1994).

Oral medication

In children the most common route for administration of medicines is the oral route, for several reasons:

■ It is safe: medicines will have a slower therapeutic effect than when administered by some other routes, so there is more time to react should side-effects

occur (for example by giving an antidote, or performing gastric lavage).

■ It is easy: most children will take medicines easily, with persuasion. No high-tech equipment is required.

■ It is cheap: oral medications are often much cheaper than other preparations of the same drug, for example intravenous drugs.

Equipment

A well-equipped paediatric drug trolley or cupboard will hold:

■ Medications
■ Medicine pots or cups, with measured volumes
■ Oral syringes: various sizes
■ Medicine spoons, again with measured graduations
■ Mortar and pestle, or tablet crusher
■ Tablet divider
■ Water (sterile water is required for babies)
■ Formulary.

Method

Most medications come in a choice of tablet or suspension form, and sometimes there is a choice of flavours and strengths. If suspensions are unavailable, tablets can be crushed and mixed with water, using either a mortar and pestle, or a tablet crusher (see Fig. 1.1). Advice should be sought from the pharmacist about whether such methods are suitable and what diluents are appropriate.

Some suspensions are very sugary, or the medication itself can cause damage to gums and teeth if used over a prolonged period (e.g. phenytoin). Rinsing the mouth with water after administration and good mouth hygiene are essential.

Some tablets cannot be crushed or dissolved, for example those with enteric coating, or slow-release tablets. Care should be taken if dividing tablets to ensure as accurate a dose as possible.

Medicines can be administered either by spoon, syringe or cup. Spoons and cups are cheap and simple, but syringes can be useful if administering non-standard volumes, or for babies. Care must be taken not to force the syringe into the mouth or between the teeth, as trauma can result. Special oral syringes are available with connectors which cannot be fitted to intravenous equipment, thus making the risk of administering oral drugs through the intravenous route less likely.

Babies.   Hold the baby firmly on your lap in a semi-reclining position. Encourage the baby to open his mouth, and place the syringe onto his tongue. Gently

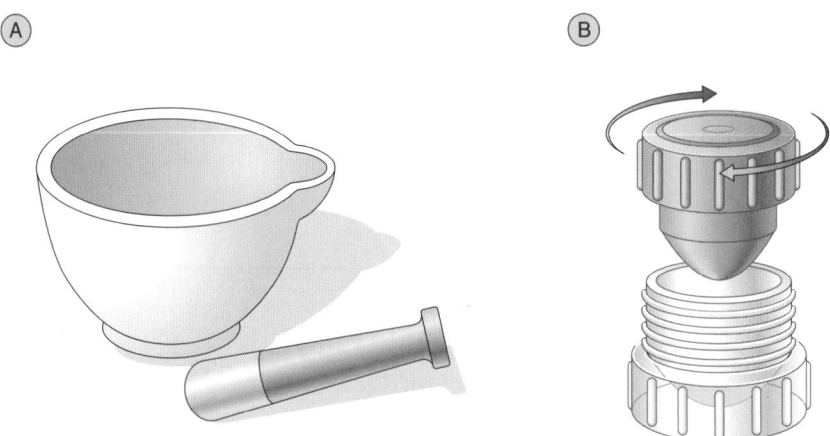

Figure 1.1
(A) Pestle and mortar;
(B) Tablet crusher.

introduce the suspension into the baby's mouth. Depressing the baby's tongue slightly with the syringe will encourage the baby to suck and swallow without choking. Gently stroking his cheeks or under his chin may also stimulate a suck reflex.

Toddlers. Because toddlers cannot understand why they must take their medicine, they may need plenty of encouragement, reward and reassurance. Some will swallow their medicine quite happily from a spoon or cup, and may enjoy using a syringe. It helps if the taste is pleasant and they are rewarded with cuddles and attention. Toddlers can be encouraged through play and fun. If they refuse, a confident, firm tone of voice may help persuade them that cooperation is worthwhile. If all else fails, a firm hold around the arms and a no fuss, matter-of-fact insistence can sometimes succeed, although it can be self-defeating as the medicine is likely to be spat out, and care must be taken to ensure that the child does not choke. Parents often 'hide' the medicine in a drink such as a milk shake, but this practice should be discouraged as it is impossible to tell how much medicine the child has had if the drink is not finished, and children may feel betrayed if they discover the deception, and refuse to drink at all. It is perfectly acceptable, however, for the taste of certain drugs to be disguised with a spoonful of jam, yoghurt or honey.

Older children. Children learn to swallow tablets at different ages, and this does require some coordination, but learning to swallow tablets is a skill worth encouraging, as tablets can be far easier to swallow and taste less bitter than suspensions. Swallowing tablets, rather than babyish suspensions, can also represent a welcome sign of growing up and learning new skills, especially important for children with chronic illness who may struggle to develop into independent adults.

Children with nasogastric or gastrostomy tubes (see Enteral Feeding, p. 115). Most 'oral' medications can be given through this route. This can be especially convenient when many unpleasant medicines are to be given. If the medicine is particularly viscous, or if it has partially dissolved granules, care should be taken not to block the tube. The tube should be checked for position as for a feed. It should be flushed with water between and after each separate drug (Williams 1989). *Note:* Sublingual medicines (e.g. nifedipine) *cannot* be given via this route.

Intravenous medication

(See also: Aseptic Non-touch Technique, p. 39; Central Lines, p. 83; Intravenous infusions, p. 151; Venepuncture and Cannulation, p. 311.)

Intravenous medication may be given by intermittent bolus injection, intermittent infusion, or continuous infusion. The choice of technique will depend on the pharmacological characteristics of the medication (half-life, preferred plasma levels, etc.) and the lifestyle of the child (intermittent bolus injections may be preferable to continuous infusion in children who are at school, for example).

Intravenous medication has the following benefits:

- It can sustain high plasma drug levels.
- It can be used in an emergency when a child cannot swallow, and will have an immediate effect.
- The drug will reach the 'target' rapidly when transported in the bloodstream.
- The drug can be absorbed if gastrointestinal absorption is impossible.

- It requires fewer needles than other forms of injections as it uses an in situ cannula, and is therefore less traumatic.
- The intravenous route is the preferred route if the child is critically ill.

However, intravenous medication also carries with it the following potential complications:

- Anaphylaxis
- Once injected, reversal is almost impossible unless an antidote exists
- Contamination: microorganisms, foreign matter (e.g. latex from a rubber bung, drug precipitate)
- Extravasation (or 'tissuing', as the vein walls break down)
- Phlebitis (inflammation of the vein, causing localised pain)
- Air embolism
- Incompatibility if several infusions/bolus drugs are given at the same time
- Needlestick injury to child or nurse
- Fluid overload.

Equipment

The following should be available to the nurse administering intravenous medication:

- Clean surface: trolley, table top, etc.
- Medication
- Reconstitution solution if needed (see below)
- Sterile saline or heparinised saline for flush (see below)
- Needles
- Syringes
- Alcohol swabs
- Giving sets, connectors, bungs and lines: a large variety of types and sizes are available
- Gloves
- Infusion pump or syringe pump
- Medication chart
- 'Drug additive' or 'date and time' labels for line, syringe or burette.

Normally, intravenous medication will be given in an environment where emergency and resuscitation equipment is available.

Because of the risk of anaphylaxis, adrenaline should be available to nurses administering intravenous injections. Community nurses will usually carry packs of adrenaline, but must ensure that they are covered by local policy to administer it in an emergency without a prescription or medical supervision.

Method

Reconstitution, dilution and length of infusion will all vary according to the drug being used. Nurses should refer to drug information sheets as a first point of reference, as these will often be the most up-to-date source of information, but recognised paediatric formularies (e.g. Royal Liverpool Children's Hospital (Alder Hey) 1994, Guy's, Lewisham and St Thomas' NHS Trust 1993) should be used as further guidance.

Administration (see also Intravenous infusions, p. 151) Many drugs require reconstitution. Some pharmacy departments offer a reconstitution service or CIVAS (centralised intravenous additives services) especially for cytotoxic or other potentially toxic drugs. In such a service drugs are prepared under strict aseptic conditions, using lamina flow chambers. CIVAS reduce waste, and therefore expense, and have the clinical benefits of reducing the incidence of phlebitis, extravasation, contamination, and drug errors (Rodkin 1987, Williams 1996). However, there will still always be circumstances when drugs are reconstituted on the wards. This must be done in a clean environment, using a sterile technique and equipment.

Medication may be added to a volume of fluid for infusion via bag or burette, or directly into the intravenous tubing or cannula through a bung near the entry site. If infusion lines are used, the amount of prime solution required should be considered when calculating the drug volume.

Doctors may sometimes administer medication directly into the vein through a hypodermic or 'butterfly' needle. This latter technique would normally only be used in an emergency, or on induction of anaesthetic.

Flush solutions are used in the following circumstances:

- to check before intravenous administration whether the line is patent
- between sequential injections or infusions, to ensure that incompatible drugs do not mix
- at the end of administration to ensure that no drug remains in the line, and to ensure that the vein remains patent.

In larger cannulae, saline is as effective, and cheaper than heparinised solutions, which should be reserved solely for small neonatal cannulae and some central and long lines (Danet & Norris 1992, Kotter 1996, Le Duc 1997).

Intravenous pumps should always be used to deliver infusions. There are many different types and makes of pump on the market. The nurse must ensure that she is familiar with each type of pump in use on her ward; evidence suggests that many drug errors occur because of staff's unfamiliarity with equipment (MDA 1995).

Intramuscular medication

Intramuscular injection is nowadays avoided where possible in paediatric practice, unless other routes are not available or are impractical. Some immunisations and vaccinations are administered intramuscularly. The route is considered unsuitable for administration of pain control, as the medication will take some time to be absorbed, so will not give immediate effect. The procedure is unpleasant and frightening so children may refuse it, even if they are in pain, and it is difficult to provide continuously steady plasma levels, causing peaks and troughs in therapeutic effect.

Equipment
- Medication and reconstituent solution if needed
- Medication chart
- Needle and syringe (see below)
- Alcohol swab (see below)
- Dish or tray

Method
Because the route is now less often used, paediatric nurses are less confident in the procedure. It is important, however, that nurses understand the safest and most effective sites for intramuscular injection, and are competent and practised in the technique.

Explanation should be given to the child and family about what is to happen, and why. A matter-of-fact, honest approach is best with children, for example, 'Yes it will hurt, but it will soon be over.' Local anaesthetic cream may block superficial pain, but deep muscular pain, stiffness or soreness may still occur.

The skin should be cleaned with an alcohol swab. The nurse should have clean hands and wear gloves, and the equipment must be sterile.

The needle should be sharp. It should be inserted at 45 or 90 degrees, depending on muscle bulk (Skale 1992). The depth of the injection can be assessed by squeezing the muscle bulk upwards and 'eyeballing' the estimated depth. The needle should not touch bony structures, but should be long enough to penetrate deep muscle. The needle should be aspirated to ensure a blood vessel has not been punctured, and then the fluid injected. The speed of the injection is a matter of personal preference; while some children prefer a short sharp shock and getting it over with, a slower injection can be gentler and less startling for anxious children if they are able to stay still.

The choice of needle will depend on the size of the muscle chosen, and the viscosity of the fluid. If the fluid is very viscous, it may be less painful to select a larger-bore needle, as the pressure of fluid being expressed will be less.

The volume of fluid should be limited for each site. Skale (1992) recommends 0.5 ml as maximum for an infant, 1 ml for a toddler, and 1.5–3 ml for a school child or adolescent. The choice of site should be documented and, if regular injections are to occur, an injection site chart should be used to ensure rotation.

However well prepared small children are, they are likely to squirm, cry out, or try to fight off the nurse. For this reason the nurse should always have assistance. It is important to reassure the child that his reaction is quite normal and that he is not being naughty, to offer lots of praise and congratulate him for his bravery. Bravery certificates are a welcome reward for most children.

Common sites (Skale 1992, Tortora & Agnostakis 1990)
Deltoid muscle (Fig. 1.2A).   This muscle is often shallow in children and babies, but can usefully be used for injections of small amounts of fluid. The muscle is easily accessible, and it is possible to hold most babies and children safely while accessing the site. It is a site often used for immunisation.

Vastus lateralis and rectus femoris muscles (Fig. 1.2B). The muscles on the front and side of the thigh are often the most bulky in infants and free of major nerve structures.

Gluteus medius muscle (outer upper quadrant of buttock; Fig. 1.2C).   This muscle is often undeveloped in babies who have not yet started to walk, and therefore should be avoided till a child has been walking for some time. There is a risk of trauma to the sciatic nerve.

Complications
- Haematoma
- Pain
- Nerve damage
- Fibrosis of muscle
- Needle phobia

Subcutaneous medication

Subcutaneous injection or infusion is a common procedure in paediatric practice. The most common reason

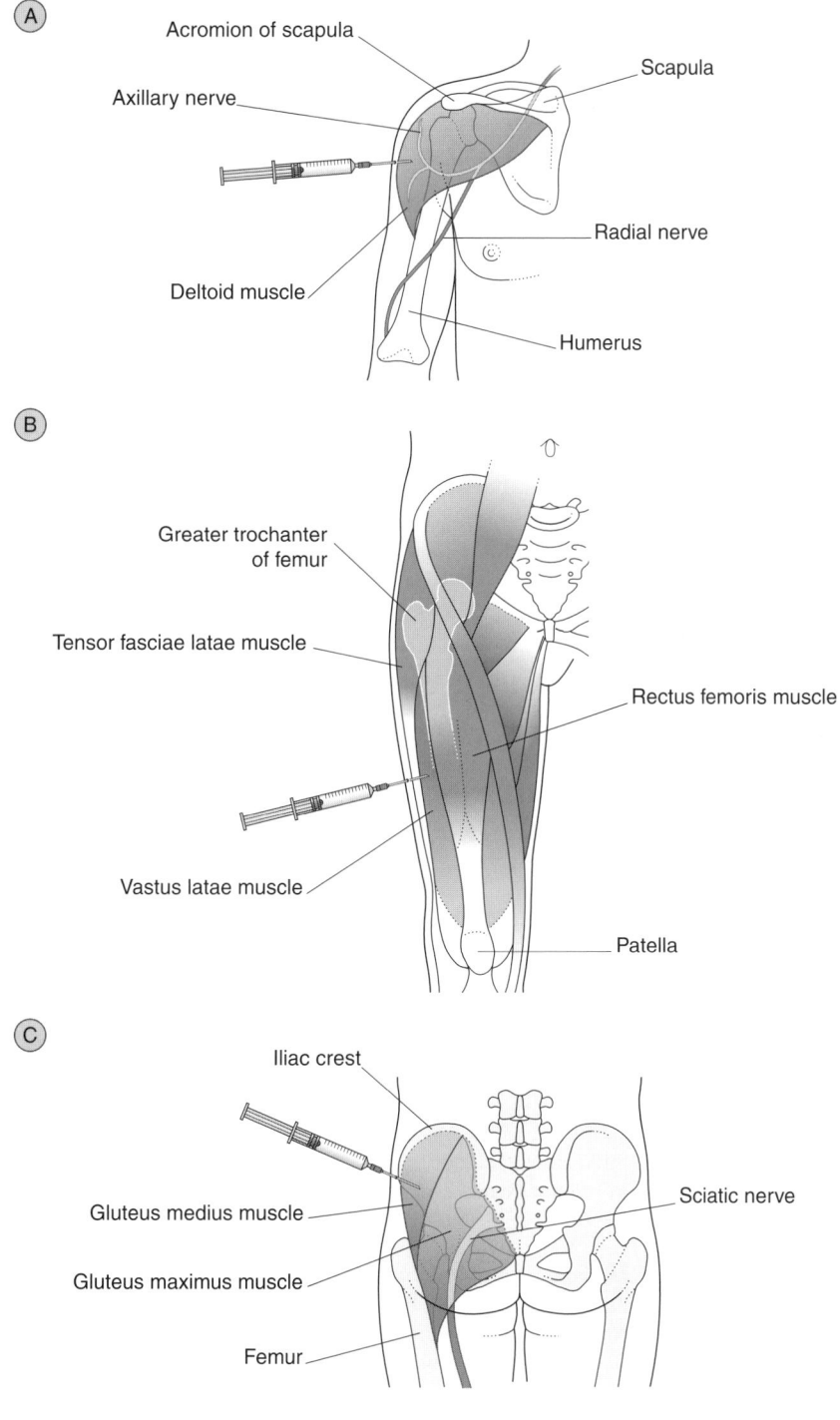

Figure 1.2

Three common sites for intramuscular injections: (A) deltoid region; (B) lateral surface of the thigh; (C) buttock.

for subcutaneous injection is to administer insulin or heparin, and for some immunisations and vaccinations. Subcutaneous injections will be absorbed slowly, though with different speed, from different sites. Continuous subcutaneous infusion of analgesics is becoming more common and can provide effective steady pain relief.

Equipment and method

It is important for nurses to distinguish between insulin syringes, which come graduated in 50 or 100 units, with an integral half-inch needle, and normal 1 ml syringes with separate gauge needle. There is scope for error if the different graduations on each system are misunderstood.

Devices such as injection pens or jet injectors are now commonly used by diabetics, and make the injection quicker and easier for the patient. Nurses using such devices must be familiar with the manufacturers' instructions.

Common sites for injection for diabetics who inject regularly are the upper thigh, abdomen, upper arm, and buttocks, because of their deep fat layer and their accessibility. Sites should be rotated, and in hospital this should be documented. If the site is used too often, it will become fibrosed. This can be quite tempting for children, because fibrosis causes numbness and therefore reduces pain, but fibrosis will decrease the efficiency of insulin absorption.

If the child is unused to injections, local anaesthetic cream can be used, but most frequent injectors do not need this.

In hospital the skin is usually cleaned with an alcohol swab; at home this is not necessary, as long as the skin is socially clean. The skin should be pinched up, and the needle is inserted into subcutaneous tissue at 90 degrees. The needle should be inserted to its full length in pre-school and older children. It is not necessary to aspirate the needle; just inject the fluid slowly. The needle should be withdrawn gently. It should not be necessary to press or rub the skin (BDA 1996/97).

Subcutaneous infusions can be used to administer analgesia, especially in palliative care situations. This route causes fewer side-effects than when opiates are infused through the intravenous route. Subcutaneous infusions can be administered through butterfly needles, or purpose-designed subcutaneous infusion cannulae. Portable infusion sets are used to ensure that the child has as free a lifestyle as possible. The needle or cannula should be resited every 2–7 days (Jody et al 1993).

Intraosseous administration

This technique is used primarily in emergency situations, especially when veins are collapsed due to shock. Quick and easy access to the circulation can be gained. The APLS (1993) guidelines recommend that the route be used if venous access fails, or if it will take more than 2 minutes to achieve in life-threatening situations. Insertion of the needle is made by a doctor.

Equipment and method

Specially designed 18 gauge needles with trocars are now available and are commonly held as a routine item on crash trolleys. The needle is inserted aseptically (if time allows) into the upper tibia or lower femur, though other sites can be used. The needle is secured with a sterile dressing, and bolus injections or infusions given, using the same connectors as for intravenous injections or infusions.

Epidural infusions

Continuous epidural infusions, and indeed other forms of spinal nerve block, are becoming more commonly used in older children, as they provide effective major pain relief without the side-effects of systemic opiates. The catheter is usually sited preoperatively in theatre under anaesthetic, by the anaesthetist or surgeon. Epidural infusions should be supervised by nursing and medical staff experienced and knowledgeable in their use. They should be used in conjunction with regular pain assessment.

Epidurals may use a local anaesthetic agent (such as bupivacaine hydrochloride) and/or opiates for analgesia. If opiates are used, the patient should be observed closely for signs of respiratory depression. Other side-effects of opiate epidural analgesia include vomiting and nausea, or excessive sedation. Naloxone should be available. If analgesia is insufficient, a technical cause such as local leakage or catheter disconnection should be sought before automatically increasing the infusion.

The nurse should observe for urinary retention as a result of local anaesthetic or opiate.

Side-effects common in older patients with epidurals, such as hypotension and lower limb paraesthesia, may be caused by an epidural haematoma. They appear to be less common in children, but nurses must nonetheless remain alert for such signs (Campbell & Glasper 1995).

Rectal medication

The rectal route is used when drugs cannot be absorbed orally, or when a local effect is required. Absorption is less reliable than via the oral route, as drugs may be expelled before absorption. Diarrhoea or impacted faeces are contraindications for the use of this route.

In some countries the rectal route is commonplace (for example in France). However, in the UK there is a reluctance to administer via this route, perhaps owing to cultural or sexual taboos about anal penetration. Because of this concern, nurses must exercise great sensitivity in using this route, especially with older children and adolescents who may be totally unaware that this technique exists. Consent should be sought where possible, especially if the suppository is to be inserted in the recovery room or while the child is sedated, and a chaperone, preferably the parent, should be present.

Equipment
- Medication chart
- Gloves
- Dish containing:
  - Suppository
  - Lubricating gel
  - Swab or tissue

Method
The child should be on his side, with his legs curled up in a fetal position. With babies it is possible just to lift the legs and flex the knees, as for changing a nappy. Gloves should be worn for this procedure. The suppository should be lubricated with water-soluble jelly and gently inserted just beyond the anal sphincter. The little finger should be used with babies, and the finger should hardly need to be inserted. It is helpful to hold the buttocks together for several minutes to prevent immediate expulsion of the suppository.

Inhaled medication (see Inhalational Devices, p. 143)

Ear drops (see Ear Care, p. 99)

Eye drops and ointment (see Eye Care, p. 103)

Topical medication (see Skin Care, p. 255)

COMMUNITY PERSPECTIVE
The role of the CCN may range from supporting parents giving oral medication to administering complex drug regimes herself.

If it is necessary for the CCN to carry drugs, these should be transported in a sturdy container or cool box. If drugs have to be left in the car between visits, care must be taken to leave them unobtrusively in a securely locked car. Controlled drugs must be kept in the possession of the nurse, and cytotoxic drugs in special carrying cases, clearly labelled (RCN 1994).

Drugs must be stored at the recommended temperatures. It may be necessary to supply the family with a drug refrigerator or freezer.

The RCN have produced a comprehensive document *Administering Intravenous Therapy to Children in the Community* (RCN 1994). Nurses administering i.v. drugs in the home would be well advised to read this. As nurses are increasingly asked to undertake pioneering clinical work in the home, each practitioner must consider her own accountability.

All drugs must be administered according to local policy. Control of Substances Hazardous to Health (COSHH) regulations (HSE 1988) apply in the home and the CCN is responsible for ensuring safe practice. This may include providing protective clothing for the administering nurse or parent and provision of spillage kits as appropriate.

The safety of the home environment for the preparation and administration of i.v. drugs will need to be assessed. Some homes may prove to be unsafe, either through inadequate standards of hygiene or lack of space, but this is the exception. The nurse will need to be able to create an aseptic field (see Aseptic Non-touch technique, p. 39).

Where parents are undertaking administration of drugs by injection, it is the responsibility of the CCN to ensure that appropriate training, supervision and written guidelines are in place. These must include information about side-effects and possible complications of therapy, including anaphylactic rescue.

Anaphylaxis kits containing adrenaline, chlorpheniramine and hydrocortisone should be carried by the nurse. The kits should include standing orders for administration agreed by the hospital. These drugs should be written up in the child's documentation by the hospital or GP.

COMMUNITY PERSPECTIVE (Contd.)

Wherever possible, two people should check intravenous drugs. The parent or an older child may be involved. However, preloaded syringes, prepared in a hospital pharmacy, are preferable.

When electrically powered syringe drivers or i.v. pumps are used, it is necessary to ensure that they are capable of running on their own batteries, in case of power failure. Parents should know what they should do if the pump/driver fails to work, as it may be unrealistic to have spare pumps available. All equipment should be serviced regularly.

When opioids are administered subcutaneously by syringe driver or intravenously via a pump, it may be necessary to have naloxone in the home, as an antidote to respiratory depression. This is unlikely to occur as the majority of children on opioids are terminally ill and will have had their dosages increased gradually.

Any clinical waste should be disposed of according to local policy.

Parents must know who to contact at any time should they have problems and the CCN must be aware of any potential problems that may occur with any of the devices in use, or the medication being administered.

Do and do not

- Do be careful.
- Do allow sufficient time.
- Do not become rushed or distracted.
- Do not 'short cut' correct checking procedures.
- Do check with the doctor or pharmacist if unsure.
- Do check that the correct patient receives the correct dose of the correct medication, at the correct time, via the correct route.

References

Advanced Paediatric Life Support Group (APLS) 1993 Advanced paediatric life support: the practical approach. BMJ Publishing Group, London

Bayne T, Bindler R 1988 Medication calculation skills of registered nurses. Journal of Continuing Education on Nursing 19(6): 258–262

British Diabetic Association 1996/97 The ABC of injecting. In: Balance for beginners

Campbell S, Glasper E A (eds) 1995 Whaley and Wong's children's nursing. Mosby, London

Danet G D, Norris E M 1992 Paediatric IV catheters. Efficacy of saline flush. Pediatric Nursing 18(2): 111–113

Dillner L 1992 Illegible writing kills patients. British Medical Journal 305(12 Sept): 604

Fradd E 1990 Sharing accountability. Paediatric Nursing 2(3): 6–8

Guy's, Lewisham and St Thomas' NHS Trust 1993 Paediatric formulary, 3rd edn. Guy's, Lewisham and St Thomas' NHS Trust, London

Health and Safety Executive (HSE) 1988 Control of substances hazardous to health regulations. HMSO, London

Health Select Committee 1997 Fifth report of session 1996/7. Hospital services to children and young people. Paper 128.1. Stationery Office, London

Jody A, Charnow N A, Fandek P H, Johnson G A, Sloane (eds) 1993 Medication administration and intravenous therapy. Springhouse, Pennsylvania

Kotter R W 1996 Heparin vs saline flush for intermittent intravenous device maintenance in neonates. Journal of Neonatal Nursing 15(6): 43–47, 55–59

Le Duc K 1997 Efficacy of normal saline solution vs heparin solution for maintaining patency of peripheral intravenous catheters in children. Journal of Emergency Nursing 23(4): 306–309

McCall Smith A 1992 Consent to treatment in childhood. Archives of Disease in Childhood 67(1): 1247

Manley G, Sheiham A, Eadsforth W 1994 Sugar coated care? Nursing Times 90(7): 34–35

Medical Devices Agency (MDA) 1995 Infusion systems. Device Bulletin DB9503. MDA, London

Rodkin S 1987 Monitoring of phlebitis during and after CIVA trial at Wellesley Hospital. Official Journal Of the Canadian Intravenous Nurses Association 3(2): 11

Royal College of Nursing Paediatric Community Nurses' Forum 1994 Administering intravenous therapy to children in the community. RCN, London

Royal Liverpool Children's Hospital 1994 Alder Hey book of children's doses, 6th edn. Royal Liverpool Children's Hospital, Liverpool

Skale N 1992 Manual of paediatric nursing procedures. J B Lippincott, Pennsylvania

Sutherland K, Morgan J, Semple S 1995 Education and accountability: self administration of medicine. Nursing Times 91(23): 32–33

Tortora G J, Agnostakis P 1990 Principles of anatomy and physiology, 6th edn. Harper Collins, New York

United Kingdom Central Council for Nursing, Midwifery and Health Visiting (UKCC) 1992 Standards for the administration of medicines. UKCC, London

Williams A 1996 How do you avoid mistakes in medication administration? Nursing Times 92(14): 40–41

Williams P J 1989 How do you keep medicine from clogging feeding tubes? American Journal of Nursing 89(2): 181–189

Further reading

United Kingdom Central Council for Nursing, Midwifery and Health Visiting (UKCC) 1992 The scope of professional practice. UKCC, London

2

Aseptic Non-Touch Technique

Introduction

Children's nurses need to perform many practical skills 'aseptically'. The administration of intravenous medications and the management of wounds are two of the most common types of aseptic procedures. Both involve situations where the child's natural defence systems have been breached and need protecting by safe nursing practice. The aseptic non-touch technique was designed for intravenous therapy by combining existing concepts and terminology (Rowley, unpublished work, 1996); however, the principles can be applied to other invasive procedures such as wound cleaning or inserting a nasogastric tube.

Learning outcomes

The aim of this section is for the nurse to:

- understand the principles of achieving asepsis
- apply the principles of aseptic non-touch technique to any particular aseptic procedure
- understand why it is important to use the correct, and thus achievable, terminology when referring to aseptic techniques.

Terms used

Infective precautions. Equipment used to help maintain asepsis, e.g. gloves, sterile towels, etc.

Key parts/key sites. Those parts or sites that, if contaminated by infectious material, increase the risk of infection. In i.v. therapy, key parts are usually parts of equipment which come into direct or indirect contact with the liquid infusion.

Aseptic non-touch technique (ANTT). An aseptic non-touch technique prevents direct and indirect contamination of key parts and key sites by a non-touch method and by other appropriate infective precautions.

General principles of aseptic non-touch technique

Always wash hands effectively.
Never contaminate key parts or key sites.
Touch non-key parts with confidence.
Take 'appropriate' infective precautions.

Factors to note

Terminology

The aseptic non-touch technique is a technique that maintains asepsis and is non-touch in nature. This is an important fact to appreciate, as other terms, such as 'sterile' and 'clean technique', are often used inaccurately and can confuse practitioners (see Box 2.1).

Important components

Handwashing. Handwashing is a central component of the aseptic non-touch technique. A number of scien-

---

Box 2.1 **Terminology should accurately reflect practice**

Sterile techniques – are not achievable
The word sterile means 'free from microorganisms' (Weller 1993); therefore, owing to the natural multitude of microorganisms in the atmosphere, it is not possible to achieve a true sterile technique for procedures in typical ward and home environments.

Aseptic techniques – are achievable
For infections to occur in the bloodstream (in i.v. therapy) or local sites (in wound care etc.) key parts or sites must be contaminated by a sufficient number of virulent, pathogenic organisms (Hendrick 1988). Therefore, a technique that prevents this level of contamination is safe. Such a technique is most accurately termed an aseptic technique, as the word asepsis means, 'freedom from infection or infectious (pathogenic) material' (Weller 1993).

Non-touch techniques – are paramount
Pathogenic organisms can not always be removed by effective handwashing (Church 1986). Additionally, handwashing is not always effective (Pritchard & David 1994). Therefore, a non-touch technique is perhaps the single most important component in achieving asepsis. Additionally, the term aseptic non-touch technique is both accurate and achievable.

tific studies have demonstrated the ability of some organisms to survive on the hands of health care workers (Adams & Marrie 1982, Bauer et al 1990). On such evidence it is not surprising that handwashing remains the most significant single procedure in preventing cross-infection in hospital (Maki et al 1973).

Although bacteria can be reduced by effective hand-washing, they will re-establish quickly over the entire hand surface in the warm and damp environment created beneath gloves (Gould 1991). This is an important fact, as a study by Stringer et al (1991) highlighted that lack of handwashing after glove removal was the most frequent breakdown in universal barrier precautions. Washing the hands both before and after a procedure, as demonstrated by Lawrence (1994), is a vital prerequisite of the aseptic non-touch technique (see Control of Infection p.13).

Aseptic fields.   The nurse must decide what kind of aseptic field is required to maintain the asepsis of equipment and key parts. The provision of sterile towels, dressing packs, etc., for all procedures is overly extravagant. For the majority of aseptic procedures, one is maintaining the asepsis of only one or two small key parts or sites. This can be achieved simply and effectively by a non-touch method and ad hoc aseptic fields (e.g. using the inside of equipment packaging).

Environmental/air contamination.   Airborne infections in hospital account for only 10% of all endemic infections (Eickhoff 1994), therefore, the potential for harmful contamination of key parts and sites by air is insignificant compared to contamination by direct contact. The nurse can reduce the potential for environmental infection by taking sensible measures, i.e. not practising aseptic procedures at the bedside immediately after activities like bed making and wound dressing, when airborne bacteria are at their highest level.

Gloves – should they be worn and what type?

Choosing among sterile, non-sterile or no gloves at all has become a contentious issue in i.v. therapy. The aseptic non-touch technique recommends the use of non-sterile gloves for nearly all aseptic procedures. The rationale for this is based upon the following information:

- There is no substantial evidence demonstrating that any particular type of glove reduces the incidence of infection.

- Even sterile gloves cannot always be considered 100% sterile, owing to a small but significant micropermeability (DeGroot-Kosolcharoen & Jones 1989).
- Key parts and sites should not be touched either by gloved or ungloved hands, so there should be no reason to wear sterile gloves.
- The control of substances hazardous to health (COSHH) regulations (HSC 1988) recommend protective clothing such as gloves for all procedures involving potentially hazardous substances (i.e. all drugs).
- The wearing of gloves for all procedures involving potential exposure to body fluids such as blood and urine was recommended by the Expert Advisory Group on AIDS (1990) and by the Center for Disease Control (1984).
- Ojajarvi (1990) established that colonisation of skin by transient bacteria is likely to result when skin is repeatedly moist or damaged. Shredded skin caused by such damage can transmit bacteria via the contact route (Gould 1991). Practitioners often have moist and damaged hands due to frequent washing and drying. Gloves may serve as a barrier to prevent de-scaling of bacteria on to key parts and key sites.
- It has been reported that excessive precautions contribute to a false sense of security (Lund & Caruso 1993). This is supported by observations of staff who thought it acceptable to touch key parts when wearing sterile gloves (Rowley, unpublished work, 1996).

Healthy, sick, and handicapped children

The definition and principles of the aseptic non-touch technique are not dependent on the diagnosis of the child. However, whereas the principles should always remain constant, infective precautions may change depending on the type of procedure or condition of the child. This is not to say that nurses should categorise perceived high-risk groups like immunosuppressed children and always insist on using a high level of infective precautions for all procedures. In many cases this would be an unnecessary waste of resources. According to Jones (1987), an ideal aseptic technique for intravenous catheter care is one that is safe and effective yet requires a minimal amount of time and equipment. Choosing appropriate infective precautions for any particular procedure is achieved by an effective assessment of risk. If the nurse considers that he cannot maintain the asepsis of key parts and sites by a non-touch method, he must take further steps to minimise the risk of contamination. This might entail the use of extra precautions such as forceps or sterile gloves.

Method

The exact method one uses to perform an aseptic technique will vary depending on the procedure. However, the basic practice and principles of the aseptic non-touch technique must underpin and complement all practices where asepsis needs to be maintained. There are two stages to the aseptic non-touch technique:

- Stage 1: – risk assessment
- Stage 2: – choice of infective precautions.

Stage 1: risk assessment

The nurse can assess the degree of risk by considering the following factors by way of a brief assessment.

- Technical difficulty of procedure:
  simple/difficult
- Environment:
  clean/dirty
- Time key parts/sites are exposed:
  short/long
- Number of key parts/sites exposed:
  few/many
- Condition/behaviour of child:
  immunocompetent/ suppressed, calm upset.

Stage 2: choice of infective precautions

After considering the factors listed in the risk assessment, the nurse asks himself what infective precautions and equipment he needs to utilise to maintain the asepsis of the key parts.

Equipment

It is impossible to provide a definitive list of equipment for all aseptic procedures. It is, however, possible to break down any aseptic procedure into five broad stages (Fig. 2.1) which require either a specific action, or a choice of infective precautions. It can be seen that components 1, 4 and 5 are compulsory for all procedures. However, for some procedures the nurse must make choices regarding the use of gloves and aseptic field. These will differ depending on how difficult each procedure is, i.e. the degree of risk involved. Table 2.1 provides three case scenarios highlighting the risk assessment and the subsequent choices the nurse made regarding infective precautions.

Observations and complications

If key parts or key sites are inadvertently contaminated, remedy the situation by cleaning with appropriate agents or by changing equipment.

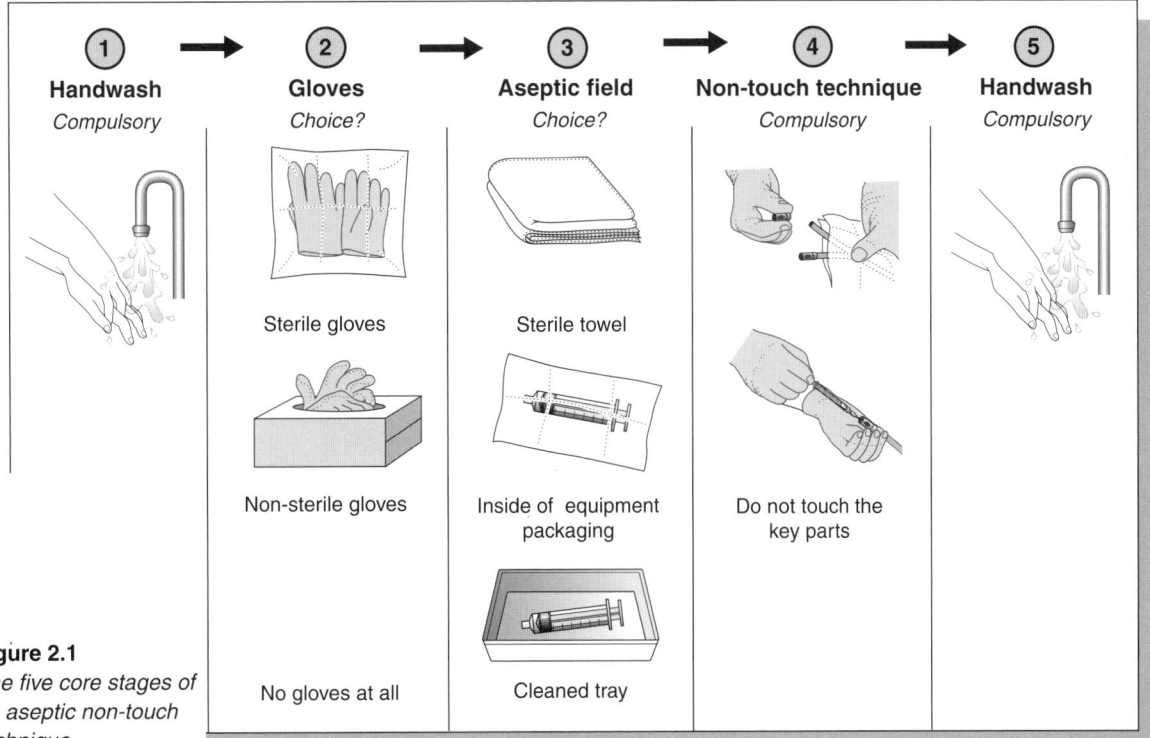

Figure 2.1
The five core stages of an aseptic non-touch technique.

Table 2.1   **Examples of risk assessment and subsequent choice of infective precautions**

Procedure	Risk assessment		Choice of infective precautions		Rationale
Injecting drugs into the central line of an immunosuppressed child	Technical difficulty of procedure Environment Time key parts/sites are exposed Number of key parts/sites exposed Status/behaviour of child	Simple Clean Short Few Immuno-suppressed	Pre-handwash Choice of gloves Choice of aseptic field Non-touch technique Post-handwash	Compulsory Non-sterile Ad hoc (cleaned tray) Compulsory Compulsory	This is a common procedure. The nurse was able to maintain the asepsis of the few key parts by a non-touch method, therefore, the fact that the child was immunosuppressed was not relevant
Removing stitches from the wound of an immunosuppressed child who is upset by the procedure	Technical difficulty of procedure Environment Time key parts/sites are exposed Number of key parts/sites exposed Status/behaviour of child	Difficult Clean Long Few Immuno-suppressed/upset	Pre-handwash Choice of gloves Choice of aseptic field Non-touch technique Post-handwash	Compulsory Sterile Sterile paper Compulsory Compulsory	The child was upset, making this a difficult procedure which needed to be completed as quickly as possible. Using forceps was difficult and took too long. The nurse chose to use his hands to hold the stitches. On an immunocompetent child with a dry and healed wound, he may still have chosen to wear non-sterile gloves. However, in this case he chose to wear sterile gloves because the child was immunosuppressed and direct contact with the wound presented a greater risk of contamination
Injecting drugs into a buretted i.v. line for an immunocompetent child	Technical difficulty of procedure Environment Time key parts/sites are exposed Number of key parts/sites exposed Status/behaviour of child	Simple Clean Short Few Immuno-competent	Pre-handwash Choice of gloves Choice of aseptic field Non-touch technique Post-handwash	Compulsory Non-sterile Ad hoc (cleaned tray) Compulsory Compulsory	This is a common and simple i.v. procedure. A sterile paper towel was not necessary for the aseptic field because the nurse used the inside of the equipment packaging and made sure that he connected key parts as soon as they were opened (i.e. the needle and syringe were connected immediately, protecting the key parts before they were placed on the cleaned plastic tray (Rowley 1997). For the actual procedure itself, the nurse only had to concentrate on maintaining the asepsis of the needle and the cleaned injectable bung of the burette

```
┌─────────────────────────────────────────┐
│ COMMUNITY PERSPECTIVE                    │
│ The principles remain the same within    │
│ the home environment.                    │
│                                          │
│ CCNs need to be aware that handwashing   │
│ facilities may be inadequate in some     │
│ homes and they will therefore need to    │
│ carry appropriate hand-cleansing         │
│ equipment and disposable towels.         │
│                                          │
│ A simple way to form an aseptic field is │
│ to clean a plastic tray with an alcohol  │
│ solution immediately prior to the        │
│ procedure.                               │
│                                          │
│ In situations where the families perform │
│ aseptic procedures, the CCN will need to │
│ ensure that they understand the          │
│ rationale for, and methods of achiev-    │
│ ing, aseptic non-touch techniques as     │
│ part of main- taining a safe             │
│ environment.                             │
│                                          │
│ In some instances it may be appropriate  │
│ for the CCN to arrange for disposal of   │
│ clinical waste, according to local       │
│ policies.                                │
└─────────────────────────────────────────┘
```

Do and do not

- Do not confuse your practice, for example by trying to keep one hand 'clean' and the other 'dirty', as this will only make things more difficult.
- Do touch non-key parts with confidence – this will make the procedure easier.
- Do concentrate on the key parts and key sites. As long as they are not touched or contaminated by you or anything else, you are practising safely.
- With time you will develop your own handling technique. As long as it meets the principles of the aseptic non-touch technique, you are practising safely and efficiently.
- Do clean away from the wound in wound care. Only uncontaminated gauze, forceps, gloves, etc. should make direct contact with the wound.
- Do not use unnecessary infective precautions as this only wastes time and resources.

References

Adams B G, Marrie T J 1982 Hand carriage of aerobic Gram-negative rods by health care personnel. Journal of Hygiene 89(1): 23–31

Bauer T M, Ofner E, Just H M, Just H, Daschner F D 1990 An epidemiological study assessing the relative importance of airborne and direct contact transmission of microorganisms in a medical intensive care unit. Journal of Hospital Infection 15(4): 301–309

Center for Disease Control (CDC) 1984 Nosocomial infection surveillance. Center for Disease Control: Surveillance Summaries 35: 17SS–29SS

Church J 1986 Spread of infection: direct contact. Nursing 3: 136–137

DeGroot-Kosolcharoen J, Jones J M 1989 Permeability of latex and vinyl gloves to water and blood. American Journal of Infection Control 17(4): 196–201

Expert Advisory Group on AIDS and the Advisory Group on Hepatitis 1998. Guidance for Clinical Health Care Workers: Protection against infection with blood-borne viruses. HMSO, London

Expert Advisory Group on AIDS 1990 Guidance for clinical health care workers: protection against infection with HIV and hepatitis viruses. Recommendations of the Expert Advisory Group on AIDS. HMSO, London

Gould D 1991 Skin bacteria. What is normal? Nursing Standard 18(5): 25–28

Health and Safety Commission (HSC) 1988 The control of substances hazardous to health: approved code of practice. SI 1657. HMSO, London

Hendrick E 1988 Infectious waste management: will science prevail? Infection Control and Hospital Epidemiology 9: 488–490

Jones P M 1987 Indwelling central venous catheter related infections and two different procedures of catheter care. Cancer Nursing 10(3): 123–130

Lawrence T 1994 Central venous line audit. Paediatric Nursing 6(4): 20–23

Lund C, Caruso R 1993 Nursing perspectives: aseptic techniques in wound care. Dermatology Nursing 5(3): 215–216

Maki D G, Goldman D A, Rhama F S 1973 Infection control in IV therapy. Annals of Internal Therapy 79: 869–880

Ojajarvi J 1990 Effectiveness of hand washing and disinfection methods in removing transient bacteria after patient nursing. Journal of Hygiene 85: 193–203

Pritchard P, David J 1994 The Royal Marsden Hospital manual of clinical nursing procedures, 3rd edn. Blackwell Science, Oxford, ch 4

Stringer B, Smith J A, Scharf S, Valentine A, Walker M M 1991 A study of the use of gloves in a large teaching hospital. American Journal of Infection Control 19(5): 233–236

Weller B (ed) 1993 Encyclopedic dictionary of nursing and health care. Baillière Tindall, London, p 81

3

Assessment

Introduction
The ability to assess the child accurately and interpret, record and report the findings are essential skills for any paediatric nurse.

Learning outcomes
By the end of this section you should be able to:

- explain the principles underlying assessment of the child
- list the essential components of an assessment
- describe how to observe and record vital signs in children
- recognise when vital signs do not fall within expected limits for a child's age, condition and developmental level.

Rationale for assessment
A child's condition can change rapidly and without warning. Observation and assessment by a skilled paediatric nurse can detect subtle differences in a child that may warn of imminent deterioration. In addition, children often cannot tell you about how they are feeling or what are their precise needs. Careful and thorough assessment is essential to ensure that the care planned and provided is appropriate to the needs of the individual child, whether ill or healthy.

Factors to note
Good assessment is based upon thorough observation and effective questioning to elicit as much accurate information as possible. Most nursing models provide assessment tools to guide the practitioner in making the assessment. The best source of information about the child will be his parents (and the child himself, if old enough). They are the ones who have the most detailed and intimate knowledge of their child. Questioning needs to be sensitive so as not to cause undue embarrassment or alarm to the child and parents.

Assessment can take many forms. Formal assessment (as described here under 'Method') is undertaken when the nurse first encounters the child and family. Recording of vital signs will provide baseline figures by which the child's progress can be monitored. From these baseline observations on admission, both improvements and deterioration can be recorded. Aside from formal assessment, a skilled children's nurse will be constantly assessing the child informally. For example, he will be observed when interacting with his parents, when playing on his own or with others, when being examined by medical staff or when the nurse is nearby undertaking other tasks. Assessments are constantly made as a result of these observations.

Sick infants
Observation and assessment are vital, but remember that a sick infant needs rest and sleep to help his recovery. Many sick infants will exhibit distress, stress and a deterioration in their condition when handled. In these babies, taking recordings using equipment such as blood pressure monitors as part of your assessment can cause more harm than good.

- Reduce the frequency of your recordings, keeping the need to handle the infant to an absolute minimum.
- Plan your care so that you do not have to disturb him unnecessarily.
- When you do have to disturb him for a reason such as taking his temperature, carry out other care at that time instead of later, e.g. change his nappy.
- Use your eyes to look carefully for any visual evidence of changes in the infant's condition.
- Utilise non-invasive equipment such as a pulse oximeter or ECG monitor to reduce the frequency with which the infant must be handled.

The infant to 3-year-old child
This age group can be particularly uncooperative when you are trying to observe their vital signs. They do not understand what you are trying to achieve and may struggle vigorously against the squeeze of a blood pressure cuff being inflated. The 9-month to 3-year olds in particular seem to object strongly to being held in one

position even when it is not painful, e.g. when a mercury thermometer is in position under their arm or you try to hold the arm to take a pulse recording. Distraction can be helpful (see Appendix 1: Play, p. 329).

Guidelines

The importance of involving both children (where age and developmental ability allow) and their parents has been highlighted. Building relationships with parents will enable you to gain as much information as possible and help gain the child's cooperation to assist you when trying to measure his vital signs. For example, some children delight in being able to push switches on electronic equipment such as a blood pressure machine. However, if encouraging this kind of involvement, it is important to teach them not to play with any machinery unless an adult is present. This is in order to prevent children tampering with each other's intravenous infusion pumps.

Parents and older children can be taught to measure vital signs and act on results in some circumstances (e.g. giving paracetamol when their child develops a fever to prevent a febrile fit). Be aware, however, that their knowledge may not always extend to accurately interpreting the results of their observations. They must understand how and when to report their results so that they can be acted upon where necessary.

Respiration

Much can be determined from observing the respiratory pattern of both the infant and the older child. It is a measurement which requires no active intervention and can indicate a wide range of changes in a child's condition, from increasing oxygen requirement to increased or decreased pain and anxiety. Simply observing the rate of breaths per minute is not sufficient. The child who is relaxed and breathing steadily and at a rate appropriate for his age and size is probably reasonably stable. The child who is holding himself rigidly with nasal flaring, a retracted neck and rapid, shallow breathing is definitely unwell.

Respiratory distress can be observed not just in the rate and depth of respirations, but also in the amount of effort expended.

- Is he using accessory muscles of respiration, e.g. the intercostal muscles?
- Is he using his shoulders to breathe?
- Is there any evidence of nasal flaring or tracheal tug (the effort involved in breathing makes the trachea

move and this can be seen as the skin at the base of the throat being tugged when the child inhales)?
- Is his breathing noisy, wheezy or is he making any vocal noises such as stridor or grunting?

All of these problems indicate increasing severity of breathing difficulty and must be reported.

Pulse oximetry and oxygen saturation

The child or infant who presents with any kind of respiratory distress should have a baseline recording of arterial saturation of oxygen (SaO_2) taken with a pulse oximeter. In the healthy infant or child the percentage saturation of oxygen should be 95–98% (Sims 1996). Pulse oximetry is a non-invasive, painless and reliable technique for measurement of the SaO_2 (Hanna 1995). When used properly, it will detect hypoxaemia before clinical signs become evident (Hanna 1995). A sensor (or probe) is placed around a fleshy part of the body, e.g. a fingertip in the older child, around the nailbed of the toe in the infant or around the ball of the foot in a neonate under 3 kg in weight. Exactly which sensor to use depends on where on the body it is sited and the child's weight. The sensor packaging will clarify the weight range of child for which it is to be used.

The sensor emits red and infrared light and has a photo-detector which detects the amount of light which is absorbed by the tissues. The different colours of oxygenated and deoxygenated blood absorb different amounts of infrared light. This information is then converted into an average value which is displayed as a percentage saturation. Pulse oximeter measurements have been shown to correlate closely to arterial blood gas values (Coull 1992).

Limitations. There are limitations to the use of an oximeter. For example, if the child's peripheral perfusion is poor (the blood supply to the extremities may be reduced under some circumstances, e.g. when the child is shocked), the readings may be inaccurate. The sensor cannot read accurately if there is excessive motion. The sensor cannot detect the difference between haemoglobin molecules saturated with oxygen and those saturated with other gases such as carbon monoxide (Carroll 1993). It is therefore not safe for use in cases of carbon monoxide poisoning. Accuracy of pulse oximetry can also be affected by the presence of direct, bright light on the sensor.

If the machine records an abnormal saturation, first look at the child. Do his physical signs fit with what the machine is telling you? Remember, though, that the main reason why the oximeter is used is because it can detect changes before clinical signs become evident.

However, if things do not seem to tally, check next that the machine is recording properly and that the sensor is properly in place.

Taking and recording a temperature

A child's temperature can be taken in one of four ways: in the axilla, orally, tympanically or rectally. There is evidence to demonstrate that taking the rectal temperature can cause trauma to the rectum and poses an unnecessary infection control hazard when a glass/mercury thermometer is used (Rogers 1992a).

The literature suggests that the rectal route is best avoided. Oral temperatures are usually only performed in the older child. There is always the risk of a younger child accidentally biting the thermometer. It is suggested that oral temperatures be confined to those children who are able to understand the risks associated with biting into an oral thermometer and who it is felt will cooperate and can be trusted. Do not take oral temperatures on any child under 5 years old or any child with a history of seizures.

Types of thermometer

There are a variety of thermometers now available for use. Increasingly the glass/mercury thermometer is not favoured and some would argue strongly that it is contraindicated because of:

- the length of time it must remain in situ to gain an accurate reading
- the possibility of failure to disinfect it carefully, leading to cross-infection
- the risk of trauma to the child and the hazards associated with mercury spillage if one is broken (Cutter 1994, Rogers 1992a).

However, there may, on occasion, be a role for the glass thermometer, particularly in the hypothermic child in whom most modern thermometers are less accurate (see below).

Electronic thermometers with single-use disposable sheaths are commonly used orally and in the axilla although Ogren (1990) questioned the accuracy of axillary temperatures recorded with an electronic device. They can also be used rectally.

Rogers (1992b) conducted research into a single-use clinical thermometer (Tempa-DOT). The study showed it to be a viable alternative to a glass/mercury thermometer, but questioned its cost. Acknowledgement was made that it did not record temperatures below 35.5°C.

Increasingly popular is the tympanic membrane (TM) thermometer. This takes an infrared recording of the temperature of the tympanic membrane. The tympanic membrane temperature is thought to closely reflect the core temperature as its blood supply is in close proximity to that supplying the organ of temperature control, the hypothalamus. Rogers et al (1991) conducted research to evaluate the TM thermometer against an electronic thermometer used orally, rectally and in the axilla. Their conclusions were that the TM thermometer was a great time saver and produced a reading most similar to the electronic rectal reading – an indication of core temperature. Barber & Kilman (1989) found the TM thermometer very popular with patients, parents and nurses. It is a very quick, simple procedure to take a temperature using one of these devices. First, a disposable cover is placed on the end of the probe (Fig. 3.1). Secondly, the probe is placed into the external auditory canal. The button to activate the thermometer is pressed. After an average of 10 seconds, the device bleeps to indicate that the temperature recording is complete. The thermometer is removed from the ear and the reading is recorded from the digital read-out on the thermometer. See Figure 3.2 for a picture of the tympanic membrane thermometer in use.

Whenever an abnormal temperature is recorded, always consider the method used to record it in the first place. For example: You note a low temperature which was obtained from an axillary recording. Check first if this

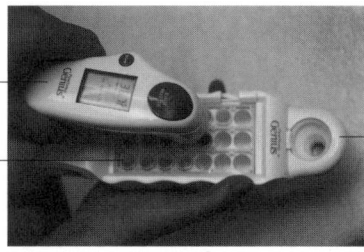

Figure 3.1
Putting a disposable probe cover on a tympanic membrane thermometer.

Tympanic membrane thermometer

Disposable probe covers stored on base unit

Base unit to which thermometer returned for charging

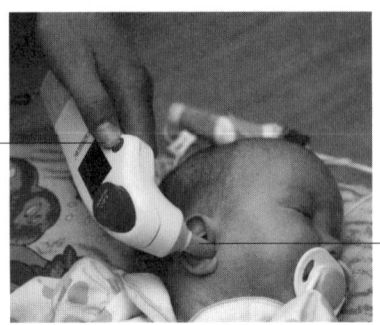

Scan button.
Press when tip of
probe is in position.
Machine will bleep when
temperature recorded
(approximately 2 seconds)

Tip of thermometer probe
gently placed into
external auditory canal
until seal made

Figure 3.2
*The tympanic
membrane
thermometer in use.*

is a true core temperature: it may be necessary to take
the child's temperature tympanically, orally or rectally.
If the core temperature is also low, then consider what is
going on. Low temperature could be due to environmental factors (not enough clothing, cold room temperature), but it could indicate peripheral shutdown due to
shock. Hypothermia (very low temperature) is a well-
recognised problem in premature infants and infants of
low birthweight.

Pyrexia (fever) is most likely to be due to infection,
which may be localised, e.g. otitis media, or could be
systemic, e.g. septicaemia. Occasionally it can have a
rarer cause such as brain tumour or Kawasaki disease.

Taking and recording blood pressure

It can be very difficult to gain an accurate blood pressure
(BP) reading in an infant using a conventional sphygmomanometer. It is extremely hard reliably to hear the
child's pulse beat in his cubital fossa (de Swiet et al 1989)
and he is unlikely to cooperate and hold completely still.
For this reason, an electronic machine which measures
blood pressure by oscillometry is recommended for use in
infants and younger children. However, it is important to
remember the limitations of such equipment. The accuracy of an electronic blood pressure machine is adversely
affected by movement in the patient. Unless very sick or
well sedated, few children (particularly the younger ones)
will hold still for the duration of the procedure. In addition, accurate recordings will only be obtained if the correct size of cuff is used. Once you have recorded the BP,
consider whether it is higher or lower than expected. A
lowered BP could indicate a degree of shock. Question
why the child might be going into shock. For example,
might it be because of sepsis or could he be bleeding
internally?

A raised BP could be because the child is in pain or experiencing rising intracranial pressure. The latter would be a

particular concern if he simultaneously demonstrated a
falling pulse rate. As with temperature, a single abnormal
recording must be re-checked.

Equipment
- Paperwork on which to record the findings made
  during assessment
- Thermometer
- Disposable sheath for thermometer if not a single-
  use device
- Blood pressure machine – electronic or manual
  depending on the age of the child
- Blood pressure cuff of the right size for the child's
  weight and arm circumference – see step 9 below
- Weighing scales appropriate to the size and age of
  the child
- A stethoscope will be needed if an apex beat is to be
  recorded
- A pulse oximeter will be needed if arterial oxygen
  saturation (SaO_2) is to be assessed
- A pulse oximeter sensor which is of the right size
  according to the child's weight (see sensor
  packaging) and the part of his body (e.g. toe, foot,
  finger) on which it is to be placed

Method
1. Be prepared before you start. Gather together all the
   equipment you could possibly need in order to
   avoid interrupting the assessment to fetch additional
   equipment. Try to ensure that you have adequate
   time to conduct the assessment and are not rushed.
   It will help build the family's confidence in you if
   you can give them plenty of time to talk to you.
2. Introduce yourself to both the child and family.
   Explain what you are going to do and why, to
   alleviate fear of the unknown. Explain to them that
   you will be asking questions and writing the
   answers they give you in the paperwork.

3. Briefly assess the child's overall condition. Is it safe to postpone getting baseline observations such as oxygen saturation, or is it necessary to obtain the information straight away? If possible, allow the child and his parents to settle in for a while. Try to gain his parents' confidence before you attempt to approach him. He will be more likely to cooperate if he sees that his parents trust you. Be aware of the best time to approach the child directly to undertake measurements and observations and to weigh him. If he is sleeping, record his respirations. If he is obviously distressed, it may further upset him to try to record his blood pressure. If his nappy needs changing, use the opportunity to weigh him.

4. Try to conduct the assessment interview as if it were a friendly chat. Encourage a two-way exchange of information. You will be far more likely to obtain full information this way than if you simply fire question after question.

5. Your nursing assessment should enable you to gain information about all aspects of the child's life. See Table 3.5 on page 52 for explanation of the areas that should be covered and the sort of questions you should be asking to elicit the right information. Remember to distinguish between what the child is like when well and what alterations have occurred as a result of his illness. Remember to check that the factual information (name, address, contact telephone numbers, etc.) in the notes is correct.

6. Observe his respirations. The most accurate recording will be the one obtained whilst the child is unaware you are observing him and whilst he is at rest. The infant will breathe as nature intended, i.e. filling his whole lung and moving his diaphragm downwards, causing his abdomen to expand. Therefore, observe the fall and rise of his abdomen, rather than his chest, in order to count his respirations. His chest and shoulders should not move, unless there is a problem. Note the rate and depth of his breathing and the amount of effort that is expended to breathe.

7. Observe his heart rate. The best site for recording the child's pulse is dependent mostly on his age. It is extremely difficult to locate a radial pulse in an infant. Sometimes it is possible to feel a brachial pulse, but even this can be difficult to count accurately because of the small size of the infant and the rapidity of the pulse. An apex beat recording is usually the most accurate in a child under 6 months. Be aware that it takes practice to be able to count an apex beat accurately. An apex beat recording is obtained by listening to the heartbeat directly, by placing a stethoscope on the front left side of the infant's chest. Be aware that in children who have circulatory problems, it may be necessary to record their pulse rate in more than one site, e.g. apex and lower limb to detect discrepancies between the two. If measuring his blood pressure and/or oxygen saturation with an electronic device, these will usually also record the heart rate.

8. Take his temperature. Consider which site and which type of thermometer is best for the age, condition and developmental level of the child. Ensure that training has been given in the use of whichever device is to be employed.

9. Take his blood pressure. De Swiet et al (1989) made the following recommendations:
   a. Determine which size of cuff is needed. A minimum of three sizes are necessary to cover the age range 0–14 years of age: 4×13 cm, 8×18 cm and 12×35 cm. Most cuffs are marked with a range finder which will give some idea if the correct size is being used. The widest possible cuff which can be applied to the arm should be used and the length of the inflation bladder should be at least two-thirds of the circumference of the arm.
   b. Try to take the recording when the child has been sitting or lying quietly for at least 2 minutes.
   c. Decisions about the child's management should never be made on the basis of a blood pressure recording taken on a single occasion.

10. Weigh him. An accurate weight is vital as so much of the child's treatment may be calculated upon his weight; for example drug dosages and fluid and nutritional requirements. Ensure that if electronic equipment is available, adequate training in its use has been given. Ideally, all weights should be taken with the child nude, remembering to preserve his privacy and dignity. Remember to note if he has anything which may add to his body weight, e.g. splints and cannula with intravenous tubing, nasal cannula, etc.

11. If there are any signs of respiratory distress, or he has a respiratory illness, record his oxygen saturation with a pulse oximeter. Having chosen the right size sensor for the child's weight and the site where it is to be used, explain what you are about to do to alleviate fear of the unknown. Place the sensor and turn on the machine. Set the upper and lower limit alarms for pulse rate and oxygen saturation. Ensure that the sensor is picking up a

good signal as indicated by stability of the visual waveform and/or a regular pulse rate. Observe his colour. Decreasing oxygen saturations require urgent action and must be reported.

12. Record the observations on the paperwork. Assess whether or not action needs to be taken as a result of your observation. Is the recording within expected limits? If not, or if you are unsure whether or not the recording falls outside expected limits, report the result to a more senior nurse.

See Tables 3.1–3.4 for average values in children who are well.

Observations and complications

Observations

Careful and subtle observation of the child and the child with his family can be informative. How does he handle his toys – is it developmentally appropriate, e.g. pincer movements to grasp a small object in a 12-month-old (Sheridan 1975)?

How does he react to his parent? Do they make eye contact; does he appear to listen to her; do they respond to each other? How does he react to you?

As a child is undressed for weighing, observe his overall appearance. Is he clean or dirty, well groomed or of unkempt appearance? Has he got abnormal bruising or unusual marks? Relate his appearance to what you know of his social situation. A child may be dirty but obviously happy, developmentally normal and well loved. Maybe parenting skills need to be taught; perhaps cleanliness is not of importance to his family, or facilities are not readily available.

Your observations can reduce the number of questions you have to ask or prompt you to ask specific questions if you see something which gives cause for concern.

Table 3.1 **Normal respiratory rates**

Age of child	Respiratory rate in breaths per minute
Newborn	30–60
6 months	30–45
1–2 years	25–35
3–6 years	20–30
> 7 years	20–25

Reproduced by kind permission from Hull & Johnston 1993.

Table 3.2 **Normal temperature**

Age of child	Core temperature in degrees centigrade (°C)
< 6 months	37.5
7 months–1 year	37.5–37.7
2–5 years	37.2–37.0
> 6 years	36.6–36.8

After Wong 1995.

Complications

There are few risks associated with assessment or taking observations. The biggest problem arises when the individual performing the task does not recognise the importance of the results obtained, misinterprets the results and takes an inappropriate action in consequence, or does not act on them at all.

Table 3.3 **Normal heart rates**

Age of child	Heart rate in pulse beats per minute	
	When child awake	When child asleep
Newborn	100–180	80–160
< 3 months	100–220	80–180
3 months–2 years	80–150	70–120
3–10 years	70–110	60–100
10 years–adult	55–90	50–90

Reproduced by kind permission from D L Wong 1995, *Paediatric quick reference*, 2nd edn. Mosby, St Louis.

Table 3.4 **Normal blood pressure values**

Age of child	Systolic blood pressure in mmHg	Diastolic blood pressure in mmHg
Neonate	60–85	20–60
Infant (6 months)	75–105	40–70
Toddler (2 years)	75–110	45–80
School age (7 years)	75–115	45–80
Adolescent (15 years)	100–145	60–95

After Hull & Johnston 1993.

Note: Blood pressure values are expressed as a range, because there are variations according to sex and the child's position on the centile charts for growth.

The nurse must:

- first, have an idea of whether or not the information obtained is normal or abnormal
- secondly, be able to assess if the result obtained was due to malfunction or misuse of equipment (if used)
- thirdly, know how to act on the results – what must be done and/or who must be informed.

Failure in any of these three areas could adversely affect the child.

There is an actual risk associated with taking rectal temperatures, namely that of trauma to the rectum (Rogers 1992a). This would be recognised by the presence of blood on the thermometer and from the rectum and the infant would be in pain. If a perforation or trauma is suspected, it must be reported immediately to the medical staff.

If a pulse oximeter sensor is used for prolonged periods, there is a risk of pressure sores (Carroll 1993, Coull 1992), and Sims (1996) suggests that there is a risk of burning the skin if a faulty sensor is applied. Sensors must be used in accordance with the manufacturers' instructions and the site changed 8-hourly when continuous monitoring is in progress.

COMMUNITY PERSPECTIVE

Whilst assessment of the child is integral in the role of the CCN, consideration must be given to the necessity of formal monitoring of vital signs, remembering that the aim of care is to make the home as unclinical an environment as possible whilst maintaining the safety of the child.

When the child's condition requires this monitoring, the parents should be given a full explanation.

Do and do not

- Do ensure that you have been properly trained in the use of electrical equipment such as pulse oximeters and blood pressure machines.
- Do remember to *record* and *report* your information.

Table 3.5 **Questions to ask during assessment**

Area of lifestyle	Questions to ask	
	Specific to infants and children < 12 months	Applicable to all age groups
Nutrition – diet and fluids	Is he bottle/breast-fed/both? What type of bottled milk, water or juice? How often does he feed and is he fed on demand? Is he on solids yet? What sorts of solids? Is he vegetarian, on any special diet? Does he use a special bottle/teat? Some congenital abnormalities such as cleft palate may require a special bottle.	What type of diet/fluids does he take? Is he on a special diet, e.g. is he vegetarian, does he have a diet dictated by religious custom or has he any special dietary needs, e.g. gluten-free, extra calorie requirements due to poor weight gain, metabolic disorder such as phenylketonuria? What are his likes and dislikes? What utensils does he use for eating and drinking, e.g. fingers, spoon, fork, knife and fork, bottle, cup or beaker? How much assistance does he need to feed, e.g. do you feed him yourself or does he just need some help such as with cutting up food? Does the younger child finger feed?
Sleep and comfort	What is his sleep pattern like, e.g. does he wake for night feeds? When does he sleep during the day? Does he have a preferred position for sleep, e.g. on his side? (Utilise this opportunity for health education – see Positioning, Handling and Exercises, p. 217)	Does he sleep at all during the day? What time does he usually go to bed? What is his usual night time routine, e.g. does he normally have a bath or a drink before bed time? Does he have a 'comforter', e.g. a special teddy, a dummy? Does he need this to sleep at night? Does he wear a nappy at night? Are there any problems with enuresis (bed wetting)? Does he wake in the night? How do you get him back to sleep? Does he have a drink by his bedside at night? If so, what?
	Children of all ages	
Hygiene, personal care	Is his skin clean, dry, intact? Any rashes, dry patches or eczema? In an infant, is there any evidence of thrush (*Candida albicans*)? Is there any unusual bruising/scratching? Is the colour of his skin abnormal, e.g. jaundiced? Has he been in contact with any infectious disease? Is his immunisation schedule up to date? Is his mouth clean and moist? Is the infant teething? How many teeth has he and what is the state of his dentition? Are there any loose teeth? Does he brush his teeth regularly? Does he require any special skin or hair care, e.g. African and Afro-Caribbean children's hair may require moisturising, and good skin care for black skin revolves around moisturising (Action for Sick Children 1993). A child with eczema will also require special skin care. Any problems passing urine? How often does he have his bowels open, what are his stools like – colour, consistency? Has he started toilet training? What stage is he at? Does he use any special words for toileting? Does he need help to dress or is he completely independent? Any special requirements regarding dress, e.g. remaining covered at all times, religious hair coverings?	

Table 3.5 (Contd.)   **Questions to ask during assessment**

Area of lifestyle	Questions to ask
	Children of all ages
Religion and culture	Are there any special religious/cultural aspects to care, e.g. clothing, jewellery, food, hygiene? Are there religious/cultural views which may affect treatment, e.g. blood transfusion or organ donation? Do the family want us to contact a specific religious figure?
Play and development	Has he achieved the expected developmental milestones for his age? Question with regard to gross and fine motor development, vision, hearing, speech and social development What are his favourite toys? How can we best amuse him whilst he is ill? Is there any other carer involved, e.g. nursery, childminder, nanny, grandparents, foster parents? Does he attend school/nursery, which one? Who are his head and class teachers? Who is his health visitor (under-5s)? Are there any special friends with whom he would like to keep in close contact?

References

Action for Sick Children 1993 Health for all our children. Achieving appropriate health care for black and minority ethnic children and their families. Action for Sick Children, London, p 13

Barber N, Kilmon C A 1989 Reactions to tympanic temperature measurement in an ambulatory setting. Pediatric Nursing 15(5): 477–481

Carroll P 1993 Clinical application of pulse oximetry. Pediatric Nursing 19(2): 150–151

Coull A 1992 Making sense of pulse oximetry. Nursing Times 88(32): 42–43

Cutter J 1994 Recording patient temperature – are we getting it right? Professional Nurse 9(9): 608–616

de Swiet M, Dillon M J, Littler W, O'Brien E, Padfield P L, Petrie J C 1989 Measurement of blood pressure in children – recommendations of a working party of the British Hypertension Society. British Medical Journal 299(19 Aug): 497

Hanna D 1995 Guidelines for pulse oximetry use in pediatrics. Journal of Pediatric Nursing 10(2): 124–126

Hull D, Johnston D I 1993 Essential paediatrics, 3rd edn. Churchill Livingstone, Edinburgh, ch 8, p 117

Ogren J 1990 The inaccuracy of axillary temperatures measured with an electronic thermometer. American Journal of Diseases in Children 144(1): 109–111

Rogers J, Curley M, Driscoll J et al 1991 Evaluation of tympanic membrane thermometer for use with pediatric patients. Pediatric Nursing 17(4): 376–378

Rogers M 1992a Temperature recording in infants and children. Paediatric Nursing 4(3): 23–26

Rogers M 1992b A viable alternative to the glass/mercury thermometer. Paediatric Nursing 4(9): 8–11

Sheridan M 1975 From birth to five years – children's developmental progress, 3rd edn. NFER, London

Sims J 1996 Making sense of pulse oximetry and oxygen dissociation curve. Nursing Times 92(1): 34–35

Wong D 1995 Pediatric quick reference, 2nd edn. Mosby, St Louis, p 7

Further reading

Bee H 1997 The developing child, 8th edn. Addison-Wesley, New York

Hanning C D, Alexander-Williams J M 1995 Pulse oximetry: a practical review. British Medical Journal 311(5 Aug): 367–370

Hazinski M 1992 Nursing care of the critically ill child, 2nd edn. Mosby Year Book, St Louis, inside cover

Hutton P, Clutton-Brock T 1993 The benefits and pitfalls of pulse oximetry. British Medical Journal 307(21 Aug): 457–458

Phillips S 1989 Monitoring vital signs in children. Nursing (Oct): 48–49

Soud T 1992 Airway, breathing, circulation and disability: what is different about kids? Journal of Emergency Nursing 18(2): 107–116

Stoneham M D, Saville G M, Wilson I H 1994 Knowledge about pulse oximetry among medical and nursing staff. Lancet 344: 1339–1342

Toms E 1993 Vital observations. Nursing Times 89(51): 32–34

4

Bereavement Care

Introduction

'Physical care of the body after death, also known as last offices or laying out, epitomises our respect for the dead and is the final special service that we can offer' (Green & Green 1992). However, effective bereavement care is more than just the physical aspects of caring for the child after death. Psychosocial care is also of considerable importance.

Learning outcomes

By the end of this section you should:

- be aware that a child and her family may choose where she dies and is cared for after death
- be able to describe the principles of caring for the child's body after death with reference to cultural and religious customs and legal requirements
- be able to help distressed relatives and staff to follow the procedures that are necessary when a child has died
- be able to identify resources which may help family and staff begin to accept the death of a child and understand and manage their own grief process
- be able to explain under which circumstances there may be a need for a post-mortem.

Rationale for bereavement care

The death of a child is a source of profound loss and distress for the whole family and, very often, staff (Anon 1993, Brown 1993, Nelson 1995, Soutter 1994). However, carefully considered and managed care of the child and her family at the time surrounding and after death can have a positive impact on their memories (Davies 1997, Hawley 1997, Speck 1992).

Factors to note

All individuals have the right to a dignified death, surrounded by those who love them, whatever the circumstances of the end of their life. Parents should always be closely involved when a child is dying.

Will there need to be a post-mortem?

After a child has died it is important to ascertain (by discussion with the medical staff) whether there is a need for a post-mortem, because this will affect the way in which the body is cared for after death. Box 4.1 details some of the major categories relating to death of a child which indicate that the case must be referred to the coroner, by law (Regulation 51 of the Registration of Births, Deaths, and Marriages Regulations 1968). In these circumstances, the coroner will usually order a post-mortem.

Sometimes, local practice requires a post-mortem to be performed in additional circumstances to those required by law. For example, if the death was within 24 hours of admission to hospital or if the deceased was detained under the Mental Health Act (Ellis & Edwards 1995). It is important to establish what local policy and practice require. Ethically, medical staff should always obtain consent for post-mortem from parents, but it is not legally required for a coroner's post-mortem (Ellis & Edwards 1995). However, parents have every right to refuse a post-mortem that is not legally required by the coroner.

Post-mortem is a very emotive subject for families, and Ellis & Edwards (1995) stress the importance of a

---

> **Box 4.1 Deaths to be referred to the coroner (adapted from Ellis & Edwards 1995)**
>
> - There is an element of suspicious circumstances or history of violence.
> - The death may be linked to an accident (whenever it occurred).
> - The death is linked with an abortion.
> - The death may be related to a medical procedure or treatment.
> - The death occurred during an operation or before full recovery from the effects of anaesthesia or was in any way linked to the effects of anaesthesia.
> - The actions of the deceased may have contributed to his or her own death, e.g. self-neglect, drug or solvent misuse.

sensitive, positive, multidisciplinary approach to the family when seeking consent for post-mortem. Careful explanation of the need for the examination and the actual procedure should be given. It must be stressed that the body will be treated with the utmost respect and the same care as for a living patient. Parents may be concerned that the body will be disfigured by the procedure and should be reassured that suture lines on the torso and above the hair line will be the only evidence of the post-mortem and will not be unduly disfiguring. Parents should be told that they will be able to view the body afterwards and should be actively encouraged to do so.

The inability to stop a coroner's post-mortem may cause extreme distress to some families, particularly those whose religion expressly forbids such a procedure. These parents will need a lot of support, and advice should be sought from their religious or spiritual advisors. Religious views about post-mortem are detailed in Box 4.2.

When post-mortem is required, any cannulae, drains or tubing should not be removed from the body without discussion with the medical staff (Green & Green 1992). Jewish and Islamic faiths require that any organs removed from the body during a legally required post-mortem examination are returned to it for burial (Green & Green 1992).

Organ donation

In some cases, the question of organ donation may arise. Suitability for organ donation will depend on the child having no evidence of major, untreated systemic infection, malignancy (excepting primary brain tumour), chronic severe hypertension or positivity to Australia antigen (hepatitis B) or human immuno-deficiency virus antibodies (Browne & Waddington 1993). A child who is maintained on mechanical ventilation must

have met the brain stem death criteria before organ donation can occur.

Browne & Waddington (1993) suggest first approaching parents when the first set of tests has been completed and the criteria met. It may be possible to broach the subject earlier than this if it is handled sensitively by someone who is experienced in discussing the subject with parents, for example a transplant coordinator. Ensure that when parents are approached regarding organ donation someone with whom they have been able to build a relationship, for example a member of the medical or nursing staff, is present. Organ donation must always be broached sensitively and by someone who has a positive attitude towards transplantation but is not seen as biased.

If parents agree to organ donation, the transplant coordinator will help support them and explain forthcoming procedures. Parents should be aware that they can see their child after donation and indeed should be encouraged to do so after preparation. They should be warned that their child will be white, cold and, depending on which organs have been retrieved, may have large scars.

Religious objection to organ transplantation is not the inevitable consequence of the laws and beliefs of the different faiths (Browne & Waddington 1993, Green & Green 1992). However, the following examples illustrate how some find it a very difficult issue:

- Jehovah's Witnesses because other transfused blood will circulate through the organ
- Christian Scientists because they prefer the body to be inviolate and to rely on the healing power of prayer
- Orthodox Jews because of their beliefs in the sanctity of the body and physical resurrection.

Once parents have consented and the coroner has agreed, organ donation can take place.

Table 4.1 lists the organs which can be used.

> **Box 4.2   Religious/spiritual perspectives on post-mortem (Green & Green 1992)**
>
> - Religions which absolutely forbid post-mortem: Jews, Muslims, Zoroastrians (Parsees)
> - Religions which strongly object to post-mortem: Christian Scientists
> - Religions which would prefer post-mortem not to occur if at all possible: Rastafarians
> - Religions which do not have specific views on the post-mortem examination: Christians, Jehovah's Witnesses, Mormons, Buddhists, Hindus, Sikhs

---

Special religious needs of the dying child and the care of the child's body after death

Information contained within this section pertaining to religious customs and death is taken from Green & Green (1992). There are several common themes between some religions relating to rituals after death. These are summarised in Box 4.3.

Other special considerations are as detailed below.

Christian families.   Many Christians will want their child to be baptised if death is imminent. If this is not possible before death, a priest may conduct a naming

Table 4.1   **Organs which can be donated from children (Browne & Waddington 1993)**

Organ	Minimum age of donor	Special requirements of donor's condition	Treatment necessary to maintain organ in good condition prior to removal
Kidney	2 years	No renal disease, good renal function	Inotrope infusion and intravenous fluids to maintain perfusion of kidneys
Liver	3 months	No liver diseases, drug abuse or alcoholism. Good liver function	—
Heart	6 months	No cardiac defect or disease. Donor's condition should be stable without excessive inotropic support	—
Heart and lung	6 months	No cardiac defect or disease or pulmonary dysfunction. No heavy smoking. Good arterial blood gases and lung compliance. Ventilation should not have been prolonged	—
Pancreas	14 years	No history of diabetes. If the liver is also being retrieved, patient must have spleen still intact	—
Cornea	Any age	No corneal scarring. No infectious eye disease	Eye care extremely important. Eyes must be closed and protected after death
Heart valves	6 months	—	Can be retrieved up to 72 hours after death

Reproduced with the permission of Stanley Thornes Publishers Ltd from *Manual of Paediatric Intensive Care Nursing*, B Carter, 1993.

Box 4.3   **Rituals surrounding care of the body after death common to the Jewish, Muslim, Hindu and Sikh religions**

- The child will not be left unattended whilst dying, nor must his body be left unattended after death.
- Cleansing of the child's body after death is only to be performed by special individuals:
  - Jewish last offices are performed by specially trained members of the community of the same sex as the dead child
  - the body of a Muslim child must not be touched by a non-Muslim, but if it is unavoidable, a non-Muslim should wear disposable gloves
  - the body of a Hindu child should preferably not be touched by a non-Hindu
  - the body of a Sikh child is cared for by family members of the same sex as the child.
- Therefore, the body of a child of any of these religions should simply be straightened, limbs straightened and the eyes closed, then covered with a clean sheet until further instructions can be obtained from the family. If a family member is not able to be present, it may be appropriate to ask if they wish a member of staff to remain with the body.
- It is important that the funeral should take place within 24 hours of death. It can be possible to arrange, even if there has to be a post-mortem.
- Any religious emblems (bracelets or necklets made from Holy thread) and jewellery on the body of a Hindu or Sikh child must be left in place on the body.

and blessing ceremony after death. In an emergency, any Christian may conduct a baptism. Baptism is important to Roman Catholics to the extent that they will allow even a non-believer to conduct an emergency baptism if a priest is not available. Roman Catholic families may also want a priest to perform the Sacrament of the Sick and Sacrament of the Dying (extreme unction). Holy Communion will be important if the child has taken his first Holy Communion.

Jewish families.   Traditionally, the body is not to be touched for 10 minutes after breathing has stopped. After 10 minutes, a feather is then placed over the mouth and nose to ensure that breathing has stopped.

Muslim families of the Islamic faith.   The dead child's extended family are likely to visit to pay respects and support his immediate family. The parents may wish the body to be placed with the face facing towards Mecca (south-east). Muslims believe that flexing the elbows, shoulders, knees and hips before straightening will help delay the onset of stiffening. Often Muslim families do not wish their child to go the hospital mortuary but arrange for the body to go straight to the mosque for cleansing or to a Muslim undertaker.

Hindu families.   A Hindu family is likely to prefer that their child dies at home and may wish a priest to be present at the child's bedside to perform holy rites. In addition to Holy thread around the child's limbs or body, the skin may be marked with paste or a sacred leaf placed in the mouth.

Sikh families.   It may be inappropriate to remove underclothing as this may have religious significance. If the child wears a turban, this must also be left in place after death. The face may be cleansed if it is dirty.

Guidelines

Family care when a dying child has to undergo resuscitation

In an emergency situation such as resuscitation, parental presence may be seen as inappropriate. In one research study, Back & Rooke (1994) found that doctors raised concerns that families would be more likely to complain if they witnessed resuscitation, e.g. complain that not enough or too much was done, nurses and doctors seemed uncaring or that inappropriate comments were made. Staff may also fear that relatives might display uncontrollable grief which could hinder the resuscitation. However, research in America (Hanson & Strawser 1992, Renzi-Brown 1989) would dispute this. Hanson & Strawser found that relatives wished to be present during a resuscitation. Throughout this 9-year

trial, staff concerns that relatives' grief could hamper the resuscitation attempts were not well founded. On the contrary, they discovered that relatives who had been present during resuscitation felt that it brought a sense of reality to their loss and helped them in their grieving process.

Excluding families from resuscitation may increase suspicion about what is or is not being done (Renzi-Brown 1989) and to quote Back & Rooke (1994), when the need for resuscitation arises, 'It seems absurd that the person who has been so involved in care is immediately ushered away to another room and not given the choice of whether or not to stay with his or her kin.'

Most research into the presence of relatives during resuscitation relates to general emergency settings, not specifically paediatrics. However, Back & Rooke (1994) found that staff were more in favour of parents being present during a paediatric resuscitation than of relatives being present during adult resuscitation. They suggest that this is reflective of parental involvement in care within paediatrics.

However, although parents should not be excluded during resuscitation, it is of vital importance that they must:

- be given the choice of whether or not to stay
- not be left on their own to witness the events
- be supported by someone who can explain what is happening to their child.

Specially trained pastoral care staff as well as nurses and doctors have been used as suitable supporters for relatives witnessing resuscitation (Hanson & Strawser 1992). In paediatrics, there may often be other relatives with the child and his parents who will also need help, support and information. Hanson & Strawser (1992) describe the inclusion of family members other than the next of kin during resuscitation, something that may need consideration.

Family care when death is expected and planning can take place

The family may wish to consider alternatives about where their child spends the last days of his life. There should be several options from which they may choose what is most suitable to their individual needs (Soutter 1994). There are three main choices: hospital, home or hospice. A hospital ward may be too noisy, busy and lacking in privacy, but some parents find comfort in being in the hospital environment. This may be due to their fears about how their child will die (Will he be in pain? Will he bleed or choke to death?). Careful discussion about their reasons for wanting to be in hospital may uncover these fears. Explanation and reassurance will help to allay them. Parents may then decide that hospital is not their first choice. Some areas are fortunate to have children's hospices where it may be possible for the child and family to spend her last hours. This can be arranged days or weeks in advance where circumstances allow, but many hospices can be of assistance at very short notice. Some hospices will care for children who have already died (for example on a hospital ward). They take the child's body into the hospice so that her family may spend some time with her in a setting which is not part of a mortuary or Chapel of Rest but more like home.

In a non-emergency situation, parents may choose who else should be present when their child is dying. Some families like to have the dying child surrounded by her whole family – parents, siblings and grandparents, uncles and aunts. Other parents may wish to be on their own with their child. The nurse may offer to tactfully refuse visitors for parents if they wish to have privacy. It can be difficult for parents to be assertive about numbers and timing of visits and visitors when their child is dying.

Other family members

Siblings and grandparents will also need a lot of support at the time of a child's death. This can be a particular issue for nurses if the parents are concentrating entirely on the dying child and dealing with their own grief. Other agencies may help provide support for these groups, e.g. play therapists for siblings, religious figures to help grandparents.

When parents are not present when their child dies

If parents have not been present at the death of their child, they must be informed as soon as possible after death. This task should be performed by someone who has access to accurate information about the circumstances of the child's death and the experience and confidence to inform the relatives. It is important to be gentle but direct. Using simple language such as 'she has died', rather than euphemisms such as 'she has passed away', will avoid misunderstandings and help parents to acknowledge their child's death; the first step towards acceptance (Nelson 1995). Do not be afraid of silence once the news of the death has been given. In a study of bereaved parents, Soutter (1994) was told by them that 'words were not necessary because the pain was too great and could not easily be assuaged'.

However, the same study also highlighted the comfort that was afforded to parents by the physical contact of an embrace. In some cultures, relatives are expected to show their grief by wailing and keening. This can be very noisy and possibly cause distress to staff and any other patients or relatives who may be near by (in a hospital setting). Explanation that this is their way of expressing their grief should be given.

Bereavement care after a child has died

Parents.   Invite parents and family to help with washing and dressing their child after death. This need not be rushed. Some parents will not want to be involved; others may welcome the opportunity (Browne & Waddington 1993). When parents wish to be involved, be sensitive as to whether or not your presence is required. Gentle explanation should be given to parents who choose to be involved. They should know that as their child is moved, air may escape from her lungs and result in a noise which may sound like a groan. They should also be aware there may be leakage of body fluids and that her blood will pool according to gravity and may make her skin appear a strange colour.

Support beyond the time immediately following death. Brown (1993) stresses the vital importance of advice, counselling and support for bereaved parents. Care and ongoing support for bereaved parents is becoming more widely available with ever increasing numbers of bereavement groups established. Examples of national groups are those such as the Compassionate Friends, SANDS (the Stillbirth and Neonatal Death Society), the Child Bereavement Trust and the Child Death Helpline. There are also many groups related to specific illness such as the Children's Liver Disease Foundation and SPOCC (Society of Parents of Children with Cancer). Often, there are local groups established in response to an identified need, such as the Forget-Me-Not Club described by Walters & Nelson (1997). It is useful to have a resource which lists all the available agencies, for example the Contact-a-family Directory. Parents should not be pushed into counselling. In the early stages of grief, they may not yet feel able to address counselling. They should also be told that access to counselling can be at any time, even years after the death of their child.

Siblings and friends of the child.   Although the need to support parents is now well recognised, help for siblings or the dead child's friends may not be so readily available. Simmons (1992) describes how, as a school nurse, she encountered bereaved children who were not receiving adequate support to help them deal with their grief.

It is important that these children are not forgotten. The school nurse, health visitor and relatives such as the grandparents and aunts and uncles may be enlisted to help support these children if there are no established bereavement groups for their benefit.

Staff.   Brown (1993) and Anonymous (1993) highlight the issue of 'who cares for the carers' and suggest that all nurses involved in the death of a child should be offered some sort of counselling, if only to evaluate the impact of the event. However, surely this sentiment should be extended further. The whole multidisciplinary team cares for a child and the whole multidisciplinary team may therefore be affected by the death of that child. The possibility of a multidisciplinary forum, facilitated by a trained counsellor to discuss feelings surrounding the child's death should be considered. Suitable facilitators may be found from the clinical psychology department, the clergy or occupational health service. It is also important to be aware if there are any members of the team who might require individual support.

Equipment needed for caring for a child after death

- Warm water for washing the child
- Soap
- Towels
- Clean nappy (if child still in nappies)
- Clean clothing which can be day or night clothes according to the parents' preference
- Dressings if necessary (if there are cannulae, percutaneous lines or drains to be removed), e.g. small adhesive, waterproof plasters and gauze swabs or padding in case of leakage of body fluids from any wounds
- Spigots or plugs to cap the end of cannulae, drainage tubes, etc. if they are to be left in situ for a post-mortem
- Gauze swabs in case the child's eyes need to be covered to help them remain closed
- Clean bed linen
- Linen skip for dirty linen
- Brush or comb
- Identity band with child's name and hospital registration number or labels which concur with local policy, e.g. Notice of Death Certificate and tape or safety pin to secure it to the sheet covering the body
- Clean sheet, big enough to wrap around the child's body
- Toy to place with her body if parents request it
- Flowers, if available, may be placed in the child's hand or nearby if suitable to the child's age and sex

The following may also be needed:

- documentation to list and record the child's belongings
- scissors and a suitable container for obtaining and keeping a lock of the child's hair
- equipment for taking hand and feet prints or casts
- camera for photograph.

Photographs taken after death can be very important. Hawley (1997) describes that 'photographs taken at that time are among our most precious reminders' (of the dead child). If it is a neonate who has died, it may be the only picture of their child that the parents will ever have.

Note: Some hospitals provide bereavement packs. They may include prompts to provide mementoes such as footprints, photographs, information about how to register the death, people who could offer help and support groups.

Some hospitals have special Moses baskets, cots or prams in which to place an infant's body.

A body bag made of heavy, waterproof plastic with zip, of a size suitable to contain the body, will be necessary if the child was suffering from hepatitis B, AIDS or was HIV positive.

Method

1. Washing and laying out of the body should be considered within 2–3 hours of death. This is because rigor mortis can begin as soon as 2 hours after death, especially if the child's temperature was high at the time of death (Green & Green 1992). This may not always be the case, however, but it may be aesthetically more pleasing if the child has been washed. It is much more difficult to handle a body when rigor has commenced. Once the child has been washed, she can be given back to parents to cuddle if they wish.
2. Remove the bed clothes and straighten the body as far as possible without using force. This may not be possible if the child has a physical deformity such as severe scoliosis, or severely retracted limbs. Support the head with one small pillow. If the cot is too small for a pillow, consider using a folded, soft towel. Cover the body with a sheet to preserve the child's privacy and dignity.
3. Remove the child's clothing; observe the body for any bruising or signs of injury. Any findings should be noted in the nursing documentation. Cover the body with the sheet.
4. Clean the child's eyes if necessary and close them. If they will not close of their own accord, it may

be necessary to place dampened gauze swabs over each eye to help keep them shut. Sometimes a small piece of tape can be used, but it must be of a type which will not cause trauma to the skin when it is removed. Micropore tape would be ideal for this.

5. Clean the child's mouth carefully. Often the jaw may be slack and leave the mouth gaping. This can be distressing for parents and present a risk of leakage of body fluids. If it is gaping, it may be necessary to support the jaw (temporarily) with a small pad, e.g. a rolled face towel under the chin. It may be acceptable to use a piece of cotton bandage tied gently around the head, but again be careful not to cause any trauma to the skin. Usually, once rigor starts to establish, the mouth will remain closed, unsupported.

6. Leakage of body fluids represents a potential hazard to those who have to handle the body after death (Green & Green 1992). Therefore, empty the bladder by applying gentle pressure to the lower abdomen. If there is a lot of leakage from the bowel or vagina, ensure that a nappy or incontinence pad is used. In any child who wore nappies when alive, the parents will find nothing odd in seeing her in a nappy after death and this will cope with most leakages. An incontinence pad may be more appropriate for an older child.

7. If there is to be a post-mortem, in accordance with instructions from medical staff, lines, drains, catheters and cannulae should be left in situ (Green & Green 1992). Any drainage bags, infusion tubing, etc. must be removed and the lines, drains, catheters and cannulae spigoted to prevent leakage of body fluids.

8. If there is no post-mortem, then everything except tunnelled intravenous catheters should be removed and carefully disposed of according to local policy. Removing tunnelled catheters would cause significant trauma, which is why they should be left in situ. Any wounds left by removing cannulae, drains, etc. should be covered with waterproof tape. Any stoma or wound which could continue to leak should be covered with padding and then waterproof tape to prevent leakage. Any removable sutures or clips should be left in place.

9. If required, cut a lock of hair from the back of the child's head (where it will not be obvious that it has been removed). Take plaster casts or foot and hand prints from the child's hands and feet.

10. The child's body should then be washed all over and carefully dried. Applying a little petroleum jelly to the lips will help prevent the skin drying out and prevent any corrosion from gastric juices (Green & Green 1992).

11. If there is jewellery on the body, it is usual to remove it unless it has religious significance. If a nurse removes jewellery, it must only be done in the presence of a witness and its removal must be recorded in the documentation.

12. Make up the bed or cot with fresh linen and dress the child. Comb her hair. Place her in the bed or cot and put a toy and/or flowers with her as appropriate. Cover her with a sheet. Some areas will require that a child who has to be put into a body bag must be placed in it as soon as possible after death. If this has to be done, it is possible to leave the zip part way down so that parents may view the body, but it should be argued that there is no need for the body to be placed in the bag until it has to go to the mortuary or funeral parlour. The child is no more infectious after death than she was before and so her parents should have the right to hold and cuddle her in death as they did in life.

13. If parents are unsure whether or not to have photographs of their child, it may be a good idea to take them now. Explain to parents that even if they feel they do not want photographs now, they may subsequently change their minds. Explain that it is possible to take them and place them in the child's medical records so that they may be retrieved for the family at a later date if they do change their minds. You may not take photographs without the parents' consent.

14. Ensure that the child has a clearly legible identity name band in situ on the wrist or ankle. Some areas require there to be a name band on both wrist and ankle.

15. Tidy up. Dispose of linen, sharps and clinical waste carefully and safely to prevent injury or cross-infection and in accordance with local policy.

16. Document the child's property, noting if any jewellery was removed and reserve the property for the family to take home if they wish.

17. If parents have not been involved in the laying out of their child, it is at this point that it would be appropriate to ask them to return to spend time with their child. Encourage them to hold her and cuddle her. They should be allowed to spend as much time as they like with their child, if at all possible. Do not be afraid to cry in front of the relatives, but ensure that they do not feel that they have to support you. Be aware that in some cultures it is a mark of respect to grieve loudly and obviously after a death.

Parents should be allowed to spend as much time with their child as possible. If circumstances (e.g. on a busy ward) make this difficult, explain to them beforehand that at this stage they will have limited time. Offer them a private place where they may see their child. This may need to be the hospital chapel or holy room. Some hospitals have special viewing rooms which are decorated like a bedroom and the child's body is placed in a bed, crib or cot according to her age. Once the child has gone to the funeral director, the parents should be able to see her there without any problem. The only exception to this is if the child is in a body bag because of a potential risk of infection. Be aware that, in many cases, once a potentially infectious body has left the hospital, it can only be seen from a distance if at all, and it may be impossible for the parents to hold and cuddle their child again. In this case, it is kindest to hold the body as long as possible where her parents can still have access to her.

18. When it is time to take the child to the mortuary or the child is to be collected by the funeral director, the body should be wrapped securely in a clean, white sheet, unless the parents specifically request otherwise. If the body has to be placed in a body bag, it must be done before the body goes to the mortuary or funeral parlour. The sheet or bag should be labelled according to local policy.

19. The Notification of Death certificate must accompany the body to the mortuary and is commonly pinned to the sheet. Obviously, pins must not be used on a body bag as this would damage the integrity of the bag. Sticky tape would suffice. Some areas require a name band label to be attached to the outside of the sheet. The Notification of Death certificate must state if the child has a pacemaker in situ (it must be removed if the body is to be cremated as it is liable to explode during cremation), or if the body is potentially infectious.

20. Ensure that the parents have clear, preferably written instructions about what they must do to register the death, organise the funeral and so on. Verbal instructions may not be assimilated when parents are distressed. If there is a bereavement pack for parents, give this to them. If there is a bereavement counsellor, he will be able to support the parents through this process and will be able to help parents access support from other agencies such as bereavement groups.

21. Finally, check who has to be informed about the child's death and who is responsible for doing so. Again, bereavement counsellors may do this as part of their role. A checklist such as that illustrated in Table 4.2 may be utilised.

Observations

As previously described, the nurse should observe the child's body for unusual marks and bruising and these should be recorded. The presence of jewellery on the body or the removal of jewellery from the body should also be observed and recorded.

Complications

Complications should not arise in caring for the body as long as careful thought and preparation are exercised. Without thorough preparation, complications that could arise include:

- inappropriate handling of the body in relation to legal requirements (post-mortem), religious custom or the parents' own wishes

Table 4.2 **Checklist of those who may need to be informed of the death of a child**

Person/agency to be informed	To be informed by
Named nurse	Nursing staff
Medical records	Nursing staff
General practitioner	Medical staff
Health visitor	Nursing staff
Paramedical staff (physiotherapist, play therapist)	Nursing or medical staff
Religious/spiritual advisor	Nursing staff
Social worker	Nursing staff
Liaison nurse	Nursing staff
Community nurses	Nursing staff
Bereavement counsellor	Nursing staff
School: head, form teacher and school nurse	Hospital school/nursing staff
Siblings' school	Nursing staff
Hospice	Nursing staff

- nurses inexperienced in managing the death of a child are left without support or resources to tell them what to do
- additional distress caused to parents who were not made aware of the risk of vocal-type noises emitting from the body or leakage of body fluids
- additional distress caused to parents who are not made fully aware of the procedures surrounding the death of their child, e.g. having to wait for a death certificate leading to a delay in the funeral.

COMMUNITY PERSPECTIVE

CCNs are likely to have been involved with the families of children with life-threatening illnesses during their treatment phase and will have had the opportunity to develop a trusting relationship. They may have met members of the extended family and close friends and will therefore be aware of the family dynamics. They may also have had the opportunity to discuss the family's spiritual beliefs.

When a child enters the palliative stage of illness, the parents should be reassured that this does not mean that no active treatment will take place. Treatment options will change but symptom control in palliative care is often active treatment. A multidisciplinary approach, involving the general practitioner, the health visitor and the Macmillan nurses will be of the greatest benefit to the family. The primary health care team will be dealing with the family for many years after the death of the child. It may also be helpful for the CCN to liaise with school nurses and teachers involved with either the dying child or the child's siblings. School friends may also need help to deal with the situation.

Discussion should take place within the family as to how and where the child will be cared for. The views of siblings must be taken into account as they may be suffering quietly on their own, not wishing to add to their parents' distress by showing their heartbreak. The CCN, being aware of this, can use her counselling skills to help families to develop a more open approach. So much control has been taken away from the family because of the child's illness that it is imperative that their wishes during the last period of life are valued. It is important to remember that no two families will cope with grief in the same way.

The decision that the family reaches must be adhered to as closely as resources permit. It is not possible to guarantee that one particular team member will be present at the time of death and the family need to be aware of this. However, they can be reassured that they will be supported 24 hours a day should they decide to care for their child at home. The family need to have a list of contact numbers and be aware of who is on call. They also need to know that a hospital bed will be available for the child should they feel unable to cope at any time. This could be for respite care or longer (Thornes 1988).

It may be that the period of palliative care may continue for months before the child reaches the terminal phase. This is time that the family can be encouraged to use for very active living. A special visit to somewhere like EuroDisney organised by one of the charities for children with life-threatening illnesses, or a short walk on a sunny day near home can equally be remembered as special times by the family after the child has died. It is important that the CCN supports these family activities, encouraging those which she feels would benefit the whole family but advocating restraint about any that she feels would tax the child unduly. However, it must be recognised that some families need time on their own, away from professional input. The CCN needs to be sensitive to this and to appreciate that she may be answering her own needs, rather than the family's, if she is visiting more than they wish. This can be an import-ant time for the family to collect mementoes, photographs, video recordings, items made by the dying child, etc. It is a period of adjustment, during which the family may be able to address the reality of impending loss and decide how and what to tell younger children, including the dying child. A great deal of emotional support is likely to be required and if the CCN is giving this, she will need opportunities to off-load, be this in the form of peer support or more formal clinical supervision.

During the final period of terminal care, the CCN team will need to be available to the family at all times. Respite care in the home may be offered. Symptom management, including pain control, is vital and a team member needs to be accessible at all times, in case treatment regimes need changing or the family require help with nursing care. Regular visits from familiar faces will help to reassure the family.

The CCN will be able to offer guidance on issues surrounding the actual death of the child and the days immediately following. She will be able to discuss:

- the likely manner of death
- the importance of involving siblings and preparing for the death (Dyregrov 1996)

- the long-term benefits of those closely involved seeing and holding the body after death (Dyregrov 1996)
- that parents can wash and dress their child in favourite clothes following death, if they wish
- where the child's body should rest before the funeral: the child's body may remain at home providing certain procedures have been undertaken by the funeral director; alternatively the body can be taken to a chapel of rest and no one will think that this means they loved the child less
- how to register the death
- funeral arrangements and what form this important ritual will take. The parents can be encouraged to allow the siblings some choice. Older children who have come to terms with their impending death may have had strong views on funeral arrangements.

In the months following death, many families need to maintain contact with the professionals involved in their child's care. Bereavement visiting should continue for as long as both parties feel to be appropriate. Work with siblings can be undertaken, for example collecting together items which remind them of the dead child and putting them in a memory box. It may be years before the family are ready to place the lid on that box and it is important for them to realise that this is perfectly acceptable. This is something over which they do have control.

CCNs may be involved where children die unexpectedly, for example as a result of major surgery. The CCN may have been involved with the family prior to the hospitalisation which resulted in death. In this situation, bereavement visiting and maintaining contact may be appropriate.

Do and do not

- Do consult the parents about their wishes for their child after she has died.
- Do remember to maintain the privacy and dignity of the child at all times after death.
- Do establish whether there is to be a post-mortem.
- Do establish if there are any special religious needs associated with care of the child after death.
- Do remember that the parents may not be the only family members who require support.
- Do remember to warn parents helping to wash and dress their child after death of how the child may appear, possible noises the body may make and leakage of body fluids.
- Do be aware if there are other staff who may be

adversely affected and require support because of the death of a child.
- Do not remove lines, cannulae, etc. if there is to be a post-mortem.
- Do not be afraid to show grief and cry with parents after a child has died, but do not allow your own grief to overshadow any situation or make parents feel that they must comfort and support you.

References

Anonymous 1993 A cry for help. Nursing Times 89(4): 29–30
Back D, Rooke V 1994 The presence of relatives in the resuscitation room. Nursing Times 90(30): 34–35
Brown P 1993 Saying goodbye. Nursing Times 89(4): 26–29
Browne J, Waddington P 1993 Care of the dying child. In: Carter B (ed) Manual of paediatric intensive care nursing. Chapman & Hall, London, ch 10, p 299
Carter B 1993 (ed) Manual of paediatric intensive care nursing. Chapman & Hall, London
Davies C 1997 When a baby dies. Nursing Times 93(8): 28–29
Dyregrov A 1996 Children's participation in rituals. Bereavement Care 15(1): 2–4
Ellis J, Edwards J 1995 Part of a learning process: the paediatric post-mortem. Child Health 2(6): 244–246
Green J, Green M 1992 Dealing with death. Practices and procedures. Chapman & Hall, London, chs 13, 16–31, pp 115–123, 149–230
Hanson C, Strawser D 1992 Family presence during cardiopulmonary resuscitation: Foote hospital emergency department's nine-year perspective. Journal of Emergency Nursing 18(2): 104–106
Hawley R 1997 Seasons of grief. Nursing Times 93(8): 24–26
Nelson L 1995 When a child dies. American Journal of Nursing 95(3): 61–64
Renzi-Brown J 1989 Risk management specialist. Nursing 19(2): 43–46
Simmons M 1992 Helping children grieve. Nursing Times 88(50): 30–32
Soutter J 1994 A strategy for caring for families in bereavement. Nursing Times 90(30): 37–39
Speck P 1992 Care after death. Nursing Times 88(6): 20
Thornes R 1988 The care of dying children and their families. Guidelines from the British Paediatric Association, King Edward's Hospital Fund for London, National Association of Health Authorities, Birmingham
Walters C, Nelson P 1997 Never too late. Nursing Times 93(8): 27

Further reading

Association for Children with Life Threatening or Terminal Conditions and their Families (ACT) and Royal College of Paediatrics and Child Health 1997 A Guide to the Development of Childrens Palliative Care Services. ACT, Bristol
Dolan B 1995 A drama within a crisis – relatives in the resuscitation room. Journal of Clinical Nursing. 4: 275
Kubler-Ross E 1985 On children and dying. Collier, New York
Stewart E S 1995 Family-centred care for the bereaved. Pediatric Nursing 21(2): 181–184
Widdrington C 1992 Preparing for loss. Nursing Times 88(49): 26–28

5

Blood Glucose Estimation

Introduction

These guidelines are related to one specific method of blood glucose estimation using BM Test 1–44 reagent strips.

Blood glucose estimation may be needed for a number of medical reasons both within the acute setting and in the community.

Within the hospital the nurse may need to check a child's blood glucose level if the child is undergoing treatment which may potentially cause a rise in the blood glucose level, e.g. during the use of steroids. If the child is susceptible to hypoglycaemia or is unconscious, the blood glucose level will also be taken. The most common reason may be associated with the management of diabetes mellitus, which also involves the education of the child and his parent/guardian.

Learning outcomes

At the end of this section the nurse should:

- be able to identify when an estimate of blood glucose level is needed
- appreciate the need to use a finger-pricking device to obtain a sample of blood
- know which fingers are recommended for obtaining a capillary blood sample
- be able to use blood glucose strips BM Test 1–44 correctly, following the instructions stipulated by the manufacturer, Boehringer Mannheim
- be able to interpret the result, record it and liaise with other health care professionals when appropriate.

Rationale for blood glucose monitoring

Capillary blood glucose measurement should only be performed by staff who have undertaken a training programme and been regularly updated, as the results obtained affect the treatment of the child (Page et al 1996).

Factors to note

Educating the child and carer

In some instances the nurse will need to teach the child and the parent or carer how to monitor blood glucose levels. This may be necessary when a child is diagnosed with insulin-dependent diabetes mellitus or for children who are receiving treatment or have a condition which affects their blood glucose level, and who therefore require ongoing measurement within the home.

When children or carers are being taught a practical skill, they need to know the importance of the procedure and how to interpret the results.

It is vital to the well-being of the child and family that adequate education is provided, as studies have shown that failing to meet the needs of the family increases the stress they feel and therefore the parents are less able to support their child (Bradford & Singer 1991).

To provide an appropriate teaching programme, the nurse has to assess the child and the child's family separately before undertaking an education plan for blood glucose measurement. Even young children have the ability to learn and be competent in doing blood glucose monitoring. Play is often a fun way of educating a young child (Hatcher 1990).

Guidelines

It is vital that the principles of performing a capillary blood glucose measurement are followed both within the acute setting and during patient and carer education.

Equipment

- Blood glucose test strips BM Test 1–44
- Finger-pricking device for multiple patient use or single patient use
- Appropriate lancet for finger pricker
- Cotton wool – sterile or unsterile
- Disposable gloves
- Sharps bin
- Watch/clock with second hand

Method and rationale

1. Explain the procedure to the child (if appropriate) and the family. This will help to alleviate any anxiety they may have.

2. Prepare all the equipment as listed. This will encourage a smooth procedure.
3. Check the expiry date of the BM Test 1–44 strips. Out-of-date strips will give inaccurate results because of contamination, but as long as the strips have been stored correctly they will remain stable until the expiry date.
4. The person taking the blood sample should wash and dry her hands with soap and water to reduce the risk of cross-contamination.
5. Wash the child's hands with soap and warm water.
6. The nurse may also need to wear gloves according to hospital policy.
7. Prick the side of the finger or heel with either the child's own device or the one recommended by the hospital.
8. After pricking the finger, wipe the first drop of blood away. This first drop of blood is a mixture of blood and tissue fluid and the action of wiping promotes further blood flow.
9. Milk the finger in a downward stroke until there is a large hanging drop of blood. A large drop of blood is needed to ensure full coverage of the strip, without having to scrape or blot the blood onto the pad.

10. Apply only one drop of blood in the centre to cover both the pads without touching the strip with the finger. As soon as the blood touches the pad start timing for 1 minute. The timing is crucial as a chemical reaction starts as soon as the blood touches the pad.

    Note: Insufficient covering of the test strip will give an inaccurate result as will smearing or blotting the blood onto the pad (see Fig. 5.1).
11. After 1 minute firmly wipe off the blood with cotton wool – this may need two strokes – and continue timing for a further minute.
12. After the second minute the result may be compared to the colour chart on the bottle of strips. If the top pad has turned green, then read the top pad for the result. If the top pad remains a beige colour then take the reading from the bottom blue pad. The top pad is more accurate at a level of 9 mmol/l or above and the bottom pad is more sensitive to a blood sugar level less than 9 mmol/l (Fig. 5.2).

    If the reading is 17 mmol/l, wait a further minute before reading the result.
13. Record the result and report any abnormality to the medical staff if appropriate.

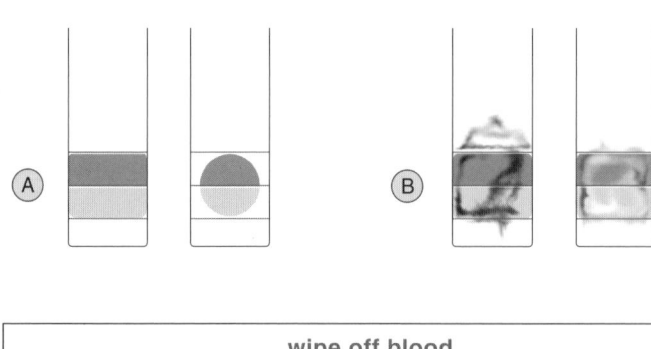

Figure 5.1
*Good technique (A)
and poor technique (B).*

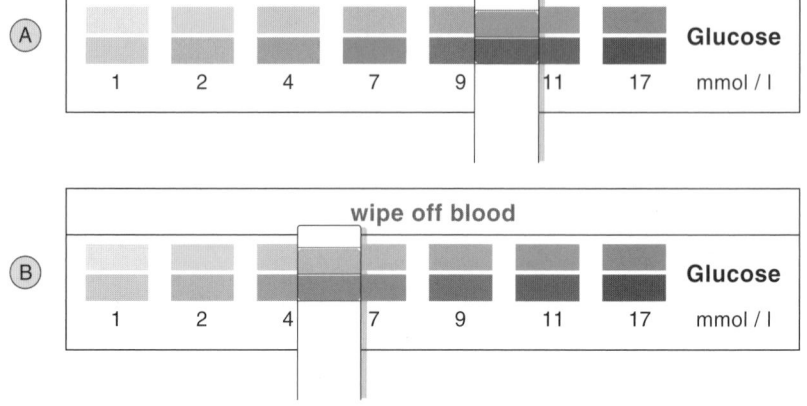

Figure 5.2
*Comparison of colour
blocks.*

14. Dispose of sharps immediately, according to local policy, to prevent needlestick injuries.

Factors to note during the procedure

- Alcohol-based wipes will contaminate the strip and give a false reading.
- Washing hands reduces the risk of cross-infection and removes any glucose from the skin.
- Warm water will also help promote blood flow to the fingers.
- A finger pricker should always be used because, owing to the measured depth of the device, it reduces the pain to the finger or heel.
- Heel pricks are needed in babies and young children to obtain a capillary sample.
- The sides of the finger should be used, excluding the thumb and index finger, as this reduces the sensation. Young children use the pincer action for picking up objects and repeatedly pricking these fingers will cause more discomfort (Fyffe 1992).
- Accurate timing is essential because if the blood is wiped off before 1 minute the result may be lower and if wiped off after 1 minute the result may be higher.
- Cotton wool is recommended as it has the correct absorbency. Tissues, gauze or paper towels will scratch the surface of the pad or remove it completely from the strip.
- Blood glucose sensors may also be used. However, the Department of Health (1987) issued a hazard warning related to inaccurate use of blood glucose meters and highlighted the need for regular training for the users, written protocols and continuous assessment of quality control to reduce the margin of error.
- Errors can be made during the visual test and therefore regular updates are needed for staff.

Observations and complications

The normal range for blood glucose level using the visual BM Test 1–44 strips should be 4–7 mmol/l.

It is important to clarify with the medical staff at what point they should be informed if the blood test result falls outside of this range; depending on hospital policy, it may be necessary to send a blood sample for estimating true blood glucose level. This will also depend on the child's condition and treatment.

Anyone who is colour blind will not be able to interpret the results.

Do and do not

- Do explain the procedure to the child and his family and the reason for the test.
- Do give the family written instructions on the procedure if they are to continue checking the glucose levels at home.
- Do explain the range that the blood glucose level should fall between, giving contact numbers for advice if the result is abnormal, if the family are to continue to monitor the blood glucose levels at home.
- Do ensure that the strips are stored at room temperature and the bottle is kept sealed at all times. Contamination is caused by moisture in the air and incorrect storage affects the readings.
- Do not change strips from one tube to another; all bottles have their own batch number and colour code on the side of the bottle. This is especially important when using a blood glucose sensor for the reading of the strip. There is also an expiry date on each bottle.
- Do not use Mediswabs as they harden the skin and cause discomfort when the finger is pricked.
- Do not cut the strips as this allows the chemicals to leak out and contaminate the rest of the strips.

References

Bradford R, Singer J 1991 Support and information for parents. Paediatric Nursing (May): 18–20

Department of Health and Social Security (DHSS) 1987 Blood glucose measurements: reliability of results produced in extra laboratory areas. Hazard warning (HN (Hazard) (87) 13). HMSO, London

Fyffe J 1992 Collection of capillary blood samples. Technical Information Bulletin Ames Education Services No. 6. Bayer Diagnostics, Berkshire

Hatcher T 1990 Learning is fun. Paediatric Nursing (March): 10–12

Page S R, Scholey K, Clarke P et al 1996 The effect of a quality assurance scheme and compulsory training programme on the performance of ward-based blood glucose measurements. Practical Diabetes International 13(5): 144–147

RCN Diabetes Nursing Forum 1991 Guidelines on the use of blood glucose monitoring equipment by nurses in clinical areas. Bayer Diagnostics UK, London

Further reading

Bannister M 1996 Promotion of diabetes self-care through play. Professional Nurse 12(2): 109–112

Marriott S 1990 Parent power. Nursing Times 86(34): 68

6

Bowel Care

Introduction

This section will concentrate on rectal washouts.

There are other forms of bowel washouts, which will be described briefly. In the majority of cases it is preferable to clear the bowel using some form of laxative. However, in cases where a mechanical obstruction of the bowel is suspected it would be dangerous to give laxatives. (Stimulating peristalsis in a bowel with an obstruction could cause a perforation.)

Bowel washouts are performed for various reasons. These include:

- preparation of the bowel for surgery or investigation
- to control faecal soiling
- to treat constipation.

Other methods of clearing out the bowel include:

- Colostomy or distal loop washout – usually performed to prepare the bowel for stoma closure or to evacuate mucus from the distal bowel in the child with a stoma.
- Colostomy irrigation (McDonald 1991) – usually performed by adults or older children as a method of stoma management, obviating the need to use a stoma pouch.
- Colonic irrigation (Fitzpatrick 1996, Van Kessel et al 1996) – usually performed daily or on alternate days on children with faecal incontinence or constipation problems.
- Antegrade colonic enema (ACE procedure) (Keily et al 1995, Mor et al 1997) – a washout performed through an appendicostomy. With this procedure the washout solution will include some type of enema solution.

Rectal washout

Learning outcomes

The aim of this section is for the nurse to:

- understand the reason for performing the washout, and be able to give an explanation to the child or carer

- be aware of the solution to be used, amount of solution and reasons for choosing the solution
- be able to perform an effective washout safely, following observation
- be aware of potential problems with the washout.

Rationale

All children, whether healthy, sick or disabled, will need comfort and support during what can be an unpleasant procedure. The more experienced the nurse is at rectal washouts, the more effective and efficient she should be.

Factors to note

One concern that nurses have is the size of the rectal tube to use. In my experience a size 10 or 12 Fr is sufficient for newborn babies and, as the washout kits supplied at our institution only fit on to rectal tubes up to size 18 Fr, we use no larger than the 18 Fr.

Children with special needs

Some children, such as those with brittle bones, have a very small abdomen; care must be taken with the amount of saline used for the washout. Medical advice should be sought.

Guidelines for infants

Equipment

- Disposable gloves
- Incontinence sheets
- Warm saline
- Rectal tube or nasogastric tube (size 10 or 12)
- Syringe (if using a rectal tube, a bladder syringe will need to be used)
- Disposable bowls
- Lubricating jelly

Method

- Explain the procedure to the parents before commencing the washout. Undress the baby, ensuring that the room is warm enough to prevent the infant getting too cold. Put on disposable gloves.

- Pour the warm saline into a disposable bowl. Draw up about 30 ml of saline into the syringe and attach the rectal tube. Prime the rectal tube with saline.
- Infants are generally more content to lie on their backs during this procedure; any position they want to assume can be accommodated.
- Lubricate the end of the rectal catheter with lubricating jelly. Locate the anus and gently insert the rectal catheter into the rectum. Slowly inject the saline into the rectum. Once it has entered the rectum, gently draw back on the syringe; if any pressure is felt stop drawing back. If no saline can be drawn back, disconnect the rectal catheter from the syringe and gently introduce the catheter further into the rectum; this will often stimulate evacuation through gravity.
- Continue the above until either the infant has passed an adequate amount of stool or the saline returning is clean. This will depend on why the washout is being performed. (If the washout is being performed on an infant with Hirschsprung's disease, it is done to deflate the bowel; therefore less saline would be needed than if the washout were being done as a means of preparing the bowel for surgery.)
- In very small babies no more than 20 ml at a time should be put into the rectum. With bigger infants no more than about 40 ml should be introduced at a time.
- The medical staff may have indicated how much saline in total should be used. If not, the total amount used is discretional, but if the infant begins to get cold owing to being undressed, the washout should be stopped .
- When the washout has ended, gently remove the catheter and wipe the infant's bottom. Put on the infant's nappy and clothes.

Guidelines for children older than infants

Equipment
- Disposable gloves
- Incontinence sheets
- Rectal washout kit (funnel with rubber tubing and connector attached)
- Rectal tube (sizes of rectal catheter that accommodate the funnel are 12–18 Fr)
- Lubricating jelly
- Warm saline
- Bucket

Method
- Gather all equipment together. Ensure that the room where the washout is to be performed is warm. This is to ensure that the child does not get cold during the procedure; being cold will make the child more uncomfortable with the procedure.
- The lower garments should be removed and the child should lie on the couch on top of the incontinence sheets. Positioning the child on the left-hand side with knees bent up to the abdomen will ensure easier insertion of the rectal tube. Explanation of every part of the procedure is important to the child and carer, as the child will not be able to see what is happening behind her. Put on disposable gloves.
- Attach the rectal catheter to the rectal washout kit. Place the bucket on the floor by the couch. Pour some saline into the funnel to prime the tube, pinching the rectal catheter so as not to lose all the saline. Lubricate the end of the rectal catheter with lubricating jelly.
- Locate the anus and gently insert the rectal catheter; about 3 or 4 inches is enough to start the washout. Lift up the funnel to allow the saline to enter the rectum by gravity. When the saline in the funnel has entered the rectum, lower the funnel and let all the saline and any stool run into the bucket.
- Leaving the rectal catheter in the rectum, refill the funnel and repeat the last step. Always note any complaint of abdominal pain; do not overfill the rectum at any time. The process can continue until the bowel is clear. However, if the child becomes cold owing to being undressed, the washout should be stopped or efforts made to keep the child warm.
- Ensure that the amount of saline put into the rectum comes back out. The catheter can be introduced further into the rectum if the lower rectum is clean.
- At the end of the washout gently remove the rectal catheter and wipe the child's bottom. It can sometimes be beneficial to ask the child to sit on the toilet to see if any more stool or saline can be evacuated.

Observations and complications
- Always use a saline solution to perform the washout. If water is used the child could absorb it and develop water intoxication.

- Always warm the saline prior to starting the washout. It has been suggested that the temperature should be 38°C. If the saline is not warmed, the child will get abdominal cramps; if the saline is too hot, the bowel mucosa can be burned.
- Always ensure that the saline entering the bowel is evacuated. This can be done by comparing the amount put in with what has returned.
- Be aware of any feelings of nausea or vomiting. If the child starts vomiting it would be wise to stop the washout. Often if children are very constipated they can feel nauseous. The medical staff should be contacted to see if an oral preparation could be given to help clear the bowel 'from above'.
- Observe any bleeding during the procedure. As the bowel has such a good blood supply it is not uncommon to have some slight bleeding from the bowel mucosa. If there is more than a slight staining of the saline the washout should be stopped and medical advice sought.

Do and do not

- Do explain the procedure to the child and carers before commencing.
- Do only use a saline solution.
- Do warm the saline before starting the procedure.
- Be aware of how the child is reacting to the washout. Most children will be upset, but if the child is extremely upset do not use others to restrain her as this could be psychologically detrimental. Some children can be better managed with oral preparations or evacuation of the bowel under anaesthetic.
- Do not put too much saline into the bowel at any one time: in small babies no more than 20 ml at a time; with older children no more at a time than fills the funnel.
- Do not use rectal washouts as a means of preparing the colon for surgery or investigations in a child with inflammatory bowel disease. These children can have a friable bowel and there could be a risk of bleeding or perforation.
- Performing washouts through an ileostomy is not advised as a general rule. Consult a stoma nurse or the medical staff if asked. One of the reasons for concern is that rapid fluid loss from the small intestine could cause shock.
- Do not continue putting saline into the bowel if none is being evacuated.

References

Fitzpatrick G 1996 The child with a stoma. In: Myers C (ed) Stoma care nursing – a patient centered approach. Arnold, London, pp 184–201

Keily E M, Ade-Ajayi N, Wheeler R 1995 Antegrade continence enemas in the management of intractable faecal incontinence. Journal of the Royal Society of Medicine 88(2): 103–104

McDonald K 1991 Colostomy irrigation: an option worth considering. Professional Nurse 7(1): 15–19

Mor Y, Quinn F M, Carr B, Mouriquand P D, Duffy P G, Ransley P G 1997 Combined Mitrofanoff and antegrade continence enema procedures for urinary and faecal incontinence. Journal of Urology 158(1): 192–195

Van Kessel et al 1996 Rectal washouts in patients with disturbed continence or disordered defaecation. Clinical results of a nursing intervention. Proceedings of Congress of World Council of Enterostomal Therapists, Hollister, USA, pp 133–134

7

Cardiopulmonary Resuscitation

Introduction

While few resuscitation situations involving children arise without warning, it remains imperative that children's nurses are skilled in the area of basic life support (Carter & Dearmun 1995, Simpson 1994). Paediatric basic life support can be defined as support of vital functions of breathing and circulation in infants and children, without the use of equipment. As accidents remain the commonest cause of death in children and as the life expectancy of children with a variety of chronic illness is increasing, the need for parents and also other members of the general public to learn basic paediatric life support is becoming increasingly important (Carter & Dearmun 1995, Whitton 1995).

Paediatric advanced life support involves the use of equipment commonly found in hospitals and could be considered as the second stage of resuscitation. However, 'if basic life support is not effectively delivered to the child attempts at advanced life support are likely to prove futile' (Simpson 1994, p. 39).

It is important to recognise that practising cardiopulmonary resuscitation using a baby or child mannequin is the most effective way of ensuring that children's nurses have appropriate skills to help an infant or child in need. In addition, these skills, in order to be fresh, require to be updated regularly.

All nurses must be aware of the emergency call telephone number and procedure for their individual clinical areas.

Learning outcomes

By the end of this section and following further reading and simulated practice the nurse should be able to:

- assess responsiveness in infants and children
- use appropriate airway opening techniques
- assess respiration by looking, listening and feeling for expired breath
- provide rescue breathing
- pulse check using appropriate sites
- provide chest compressions
- identify priorities in advanced life support.

Rationale

Commentators on both sides of the Atlantic acknowledge the importance of resuscitation as a nursing skill (American Heart Association 1994, Resuscitation Council (UK) 1997).

Basic life support is useful and is context free. It can be performed by a single rescuer and does not require the presence of resuscitation equipment.

Many children die or suffer permanent neurological impairment each year because of sudden infant death syndrome, infections or trauma. Appropriate prompt action can help avoid many of them.

Advanced life support involves the use of equipment and drug therapy. This stage normally commences once the resuscitation team arrives. However, it may be commenced before they arrive if the child does not respond to basic life support interventions.

Advanced life support will be futile if basic life support is not delivered effectively.

Factors to note

Babies and children differ from adults in a number of ways:

- The causes of their cardiopulmonary arrest are different, with adults tending to suffer from *primary* cardiac arrest, whereas children, who predominantly have healthy hearts, tend to have *secondary* cardiac arrest following a period of hypoxia often associated with an airway or breathing emergency. This fact suggests that cardiac arrest in children may be preventable if appropriate measures are taken to deal with the airway or breathing problem. The presence of hypoxia also explains why children fare so poorly following cardiopulmonary arrest. If the heart is deprived of oxygen to the point where it can no longer function, then similar effects must be seen in the brain and other vital organs (Hampson-Evans & Bingham 1998).
- Respiratory infection and sepsis are the primary causes of cardiopulmonary arrest in children under

5 years of age, with trauma being the major cause in the 5- to 14-year age group (Williams 1994).

- Babies and children differ from each other in resuscitation terms. The infant is defined as being in the first year of life and the child is defined as being from the age of 1–8 years. Those children older than 8 years, although still considered as children, may require two-handed chest compression as in adults (Resuscitation Council (UK) 1997).
- The surface area of the face is smaller in babies.
- The paediatric larynx is funnel shaped, not cylindrical. This renders the larynx more susceptible to impaction of foreign objects.
- The larynx of the child is soft and the trachea is short. The tongue of the infant or child is large in comparison and, as such, increases airway obstruction and obscures the view of the glottis (Bishop-Kurylo & Masiello 1995, Williams 1994).
- Infants have poorly developed accessory muscles and an immature bronchial tree, the diaphragm being the major muscle of respiration (Hazinski 1992).
- The pressure required for chest compression is less in babies.
- Chest compression should be commenced if no pulse is palpated in the child or the pulse rate is less than 60 beats per minute or absent in the infant. In the latter instance, time should not be wasted counting the pulse for a full minute; instead a beat of one per second is sufficient assessment.
- Basic life support should be initiated before the administration of any drugs or other intervention is considered.
- Cardiac arrest is defined as the absence of palpable central pulses. Three cardiac arrest rhythms may be identified on electrocardiograph (ECG) monitoring in children.
- Asystole, total absence of pulse, occurs in > 90% of all paediatric cardiac arrests (Simpson 1994).
- Extreme hypoxia and acidosis results in all arrest scenarios.
- Ventricular fibrillation, although rare in children (less than 10%), requires to be rapidly identified in order to institute prompt action (Simpson 1994). It is most likely to occur in children who are hypothermic, have structural cardiac disease or have taken an overdose of tricyclic antidepressants.
- Precordial thump, a blow to the chest prior to cardiac massage, may be effective if given at the start of ventricular fibrillation; however, this is only achievable in the child who is being cardiac monitored. The use of a precordial thump is controversial (Simpson 1994, Woodward 1994).

- Defibrillation takes precedence in the treatment of ventricular fibrillation. Shocks should be given in sets of three. Paediatric paddles should be used in children below 10 kilograms (European Resuscitation Council 1994).

Basic paediatric life support

Method

The following has been agreed as the basis for one-rescuer basic life support in infancy and childhood (European Resuscitation Council 1994, Resuscitation Council (UK) 1997).

- Assess the environment surrounding the infant or child; move the child if the environment is dangerous. It is also important that the nurse does not become the next victim of whatever fate befell the child. If neck injury is suspected, all attempts should be made to move the child with the spinal column intact.
- Assess the level of responsiveness by gently shaking or pinching the child's fingers or toes. Tactile and verbal stimulation should be used. Care should be taken to avoid vigorous shaking as brain injury can be caused in this way.
- If the child is unresponsive, call for help but do not leave the child alone. It is possible that this unconsciousness may cause airway obstruction. Opening of the airway may be the only resuscitative action that is required.

Opening the airway

- The airway can be opened in either of two ways:
  - Head tilt/chin lift: one hand is placed on the child's forehead, and a finger of the other hand is placed on the bony tip of the chin. The head is then tilted back and the chin lifted upwards and forward (see Fig. 7.1). It is important to avoid overextension of the neck and compression of the soft tissues under the chin as either of these can cause obstruction of the air passages.
  - Jaw thrust: this technique is the preferred choice where neck injury is suspected because it allows the airway to be opened without moving the neck. In this instance the index fingers of both hands are placed behind the angles of the jaw and the mandible is lifted upwards carrying the tongue forward. This manoeuvre may close the mouth, however, so the thumbs should be placed on the tip of the chin (Hampson-Evans & Bingham 1998).

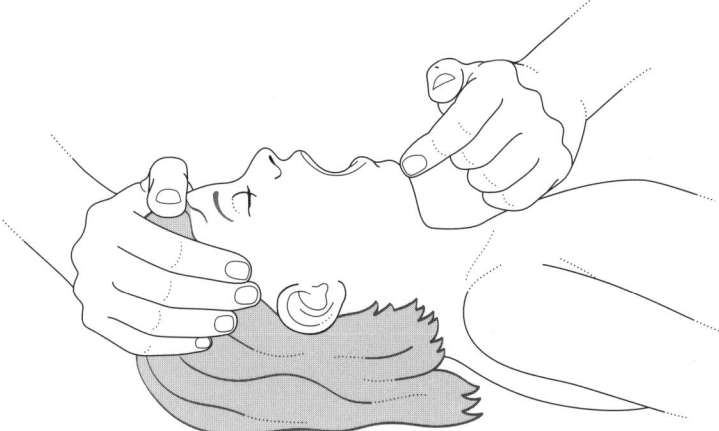

Figure 7.1
*Airway opening: head
tilt/chin lift.*

- Once the airway is open assess breathing.
- If impaction of the airway by a foreign body is suspected or witnessed, this must be removed.
- Interventions to remove the foreign object are aimed at creating an artificial cough (MacNab 1996).
- Administer five back blows (between the shoulder blades), with the child lying prone, head lower than the chest. Turn the child and administer five thrusts to the sternum. Check mouth for object and remove if seen. Do not blindly sweep the mouth. Repeat this if no object is seen, providing intermittent respirations as oxygenation/ventilation may still occur if enough time is allowed for the lungs to fill and empty. Repeat the procedure until the obstruction is cleared (Resuscitation Council UK 1997, MacNab 1996).
- Assess breathing by observing the chest for chest movement, listening for breath sounds at the child's mouth and nose, and feeling for evidence of expired breath with your cheek.
- If there is no breathing, artificial ventilation should be commenced without delay.
- For infants, deliver breaths to lungs via the mouth and nose. It has been suggested that in some infants it is not possible for an adult to effectively cover both mouth and nose for ventilation (Tonkin et al 1995), but the Resuscitation Council UK (1997) and

American Heart Association (1994) continue to recommend mouth-to-mouth-and-nose rescue breathing for the infant under 1 year old; this is further supported by Nadkarni et al (1997).
- For the child, breathing should be by the mouth-to-mouth route.
- Maintain the airway in an open position throughout ventilation.
- Deliver breaths slowly, $1-1\frac{1}{2}$ seconds each, to minimise the possibility of gastric distension and optimise filling of lungs (McCrory & Downs 1990, Resuscitation Council (UK) 1997).
- Observe the chest during rescue breathing to ensure that it rises and falls. This movement confirms the patency of the airway.
- Deliver five rescue breaths; if chest movement is not witnessed, reposition the airway. If this is unsuccessful, the possibility of a foreign body should be considered.

Checking the pulse
- Assess circulation by palpation of pulse and observing for any other signs, e.g. swallowing, moving, breathing (Resuscitation Council (UK) 1997).
- In the child, the carotid artery should be palpated.

- In the infant, palpation of the femoral artery in the groin, or the brachial artery on the inside of the middle section of the upper arm (see Fig. 7.2), are indicated as the carotid artery is difficult to locate owing to the short nature of the neck.
- If no pulse is palpated or the pulse rate is less than 60 beats per minute (in the infant), chest compressions should be commenced.
- In both infants and children, the lower third of the sternum should be compressed in the midline.
- In infants, identify this mark as follows:
  – draw an imaginary line from nipple to nipple
  – place three fingers on the infant's chest, with the top finger touching the imaginary line
  – lift the top finger away from the chest
  – the remaining two fingers are now positioned on the lower third of the sternum.
- In infants, compress by one-third of the depth of the chest (Resuscitation Council (UK) 1997).
- In the child, identify this mark as follows:
  – feel for the rib cage on the side of the chest nearest to you
  – trace upwards with your finger until you locate the xiphisternum
  – measure two finger breadths above the xiphisternum
  – position the heel of one hand at this point. Thus the heel of the hand is positioned on the lower third of the sternum.
- In the child, compress for one-third of the depth of the chest (Resuscitation Council (UK) 1997).
- In the older child, compression with one hand may not provide sufficient force. Two-handed compression may be necessary. This is more commonly associated with adults. The sternum should be compressed one-third of the depth of the chest.
- In both the infant and the child, five compressions of the chest should be followed by one breath (ratio for older children 15:2). This should be repeated 20 times. Compression at a rate of 100 per minute should be attempted.
- When 1 minute has elapsed it will be necessary to summon help, if it has not already arrived. Where possible, the child should be moved to the nearest

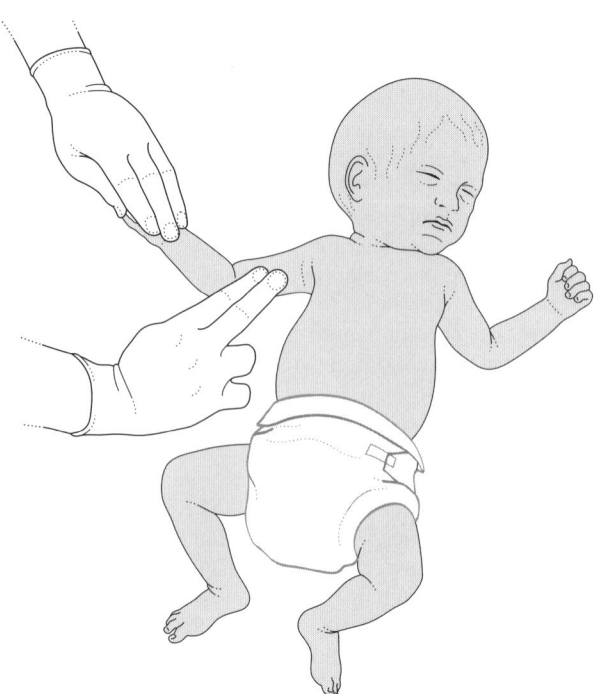

Figure 7.2
Palpation of the brachial pulse.

telephone so that help can be summoned. This facilitates a quicker resuming of the resuscitation; however, the child may have to be left momentarily.

Do and do not
- Do practise locating brachial and carotid pulses.
- Do attend to the needs of the child before telephoning. The cause of the emergency is probably airway or respiratory in nature and quick attention to this may prevent the heart from stopping.
- Do not assume that you are competent in life support because you have read about it. It is imperative that you take time to practise using appropriately sized mannequins.
- Do not blindly sweep fingers around an infant's or child's mouth. Remember that the paediatric larynx is not cylindrical but funnel shaped and it is possible that blind finger sweeps may impact an object in the larynx, causing harm.

Advanced paediatric life support

Effective basic paediatric life support is a prerequisite for advanced life support, which aims at providing continued perfusion of the coronary and cerebral arteries with oxygenated blood through the use of additional equipment and medication, thus enabling the heart to regain its effectiveness as a pump (European Resuscitation Council 1994, Hampson-Evans et al 1998).

Advanced paediatric life support inevitably will be performed and continued within the clinical setting where it is important that all staff involved are updated frequently on the techniques that are used in both types of life support, thus being familiar with paediatric practice (Bishop-Kurylo & Masiello 1995, Williams 1994).

What must be remembered is that basic life support techniques will continue despite the introduction of advanced life support.

The emergency trolley
Emergency equipment for use during advanced life support should always be readily available within all clinical areas. Although the type and style of emergency trolley will differ between clinical and community areas, the basic contents of the trolley should be similar. In comparison to emergency trolleys used within the adult setting, the trolley within the paediatric setting will carry a wide range of equipment in order to meet the needs of the wide age range and corresponding differences in body proportions of children. Box 7.1 identifies the basic requirements of the paediatric emergency trolley.

The contents of the emergency trolley should be checked on a regular basis, as per local policy, to ensure that all equipment is functional. Expiry dates should be checked on all drugs, intravenous fluids and disposable equipment; batteries and spare bulbs for the laryngoscope should also be checked.

Maintenance of airway

A secure and effective airway is essential if ventilation is to be maintained.

Equipment
- Face masks
- Self-inflating bag–valve–mask device with reservoir attached
- T-piece anaesthetic circuit
- Oxygen supply
- Oxygen tubing
- Selection of oropharyngeal airways
- Selection of endotracheal tubes
- Laryngoscope
- Blades for laryngoscope
- Zinc oxide tape for securing endotracheal tube
- Water-based lubricant jelly
- Scissors
- Suction source and catheters
- Stethoscope

Method
- Once equipment is available, change from mouth-to-mouth ventilation to the use of a self-inflating bag–valve–mask with reservoir and face mask. This is connected to the oxygen supply, thus providing a higher concentration of oxygen, which is preferential in advanced life support (European Resuscitation Council 1994).
- The face mask should provide a good seal around the nose or nose and mouth to enable optimal ventilation. A mask of an appropriate size should be chosen. The mask should fit snugly around the child's nose and mouth. A mask that is too large will allow carbon dioxide to accumulate and be delivered back to the child (McCrory & Downs 1990, Williams 1994).
- Where the child's airway cannot be maintained adequately, an oropharyngeal airway should be inserted.

Box 7.1 **Basic contents of the paediatric emergency trolley**

Airway maintenance
- Selection of oropharyngeal airways: variety of sizes ranging from infant to adult
- Endotracheal tubes: variety of sizes from infant to adult
- Laryngoscope with selection of blades straight and curved, spare handle, spare batteries and bulbs; McGill forceps
- Ventilation face masks: variety of sizes and types
- Self-inflating bag–valve–mask system with reservoir
- Re-breathing set
- T-piece/anaesthetic circuit
- Oxygen tubing, face masks, nasal prongs and portable oxygen supply
- Suction tubing, catheters and portable suction unit
- Oxygen saturation monitoring equipment

Cardiac monitoring
- Cardiac monitor electrodes
- Cardiac monitor
- Blood pressure cuffs

Drugs and intravenous fluids
- Emergency drug box containing adrenaline, sodium bicarbonate, atropine, anticonvulsant drugs, lignocaine and other drugs as per local pharmacy policy
- Saline/dextrose 500-ml bags of fluid: variety of concentrations
- Protein plasma solution
- Fluids used for intravascular volume expansion, e.g. Ringer's lactate solution

Other equipment
- Intravenous infusion equipment
- Selection of intravenous cannulae
- Intravenous cut-down set
- Intraosseous needles, spinal needles
- Syringes, hypodermic needles
- Splints
- Selection of urinary catheters and nasogastric tubes
- Stethoscope
- Silver swaddler
- Scissors
- Mediswabs
- Lubricant gel (water-based)
- Surgical tape
- Blood specimen bottles, labels

- The size of the oropharyngeal airway is determined by positioning the airway next to the child's face. A correctly sized airway should extend from the centre of the mouth to the angle of the jaw (European Resuscitation Council 1994, MacNab 1996).
- In infants, insert the airway with the convex side upwards. The tongue should be guided out of the way using a tongue depressor or the blade from a laryngoscope (MacNab 1996).

- In the child, insert the airway with the concave side upwards; when the tip reaches the soft palate rotate the airway through 180 degrees and slide over the tongue.
- Oropharyngeal airways should be used with caution. Airways that are too small will cause additional obstruction, while those that are too large may damage the posterior pharyngeal wall (Williams 1994).

- Once the airway has been inserted, bag–valve–mask ventilation should be continued.

Endotracheal intubation

Performed by experienced medical staff, endotracheal intubation remains the most effective method of securing and maintaining the airway. This should be performed as soon as possible when effective ventilation cannot be otherwise obtained (European Resuscitation Council 1994, Williams 1994). However, it must be remembered that oxygenation is the priority.

- The size of the endotracheal tube is very important. This can be estimated by a number of methods:
  - In infants, the size of endotracheal tube usually required is 3.0–3.5 mm for the newborn, while infants from 6–9 months require size 4.0 mm (MacNab 1996).
  - In the child, the size of the endotracheal tube can be estimated by use of the following equation:

$$\text{Size of endotracheal tube in mm} = \frac{\text{Age in years} + 4}{4}$$

  - Broselow tape is a specifically designed tape measure which can be used to identify the correct size of endotracheal tube (Begg 1995).
  - Another useful guideline is to use a tube of about the diameter of the child's little finger or of a size that will just fit into the nostril (European Resuscitation Council 1994).
  - These measurements provide an estimate of the internal diameter of the tube.
- Endotracheal tubes used in children less than 8 years old are normally uncuffed, as the cuff may cause damage to the soft airway tissue; also the narrow cricoid cartilage forms a sufficient seal (Williams 1994).
- Before intubation, the child is oxygenated with 100% oxygen.
- In infants and young children a straight-blade laryngoscope is normally used during insertion.
- In older children a curved-blade laryngoscope is normally used.
- The endotracheal tube is frequently inserted via the nasal route within the intensive care setting; the laryngoscope and McGill forceps are used to help visualise and direct the insertion of the tube. Once inserted, the tube is fixed in place using zinc oxide tape. This route of insertion is technically more difficult in the emergency situation.
- Once the tube has been inserted, oxygenation can be performed by attaching the re-breathing equipment directly to it, or by the use of a mechanical ventilator.

- Symmetrical chest movement and equal lung air entries should be observed and heard.

Vascular access

Speed is vital when administering fluid or drugs in the advanced life support situation. The method and equipment used for administration will vary with the type of access that is used.

Equipment
- 70% isopropyl alcohol-impregnated swabs (Mediwipes) and/or antiseptic solution appropriate to local area
- Intravenous cannulae (varying sizes)
- Syringes (varying sizes)
- Central venous cannulae
- Intraosseous cannula
- Intravenous administration sets
- Sterile dressing pack

Method

Venous access
- Where possible, peripheral venous access should be attempted; however, this is often difficult to achieve in the critically ill child.
- If central venous access is already established, this should be used, but if it is not, only peripheral access should be attempted, as attempting central access is hazardous in the emergency situation (European Resuscitation Guidelines 1994).
- If venous access is not achieved within 90 seconds, intraosseous access should be attempted (MacNab 1996).

Intraosseous access
- This is a safe, simple, rapid means of access in all children.
- An intraosseous cannula is a fine screw-like needle which is inserted into the medullary cavity of the tibia or femur using an aseptic technique.
- Fluids and drugs can be rapidly infused using this type of access; however, it is not for long-term use.

If access is impossible to obtain, some drugs, e.g. adrenaline, atropine and lignocaine, can be given via the endotracheal tube following dilution with saline. The endotracheal dose is 10 times that of the intravenous dose. Once administered, several rapid ventilations should follow (European Resuscitation Council 1994, Nadkarni et al 1997, Woodward 1994).

This route is not suitable for fluid administration.

Drugs and fluid therapy

Artificial ventilation with oxygen and fluid replacement therapy may re-establish cardiac output without the need for drug therapy. Paediatric emergency resuscitation trolleys should include a variety of crystalloid and colloid intravenous fluids. These would include saline solution in varying concentrations, Ringer's lactate solution, access to human albumin and plasma. The type of solution used is dependent on the cause of the arrest.

These drugs and intravenous fluids should be available within the emergency resuscitation trolley.

Drug therapy

The action of drugs used in resuscitation, and their metabolism, is poorly understood in children. The following examples are those recommended in the guidelines produced by the European Resuscitation Council (1994).

Adrenaline.   This is the first-line drug of choice in paediatric resuscitations (European Resuscitation Council 1994, Simpson 1994). Adrenaline will cause an increase in peripheral vascular resistance without constricting coronary or cerebral vessels. This raises systolic and diastolic pressures during cardiac compressions (Simpson 1994).

Recommended doses are as follows (European Resuscitation Council 1994, Nadkarni et al 1997, Resuscitation Council (UK) 1997):

First dose	10 µg/kg of body weight
Subsequent doses	100 µg/kg of body weight

Sodium bicarbonate.   Sodium bicarbonate has been routinely used in paediatric resuscitations for many years. The rationale for its use is the reduction of the metabolic acidosis which occurs during cardiac arrest. However, a concern with the use of bicarbonate is that it produces more carbon dioxide because of its buffering action and thus acidosis is increased.

The European Resuscitation Council (1994) now recommends that sodium bicarbonate be used sparingly and only after careful clinical consideration of profound acidosis in children who have had no response from the first dose of adrenaline.

The dose of sodium bicarbonate recommended is 1 mmol/kg and should be administered as a slow bolus (European Resuscitation Council 1994). This should

only be after effective ventilation has been achieved and adequate chest compressions given. Effective chest compressions and ventilation are equally effective in the reduction of myocardial acidosis (MacNab 1996).

Atropine.   Although there is no clear evidence that atropine is a useful drug in cardiac arrest and paediatric resuscitation, it may be considered as part of the ongoing management of haemodynamically significant bradycardia and after adequate oxygenation (Simpson 1994).

The recommended dose is 0.02 µg/kg. The maximum dose in children is 1 mg and in adolescents 2 mg (European Resuscitation Council 1994).

Glucose.   Sick children and especially infants may develop hypoglycaemia. Blood glucose should be assessed as soon as possible and treated promptly with glucose solution (Williams 1994).

Defibrillation

Defibrillation is not commonly required in paediatric resuscitation. It is the term used for the stimulation of the heart muscle using electric currents and is normally performed by experienced medical staff and appropriately trained registered nurses. Used primarily for ventricular fibrillation and pulseless ventricular tachycardia, the voltage applied is initially 2 J/kg for the first two shocks and 4 J/kg for subsequent shocks (European Resuscitation Council 1994, Williams 1994). Ventilation and chest compressions should be continued except when shocks are being delivered. Shocks should be delivered in sets of three, where necessary.

Paediatric paddles (4.5 cm) are used in children less than 10 kg in weight, with adult paddles being used for larger children.

Equipment should be readily available to all clinical areas. Often, however, the defibrillation equipment is shared between areas.

Equipment should be checked on a regular basis to ensure that it is charging and discharging properly. This should be performed by appropriately trained registered nurses. Bioengineering departments should check defibrillator equipment regularly as per local policy.

Do and do not

- Do familiarise yourself with the location of the emergency trolley and equipment within your clinical area.
- Do ensure that you know the emergency call number for cardiac arrest.

- Do ensure that you attend a regular resuscitation update. A minimum of yearly is essential.
- Do familiarise yourself with the layout and contents of the emergency resuscitation trolley.
- Do ensure that parents are supported.
- Do not panic, as chaos within an emergency situation can cost valuable time. An organised person will help focus and calm the rest of the team.
- Do not exclude parents and relatives from the resuscitation room unless it is at their request.

Summary

Resuscitation must begin immediately and not wait until equipment arrives. All personnel working with children require to learn about both basic and advanced life support. It is imperative that the children's nurse is aware of the different techniques for both basic and advanced support and is competent in both.

It remains vital that basic life support skills and techniques are well taught and updated, as ineffective delivery of basic life support will render advanced life support futile.

References

American Heart Association 1994 Textbook of pediatric advanced life support. AHA, Dallas

Begg J E 1995 A pediatric care and resuscitation cart: one community hospital's ED experience. Journal of Emergency Nursing 21(6): 555–559

Bishop-Kurylo D, Masiello M 1995 Pediatric resuscitation: development of a mock code program and evaluation tool. Pediatric Nursing 21(4): 333–336

Carter B, Dearmun A K 1995 Child health care nursing – concepts, theory and practice. Blackwell Science, Oxford

European Resuscitation Council 1994 Guidelines for paediatric life support. British Medical Journal 308(May): 1349–1355

Hampson-Evans D C, Bingham R M 1998 Paediatric Resuscitation. The European Resuscitation Council Guidelines 1998. Care of the Critically Ill 14(6): 188–193

Hazinski M F 1992 Nursing care of the critically ill child, 2nd edn. Mosby, St Louis

McCrory J H, Downs C E 1990 Cardiopulmonary resuscitation in infants and children. In: Blumer J L (ed) A practical guide to pediatric intensive care, 3rd edn. Mosby, St Louis, ch 6

MacNab R 1996 Paediatric life support. Paediatric Nursing 8(4): 28–33

Nadkarni V, Hazinski M F, Zideman D et al 1997 Paediatric life support. An advisory statement by the Paediatric Life Support Working Group of the International Liaison Committee on Resuscitation. Resuscitation 37: 115–127

Resuscitation Council (UK) 1997 The 1997 resuscitation guidelines for use in the United Kingdom. Resuscitation Council (UK), London

Simpson S M 1994 Paediatric advanced life support – an update. Nursing Times 90(27): 37–39

Tonkin S et al 1995 Nasal route for infant resuscitation by mothers. Lancet 45: 1353–1356

Whitton H 1995 Infant resuscitation in parenthood education. Health Visitor 68(11): 454–455

Williams C 1994 Paediatric cardiopulmonary resuscitation. British Journal of Nursing 3(15): 760–764

Woodward S 1994 A guide to paediatric resuscitation. Paediatric Nursing 6(2): 16–18

Further reading

Seidel J, Tittle S, Hodge D III et al 1998 Guidelines for paediatric equipment and supplies for emergency departments. Journal of Emergency Nursing 24(1): 45–48

Quinn T 1998 Cardiopulmonary resuscitation. Nursing Standard 12(46): 49–56

8

Central Lines

Introduction

A central line is inserted when a child requires frequent and/or long-term venous access. Reasons for insertion may include the administration of total parenteral nutrition, cytotoxic drugs or frequent intravenous antibiotics. These lines are usually inserted under general anaesthetic in theatre by experienced paediatric surgeons, and occasionally by experienced anaesthetists.

Learning outcomes

By the end of this section you should:

- be aware of the different types of central venous lines currently in use
- understand the reasons for their use and all aspects of their care
- understand the importance of asepsis in central venous line care
- be able to explain all aspects of the care to the child and family
- be able to recognise potential problems and deal with them appropriately.

Rationale

Central venous lines play a crucial role in the administration of treatment to many children with acute and chronic potentially life-threatening illnesses (see Table 8.1 for examples). They reduce the need for frequent venepuncture which is extremely distressing for all children, particularly the very young.

Nurses have a key role in the care of these lines. In addition to performing the practical procedures, they are responsible for the education of the child, family and those in the community who are unfamiliar with central lines. A sound policy for line care, adhered to by all involved, will help to ensure that a line can safely remain in use for as long as required.

Central venous lines and ports will be encountered by community staff as most children will go home with these devices in situ (Hollis 1992). The amount of direct involvement by community staff in the care of these lines is variable, as in many instances the parents will carry out all the care at home.

Factors to note

There are three types of central line in use in paediatrics.

Tunnelled central venous line Also known as a Broviac, or Hickman line, or often by the child as a 'wiggly'. These are skin-tunnelled Silastic catheters which are inserted, under general anaesthetic, into the subclavian or internal jugular vein (see Fig. 8.1). These lines can be single-, double- or triple-lumen with each lumen having an external clamp. The type inserted depends upon the clinical requirements of the patient.

The Groshong catheter is a similar type of line, but it has an internal valve to prevent the backflow of blood, so does not require an external clamp.

Implanted port Also known as a Port-a-Cath, Vascuport or TIVAD (totally implantable venous access device). This is a Silastic catheter, inserted into the subclavian or internal jugular vein, which is attached to a metal chamber sealed at the top with a septum of self-sealing silicone. The port (metal chamber) is positioned under the skin of the chest wall. Access to this system is via straight or angled Huber non-coring needles through the septum of the port (Fig. 8.2).

Note: Always use 10 ml or larger syringes with the ports as recommended by the manufacturers.

Non-tunnelled long line. This is a short-term venous access device more commonly used in the intensive care or high-dependency setting. These lines are not skin-tunnelled and can be inserted under local anaesthetic. They are usually held in place with skin sutures. These lines can have a single, double or triple lumen. Peripherally inserted central catheters (PICC lines) are included in this category of central venous lines.

The type of line used for a particular child will depend upon various factors:

- the age of the child
- the length of time it will be required
- what treatments it will be used for

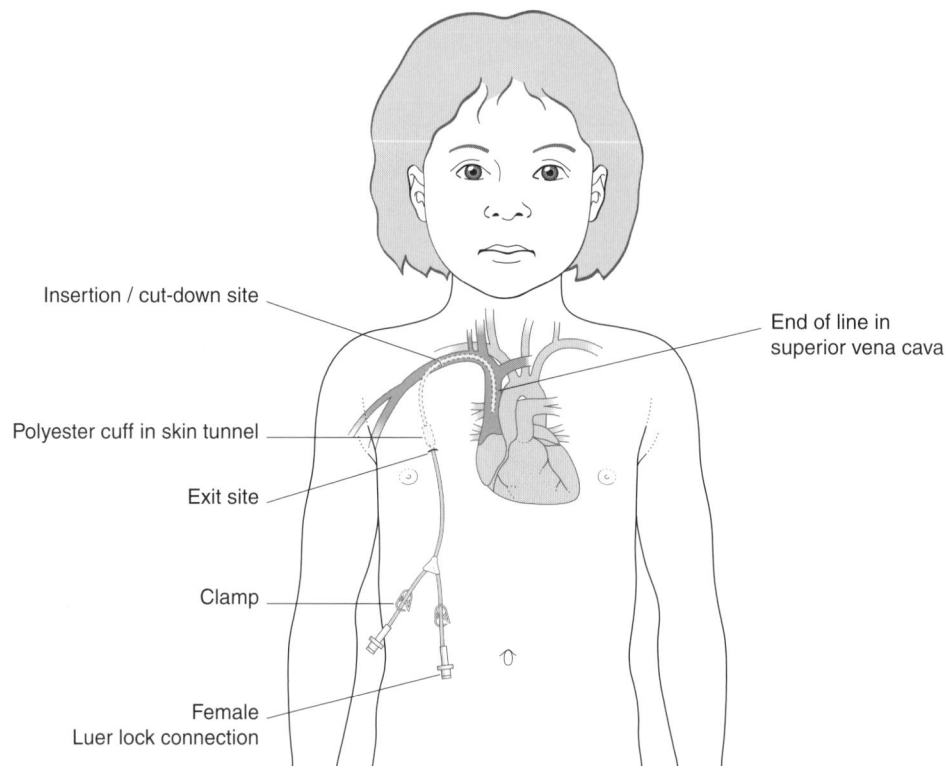

Insertion / cut-down site

End of line in superior vena cava

Polyester cuff in skin tunnel

Exit site

Clamp

Female Luer lock connection

Figure 8.1
Position of central venous line.

- how often it will be used.

Table 8.1 gives examples of conditions and the type of line used for each condition.

Preparation of the child and family for the insertion of any central line is essential. This includes information from medical and nursing staff, plus preparatory work by the hospital play specialist if available. After discussion with the child and family, it may be useful to introduce them to another child with the same type of line.

These lines can be in situ for months or even years, often in children who are immunocompromised. As they provide direct access to the child's central venous system, the major risk is of infection either to the exit site or the line itself with the potential for septicaemia. For this reason alone, strict aseptic procedures need to be maintained with all types of central line (Carnock 1996, Harrison 1997, Hollis 1992, Puntis et al 1990, Rumsey & Richardson 1995).

Table 8.1 **Types of line used for various conditions**

Central venous line			
Single	Double or triple	Port	Long line
Solid tumours	Bone marrow transplants	Cystic fibrosis	Critically ill, requiring inotropes etc.
Chronic malabsorption for TPN	Acute myeloid leukaemia	Haemophilia	
	Acute lymphoblastic leukaemia (ALL)	Beta-thalassaemia major and other transfusion-dependent haemoglobinopathies	
	Non-Hodgkin's lymphoma	ALL (low risk)	
	Neuroblastoma	Solid tumours (low-intensity chemotherapy)	

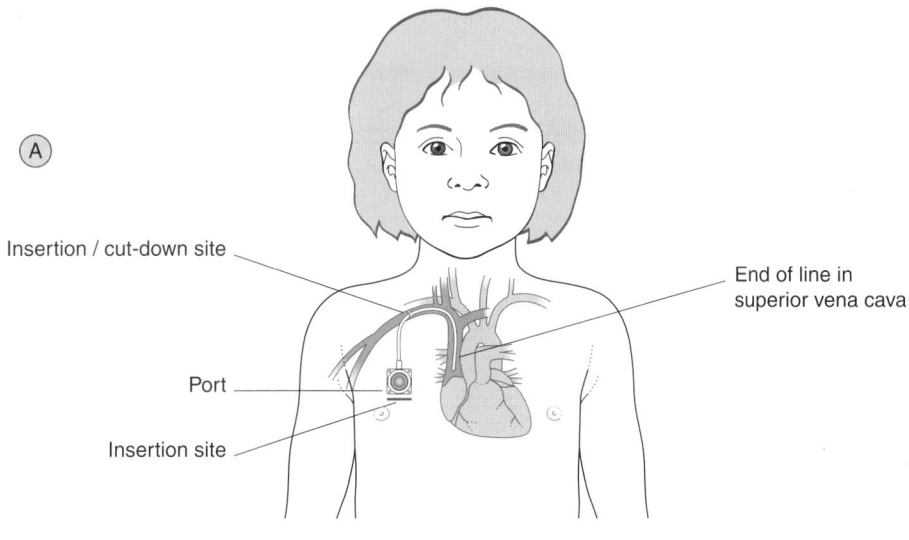

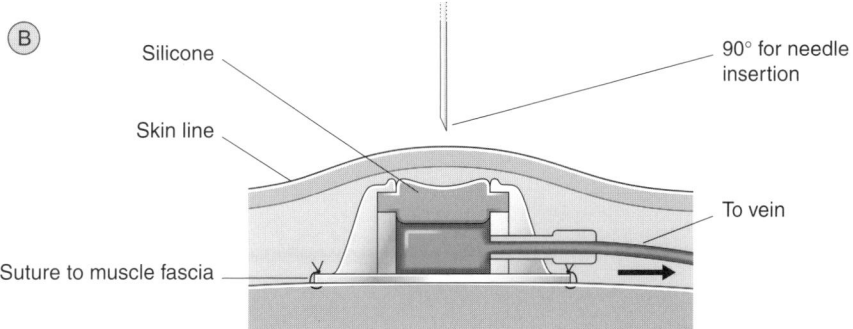

Figure 8.2
*(A) A port in situ. (B)
Cross-section of a port.*

Many children will be at home with these lines so they and their families need to follow the same procedures and be knowledgeable about potential problems and how to deal with them. Community nursing staff may also be involved in their care.

General guidelines

- All staff undertaking these procedures must be knowledgeable about and adhere to the relevant hospital policy.
- Thorough handwashing is the single most effective means of improving central line care (Lawrance 1994). In many centres sterile latex gloves are also worn when performing any procedures involving accessing the central venous system via these lines.

- Before accessing any line, it is important to check for any sign of damage to the line or attachments. It is also necessary to observe for signs of leakage of blood or fluids when accessing a line.
- When drugs are administered via the system, it must first be flushed with an appropriate solution, i.e. 0.9% sodium chloride. The line must be flushed before and after each drug, and before heparinising the system to maintain patency (see below). A small number of drugs are incompatible with 0.9% sodium chloride, e.g. amphotericin and some cytotoxic drugs. In these situations the line must be flushed with an alternative, e.g. 5% dextrose, or as indicated by the pharmacist.
- Lines which are not in use must be heparinised, i.e. flushed with a heparin solution, to maintain their

patency. The solution most commonly used is heparin 10 units per ml saline.

Central venous lines require heparinising weekly when not in use, and after every episode of access. Some lines with very small lumens will require it more frequently. Evidence suggests that weekly flushing with 0.9% sodium chloride is sufficient to maintain patency (RCN Leukaemia and Bone Marrow Transplant Nursing Forum 1995). There is considerable variation in the frequency of heparinising lines, so local hospital policy must be adhered to.

Ports require a heparin flush every 4 weeks when not in use, as recommended by the manufacturers.

Long lines are rarely not in use, being removed if no longer required. Follow individual hospital policy for heparinising these lines.

According to the manufacturer's instructions, Groshong catheters do not need heparinising. A 0.9% sodium chloride weekly flush is sufficient.

- The distal hub of a central venous line is capped with a Luer lock cap. Various systems are available and the type used will vary depending upon individual hospital preference, e.g. click-lock system, or needleless systems. The exact method of accessing the lines will therefore vary depending upon the system used. However, the basic principles will still apply.

The Luer lock cap is changed using an aseptic procedure with the line clamped at all times. The frequency of cap changes will depend on the number of occasions the line is accessed, and the type of cap used.

- Cleaning solutions for caps and exit sites also differ between hospitals, usually being determined by the consultant microbiologist based on his interpretation of current research. All are alcohol-based, e.g. povidone-iodine solution, industrial methylated spirits and Azowipes.

- Guidance must be sought from experienced nursing or medical staff if there are any problems with a line, e.g. resistance when flushing a line, or inability to aspirate blood.

Administration of bolus drugs into a heparinised central line via the cap

This applies to any type of central line.

Equipment
- Injection tray/receiver
- Prescription chart
- Drugs and diluents (if not prepared by pharmacy)
- 0.9% sodium chloride
- Heparin/saline solution (10 units heparin/ml saline)
- Syringes (10 ml syringes required for ports)
- 21G and 23G needles
- Cap-cleaning equipment, e.g. sterile cotton wool balls and povidone-iodine solution
- Sterile gloves

Method
1. Wash and dry your hands thoroughly to prevent spread of infection.
2. Check and draw up all the prescribed drugs (see Administration of Medicines, p. 29), flushing solution and heparin/saline solution using appropriate syringes and 21G needles. Discard 21G needles and replace with 23G needles, ensuring that the contents of each syringe are identifiable to prevent errors in administration.
3. Pour cleaning solution onto cotton wool balls.
4. Take the prepared equipment to the child and explain the procedure to the child and family. Expose the end of the line for easy access.
5. Open the pack of sterile gloves; wash and dry your hands thoroughly; put on gloves. (The sterile inner paper from packaging can be used as a drape if required.)
6. Ask the child or parent to hand you the end of the line.
7. Thoroughly clean the end of the cap with the cleaning solution; allow to dry.
8. Withdraw fluid from the line to observe backflow of blood, so ensuring patency.
9. Administer the drugs over the manufacturer's recommended time, flushing before and after each drug with 5 ml of the correct flushing solution.
10. Heparinise the line. Flush the line with 4–5 ml of heparinised saline, closing the clamp whilst administering the last 0.5–1 ml. Remove the syringe and needle. Continuous positive pressure ensures that the whole line is filled with heparinised saline and has not allowed aspiration of blood into the proximal end of the line. This minimises the risk of a blood clot and subsequent line blockage.
11. Ensure that the child is comfortable and the line is secured (some children wear a wiggly bag, which is a drawstring bag made of washable fabric and worn around the child's neck).
12. Clear away and dispose of all used equipment, as per hospital policy, to maintain a safe environment.

Connecting or changing an infusion set

Additional equipment
- Intravenous fluid and prescription chart
- Intravenous administration set and filter if required (some centres use 96-hour filters)

Method
1. Wash and dry your hands thoroughly.
2. Prime the administration set with the prescribed i.v. fluid.
3. Follow steps 2–6 of the previous procedure.
4. If the line is heparinised, clean the end of the cap and line thoroughly with cleaning solution and allow to dry. Withdraw 3–5 ml of solution from the line observing for blood, flush with 5 ml 0.9% sodium chloride and attach the i.v. administration set.
5. If the line is already attached to an infusion, clamp the line, clean the cap, remove the old infusion set and attach the new set. Flush with 0.9% sodium chloride only if the fluid to be administered is different from the previous one.
6. Ensure that the whole system from the child to the i.v. fluid bag is complete and secure, and that the child is comfortable. Open the clamp, set the infusion pump to the prescribed rate and commence infusion.
7. Clear away and dispose of all used equipment.

Accessing a port for use

This applies to ports only.

A variety of angled needles (Gripper) are available with an integral extension for connection to infusion sets (see Table 8.2). The size chosen will depend upon the viscosity of the fluids to be administered, whilst the length is determined by the size of the child and the amount of subcutaneous tissue over the port.

Equipment
- Dressing trolley
- Dressing pack
- Prescription chart
- Cleaning solution
- Sterile gloves
- Gripper needle of appropriate size and length

Table 8.2   **Gripper needles with extension**

Size	Length
20 gauge (0.9 mm)	0.75 inch (19 mm)
20 gauge (0.9 mm)	1.00 inch (25 mm)
20 gauge (0.9 mm)	1.25 inch (32 mm)
22 gauge (0.7 mm)	0.75 inch (19 mm)
22 gauge (0.7 mm)	1.00 inch (25 mm)
22 gauge (0.7 mm)	1.25 inch (32 mm)

- 10 ml syringes
- 21G and 23G needles
- Heparinised saline (the strength used may differ from that used with central venous lines)
- Occlusive dressing

Local anaesthetic cream (e.g. EMLA or Ametop) should be applied to the skin over the port 1 hour before the procedure to minimise discomfort.

When accessing a port, it may be necessary to hold the child securely, especially a young child. The parents and an additional nurse may be required. Preparation for this procedure by the play specialist is invaluable if available.

Method
1. Clean the dressing trolley with alcohol-based solution, e.g. Azowipes, and assemble the required equipment.
2. Explain the procedure to the child and parents; allow them time to ask questions.
3. Wash and dry your hands thoroughly.
4. Prepare a sterile field by opening the dressing pack and emptying other sterile items onto it. Pour cleaning solution into a gallipot within the sterile field.
5. Wash and dry your hands thoroughly and put on gloves.
6. Connect the injectable cap to the extension of the Gripper needle. Draw up heparinised saline solution using a syringe and 21G needle, then replace the latter with a 23G needle; prime the extension and Gripper needle; clamp the line; remove the syringe and needle, retaining all items within the sterile field.
7. Ask an assistant or the child or parent to remove the anaesthetic cream.
8. Place a dressing towel over the child's abdomen below the port.
9. Clean the raised port access site and surrounding skin thoroughly with cleaning solution, working in

a spiral from the raised centre outwards for at least 10 cm (4 inches). Repeat at least twice; allow to dry.

10. Palpate and locate the port, holding the outer edges through the skin with the fingers. Ensure that the port is secure and non-mobile. Visualise the centre of the port and insert the Gripper needle at an angle of 90 degrees to the skin, through the silicone, until it meets the metal back-plate of the port (see Fig. 8.2).

11. Via the injectable cap, insert the 23G needle and syringe. Unclamp the line, withdraw the plunger until blood is aspirated, then flush with heparinised saline clamping the line whilst administering the last 0.5–1 ml, i.e. under positive pressure.

12. Cover the Gripper needle with an occlusive dressing. It may also be necessary to pad the underside of the needle with sterile gauze if too long a needle has been inadvertently used.

13. Ensure that the child is comfortable and the line is well secured.

14. Clear away and dispose of all equipment.

Note: When a port is in long-term use, the needle must be changed weekly as recommended by the manufacturers.

Routine heparinising of a port

Equipment
As for accessing a port for use (above).

Method

1. Follow steps 1–10 of the method for accessing a port for use (above).

2. Via the injectable cap, insert the syringe with the 23G needle; unclamp the line; withdraw the syringe plunger until blood is aspirated. Flush with heparinised saline, removing the Gripper needle whilst still injecting the last 0.5 ml. Support the port with thumb and forefinger when removing the needle. (Another pair of hands is required, e.g. parent or another nurse.) This positive pressure manoeuvre prevents backflow of blood into the system, so preventing clot formation and potential occlusion.

3. Immediately wipe the puncture site with cotton wool soaked in cleaning solution, apply a plaster if requested by the child. Ensure that the child is comfortable.

4. Clear away and dispose of used equipment.

Central line dressings

There are many local variations in the method and frequency of dressings. A small study by Lucas & Attard-Montalto (1996) showed no difference in exit site infection rates between two groups, one with a dressing, the other without. Comparisons between Opsite IV3000 and either conventional film dressings (Keenlyside 1993) or sterile dry gauze (Brandt et al 1996) have also been carried out. Keenlyside found Opsite IV3000 to be highly desirable with reduced moisture accumulation and improved condition of the patient's skin. Brandt and colleagues found no significant difference in infection rates but the Opsite IV3000 was more cost-effective as it was changed weekly as opposed to a daily dressing change with sterile gauze.

Cleaning solutions have also been compared for effectiveness in preventing infections. Maki et al (1991) found that 2% chlorhexidine was the most effective for cleaning exit sites, and for handwashing.

The main reasons for using a dressing on exit sites, especially in paediatrics are:

- to prevent contamination with extraneous matter
- to promote patient comfort
- to aid the secure fixation of the central line
- to prevent small children from interfering with the line.

Care of central venous line exit site

These lines are skin-tunnelled from the entry to a major vein to the exit site on the chest wall. This exit site is a potential site of infection as it is a long-term break in the skin's integrity. As a potential source of infection, the exit site requires careful monitoring and scrupulous hygiene.

Factors to note
Most children with central venous lines will go home with them in situ (Hollis 1992). The child and parents need to be taught the importance of maintaining a clean exit site. Many parents want to learn how to do the dressing, so nursing staff need to teach them and assess their competency prior to the child's discharge. There will be some parents who do not wish to take on this responsibility, so alternative solutions need to be found. In these situations, dressings may be done on weekly clinic visits or in the home by community staff.

Equipment

- Dressing trolley
- Dressing pack containing sterile towels and swabs
- Chlorhexidine gluconate solution
- Opsite IV3000 (10×12 cm)
- Bag for disposal of used equipment
- Additional tape, e.g. Mepore, for securing the line
- Swabs if infection at exit site is suspected

Method

1. Assemble the equipment, take it to the child's bed and pull the curtains for privacy.
2. Explain the procedure to the child and family; allow time for questions and encourage the cooperation of all involved.
3. Wash and dry hands thoroughly, open the dressing pack and prepare all the equipment.
4. Remove the old dressing and discard it in the disposal bag.
5. Examine the exit site for any signs of infection, e.g. redness or exudate. Take swabs for culture if any signs of infection are present.
6. Wash and dry hands thoroughly.
7. Perform an aseptic dressing using chlorhexidine-soaked swabs. Swabs are wiped round the exit site in a circular movement, starting at the centre and working outwards for at least 5 cm. Repeat at least twice with a new swab each time; allow to dry.
8. Clean the line with another swab, from the exit site away from the child for at least 10 cm. Allow the cleaning solution to dry.
9. Coil the line and apply Opsite IV3000 over the exit site, ensuring good adhesion by applying gentle pressure over the whole dressing. If a child is sensitive to Opsite IV3000, another sterile dressing may be required.
10. Loop the hub end of the line up to the chest and secure it with another piece of tape or insert the hub into a wiggly bag if worn by the child. (If a wiggly bag is worn, we suggest that a clean bag is used each day.) Ensure that the child is comfortable.
11. Clear away and dispose of all used equipment.
12. Label swabs and appropriate microbiology forms if required.
13. Record appropriate information in the child's nursing notes.

Dressing a port in use

A dressing is only required if a port is in use for treatment. When not in use, the skin's integrity is not broken so normal personal hygiene is sufficient once the initial insertion wounds have healed.

The dressing on an accessed port need only be changed if it becomes soiled or there is clinical indication, i.e. potential infection. The recommended weekly needle change will obviously entail a dressing change as part of that procedure.

Method

The method is the same as for care of the central venous line exit site but extra care should be taken to prevent dislodging the needle.

Dressing change on a long line

A long line is generally sutured at the exit site at the time of insertion. The long line entry site is protected under Opsite IV3000 for ease of observation. This dressing can remain in place for up to 7 days, but can be changed sooner if required (Brandt et al 1996). Care must be taken not to dislodge the long line. The hub(s) should be padded to ensure the child's comfort.

The procedure for cleaning the site is the same as for central venous lines.

Observations and complications

Infection and potential septicaemia

Of the central line during placement. Sterile conditions in theatre should prevent this, but if the child has a systemic infection at the time of insertion, the lumen of the line can become affected.

Via the infusion system during use. Aseptic handling of the line and any infusions or additives should prevent infection occurring via this route. Filters can also be used, especially for total parenteral nutrition solutions with the exclusion of the lipid.

Of the exit site or skin tunnel. Scrupulous hygiene of the exit site is essential to block this route of infection. Indications of infection are redness and/or exudate at the exit site, and in some instances pain or swelling.

If an infection is suspected, i.e. the child has a fever, blood cultures and exit site swabs should be taken, then intravenous antibiotics commenced. These can usually eradicate any infection. Only in extreme circumstances are lines removed because of infection, and then only after lengthy consideration by medical staff in consultation with the child and family. These lines are very precious, especially in the high-risk patients who have them, so prevention of infection is imperative.

Occlusion

Fibrin clot within the line. This is prevented by regular heparinisation, but it is sometimes necessary to dissolve a clot by using an antifibrinolytic agent such as urokinase (5000 units).

A line that does not flush back or bleed back, and has had no obvious kinks in it, is most likely to have an occlusion caused by a fibrin clot.

Drug precipitate. This can occur if certain solutions are not infused correctly, for example etoposide, calcium, diazepam, phenytoin and total parenteral nutrition. Precipitates can be removed by using 90% alcohol or hydrochloric acid, depending upon the likely cause of the occlusion; this must *only* be carried out by experienced senior personnel (Rumsey & Richardson 1995).

Kinking of the line. This may be either externally or internally within the child's venous system. Visually check all external parts of the line for kinks first, then try altering the child's position. If the line still appears to be blocked, a chest X-ray examination may be required to check for internal kinks.

Catheter misplacement

Perioperatively. If this occurs there is a potential for pneumothorax, haemathorax, perforation of a vein or dislodgement during surgery. Any of these complications could be apparent in theatre and would be rectified there.

Postoperatively, check the X-ray picture taken after insertion with the medical staff before using the line, observe the child for any signs of chest pain, dyspnoea, cyanosis or bleeding/haematoma. Notify medical staff if any adverse signs are present.

Line accidentally pulled by the child. Check the exit site for signs of trauma or external appearance of the cuff. If the cuff is not visible or partially visible, check that the line is capable of being aspirated and flushes with no pain or swelling along the tunnel site. Inform medical staff of the situation. A slight misplacement may just require a further restraining suture around the cuff, allowing continued use of the line. A major displacement may result in the line having to be removed.

Superior vena cava syndrome

This can occur at any time because of a thrombus causing obstruction of the venous return to the superior vena cava. Signs include engorgement of head and neck veins, oedema of the head and neck and potential respiratory distress. Medical intervention is required.

Air embolism

This can occur if the line is damaged or left unclamped during a cap change. Careful handling, strict procedures, good staff and family education should prevent this. All care givers should be taught to clamp the line close to the exit site if it should become inadvertently split or cut. Report the incident immediately to senior medical or nursing staff.

Central line breakage

This can occur if, for example, the line is cut or bitten by the child. The line must be clamped above the break as explained above. Repair kits are available for all central venous lines. The repair is usually performed under aseptic conditions by experienced senior nurses or medical staff. Details of the child's central venous line should be documented in the medical notes so that the appropriate repair kit is used.

Potential complications are summarised in Table 8.3.

COMMUNITY PERSPECTIVE

The CCN is likely to be involved in the care of tunnelled central venous lines and implanted ports. Hospital visits can be minimised and inpatient time reduced if the CCN undertakes the administration of drugs and blood sampling at home or in school.

Routine flushing of lines can also be undertaken by the CCN if the family do not wish to take on this responsibility.

Although cross-infection is less likely to occur in the home environment, there are other safety aspects that need to be addressed. The CCN may have difficulty in maintaining an aseptic field when there are other siblings or pets in the household. She will also need access to an anaphylaxis kit. (See Administration of Medicines, p. 29.)

The CCN is also in a position to educate the family about the central lines, enabling them to undertake more of the care themselves if they wish.

Do and do not

- Do ensure that the line is clamped during cap changes.

Table 8.3 **Summary of potential complications**

Observation	Possible cause
Fever	Line infection/septicaemia
	Exit site infection
Line not flushing or bleeding back	Kink in line
	Fibrin clot
	Drug precipitate
	Displacement of line
Chest pain, dyspnoea, cyanosis	Pneumothorax
	Haemathorax
	Superior vena cava syndrome
Fluid leaking out of line	Damage to line, e.g. split or tear
	Connections not correctly
	attached

- Do always wash and dry hands thoroughly.
- Do always maintain strict aseptic techniques.
- Do seek expert advice or help with any problems.
- Do educate the child and family in correct line care and how to clamp the line when it is cut or damaged.
- Do not carry out any procedure for which you have not been trained.
- Do not be afraid to seek help from experienced personnel. These lines are very precious, and with good care can last a long time, greatly aiding in the child's treatment.
- Do not use syringes smaller than 5 ml as they will produce a greater pressure than that of the central line and may result in a fracture if the line is blocked.

References

Brandt B, DePalma J, Irwin M, Shogun J, Lucke J 1996 Comparison of central catheter dressings in bone marrow transplant recipients. Oncology Nursing Forum 23(5): 829–836

Carnock M 1996 Making sense of central venous catheters. Nursing Times 92(49): 30–31

Harrison M 1997 Central venous catheters: a review of the literature. Nursing Standard 11(27): 43–45

Hollis R 1992 Central venous access in children. Paediatric Nursing 4(6): 18–21

Keenlyside D 1993 Avoiding an unnecessary outcome. A comparative trial between IV3000 and a conventional film dressing to assess rates of catheter-related sepsis. Professional Nurse (Feb): 288–291

Lawrance T 1994 Central venous line audit. Paediatric Nursing 6(4): 20–23

Lucas H, Attard-Montalto S 1996 Central venous line dressings: study of infection rates. Paediatric Nursing 8(6): 21–23

Maki D, Ringer M, Alvarado C 1991 Prospective randomised trial of povidone iodine, alcohol and chlorhexidine for prevention of infection associated with central venous and arterial catheters. Lancet 338: 339–343

Puntis J, Holden C, Smallman S, Finkel Y, George R, Booth I 1990 Staff training: a key factor in reducing intravascular catheter sepsis. Archives of Disease in Childhood 6: 335–337

RCN Leukaemia and Bone Marrow Transplant Nursing Forum 1995 Skin-tunnelled catheters, guidelines for care, 2nd edn. RCN, London

Rumsey K, Richardson D 1995 Management of infection and occlusion associated with vascular access devices. Seminars in Oncology Nursing 11(3): 174–183

Further reading

Baranowski L 1993 Central venous access devices. Journal of Intravenous Nursing 16(3): 167–194

BCSH 1997 Guidelines on the insertion and management of central venous lines. British Journal of Haematology 98: 1041–1047

Hurtubise et al 1980 Restoring patency of occluded central venous catheters. Archives of Surgery 115: 212–213

Keegan-Wells D, Stewart J 1992 The use of venous access devices in paediatric oncology nursing practice. Journal of Paediatric Oncology Nursing 9(4): 159–169

Stokes D et al 1989 Early detection and simplified management of obstructed Hickman and Broviac Catheters. Journal of Paediatric Surgery 24(3): 257–262

Vidler V 1994 Use of Port-a-Caths in the management of paediatric haemophilia. Professional Nurse 10(1): 48–50

9

Chest Drainage

Introduction

Chest drainage may be observed in several practice placements, including intensive care, the neonatal unit, accident and emergency departments, as well as the general paediatric ward. It is a common practice that requires a thorough knowledge of research-based principles and pathophysiology to nurse effectively and avoid complications.

Learning outcomes

After reading this section the nurse will be able to explain:

- why chest drainage is used
- how it is set up
- how the patient is assessed and drainage monitored
- why some traditional practices are controversial
- complications that may occur.

Pathophysiology

Before learning about chest drainage, it is important to remember that:

- The lungs maintain expansion through diaphragmatic and intercostal contraction during inspiration, causing air to be drawn into the lungs by negative pressure, followed by expiration and an elastic recoil of the lungs to their original state.
- The heart is positioned in the mediastinum. If blood and secretions build up around the heart, or the lung is pushed over to the wrong side of the chest, the heart will become restricted and its function compromised. This is known as cardiac tamponade.
- The pleural cavity is a potential space, lying between the visceral and parietal pleura, the diaphragm, and mediastinum. Pressure in the space is normally negative (-4 to -10 mmHg). A small amount of fluid is secreted into the space and acts as a lubricant (O'Hanlon Nicholls 1996).

The following conditions require chest drainage:

Pneumothorax. Air is present in the pleural space. A pneumothorax may be termed *spontaneous* (frequent in neonates who aspirate stomach contents, causing alveolar rupture); *tension* (the alveoli rupture and leak air into the pleural space – this may occur in critically ill children requiring positive pressure ventilation); or *open* (through trauma) (Wyatt 1995).

Haemothorax. Blood is present in the pleural space and mediastinum. This can occur after chest surgery or trauma.

Pleural effusion. Secretions such as fluid, pus (empyema), or chyle from the thoracic duct (chylothorax) fill the pleural space, often as a complication of surgery, or a pre-existing illness (e.g. cystic fibrosis).

Guidelines

Insertion of a chest drain may be performed as an emergency by the doctor. If this is the case, there is little time to alert and prepare parents or the child for the procedure, but simple, brief explanations should be given. If the parents are not present, it is not usually possible to wait to gain their consent, as a delay could be life-threatening, but every effort should be made to contact them and inform them of the situation. If chest drains are expected as a result of surgery, children can be prepared through play, with verbal and visual explanation suitable for their conceptual understanding. There will be more time to give parents and the child fuller information. Once the tubes are in place, parents can be taught some of the nursing techniques should they wish to be involved.

The procedure is painful and distressing. Cooperation is likely only in the older child; therefore, if time allows, sedation and analgesia should be given, usually by intravenous injection. Local anaesthesia is normally used around the puncture site. If the child is ventilated, breathing against the ventilator may worsen the condition, so paralysis may also be advised.

Full resuscitation and monitoring equipment should be at hand in case of sudden collapse. The child should have an intravenous line, though in an emergency the insertion of the chest tube may have higher priority.

Equipment

Chest drain

The doctor will specify the size and type of drain, depending on the child's size and the urgency of the procedure, and whether air or serous matter will need draining. The drain could be as small as a 19–23 gauge butterfly needle or intravenous cannula, or a proprietary chest drain, ranging from 8 to 32 French gauge (Fg). These chest drains consist of a trocar inserted into a PVC catheter, with drainage eyes. Some are specifically designed for neonatal or emergency use.

Chest drainage system

There are now many systems in use on paediatric units, including the traditional self-assembly sets, and the more recent ready assembled proprietary closed versions (Fig. 9.1). All follow the underwater seal principle, and consist of tubing, a water chamber, collection chamber and suction chamber or connections (Fig. 9.2).

Other equipment

- Large dressing trolley

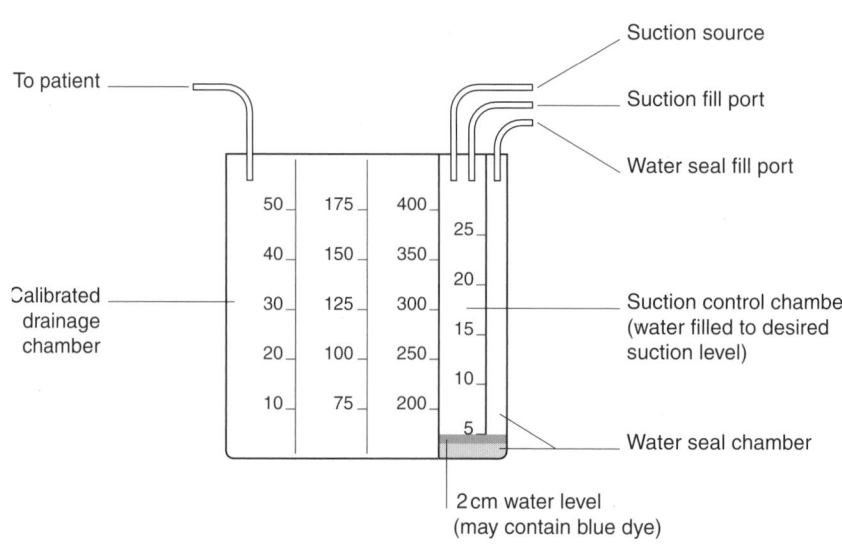

Figure 9.1
Principles of an all-in-one chest drainage unit. Note that it is the level of water in the suction chamber, not the level of suction at source, that controls the level of suction in the patient (Smith et al 1995).

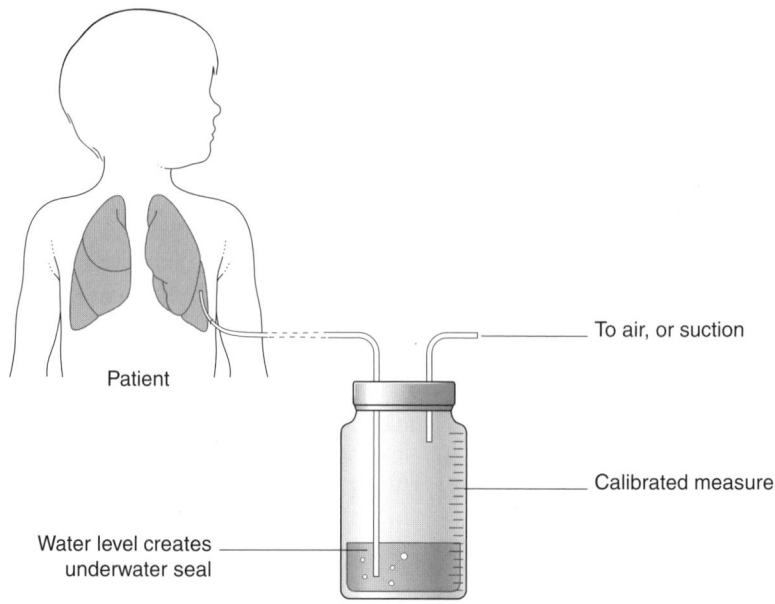

Figure 9.2
Simple underwater seal system.

- Medication as above: local anaesthetic, intravenous analgesia, sedation and/or paralysing agent
- Sterile or distilled water
- Sterile gloves
- Syringes and needles
- Dressing of choice
- Skin disinfecting solution
- A surgical dressing or cut-down pack may be helpful, and should contain the following:
  – Sterile field
  – Gauze swabs
  – Suture and needle, suturing forceps
  – Sterile scissors
  – Small scalpel
  – 2 chest drain clamps (see below)

Method: insertion of tube

Position. The child will be positioned on his back or side, depending on the chosen site for the tube and the reason for chest drainage. Because fluid follows gravity, tubes to drain secretions or blood will normally be placed posteriorly, at the lung base. As air normally rises, a tube to drain a pneumothorax will be positioned anteriorly, at the apex of the affected lung (Wyatt 1995).

In an acute emergency, the doctor may not wait for equipment to be collected and checked. The doctor will insert a butterfly needle, cannula, or trocar into the chest, and immediately submerge the end under water, so that air is drained; the water prevents re-aspiration of air into the pleural space. The air may also be aspirated gently using a syringe and three-way tap. The procedure should be performed under aseptic conditions, though again in an emergency there will be little time to prepare an elaborate sterile field (Wyatt 1995).

The nurse is responsible for preparation of the child and equipment, assisting the doctor with the procedure and maintaining asepsis, connecting the system, and comforting and observing the child.

The chest drain should be connected as soon as possible to the underwater seal drainage system, and the doctor may ask that the unit be connected to low thoracic suction; 4–5 cmH$_2$O is normal, with an absolute maximum of 20 cmH$_2$O (Carroll 1993). With the all-in-one systems, suction is regulated by the volume of water in the suction chamber (see Fig. 9.1) (Smith et al 1995).

The drainage system should at all times be at least 1 foot below the child's chest.

The drain will be sutured to the skin by the doctor. Traditionally a purse-string suture was used to ease removal; this type of suturing technique is less often used nowadays. The tubing should be securely attached to the child's skin with adhesive tape, to prevent pull on the insertion site. A dry keyhole dressing may be applied to the skin, and secured with tape, or a spray or occlusive dressing used, which allows for visual inspection of the wound.

The child should be positioned comfortably after the procedure, reassured and comforted.

Observations and complications

The child's condition should be observed throughout the procedure and thereafter, especially in the first minutes and hours following insertion, when physiological changes may occur. The frequency of observation will depend on the child's condition, but in the first hour it may be quarter- to half-hourly.

Observation should be systematic, starting with the child, then the equipment. All observations should be recorded.

The child

- Respiration: rate, colour, distress or recession, oxygen saturation.
- The child's general condition and colour: these should improve very soon after the chest drain is inserted.
- Vital signs of heart rate and blood pressure. A fall in blood pressure or rising heart rate may indicate cardiac tamponade, or recurring pneumothorax, and should be reported immediately.
- Listen to the child's breath sounds, using a stethoscope. Observe for air entry and any quiet areas.
- Arterial blood gases. Depending on local policy, blood for this test may be taken by the nurse or doctor. Frequency of blood gas analysis should be discussed with medical staff.
- Temperature should be monitored regularly to identify infection.

The equipment

- Identify and label the drains. The child may have more than one, especially after surgery, and it is important to understand their position and intended purpose.
- Observe the insertion site and dressing. There may be signs of fluid or air leakage, or the skin around the site may feel crackly. If so, surgical emphysema may be present and should be reported to the doctor (O'Hanlon Nichols 1996). The dressing should be left in place if clean and dry.

- Observe the chest tubes. The connections should be secure. Some units use sticky tape to ensure that they do not become accidentally separated, though be aware that sticky tape may actually conceal a loose connection. The tubing should be free and unkinked. Excess tubing should not hang in dependent loops from the bed, as this can increase resistance and lessen effective drainage; instead it should be positioned in flat loops on the bed.
- Observe the colour of the drainage, and presence of blood. (Some bloody drainage can be expected immediately after surgery or insertion of a chest drain.) Check the volume of fluid drained. It is usual to mark the level of fluid on the collecting chamber, along with the time and the nurse's initials. The level should be recorded on the fluid balance chart, in accordance with local policy, remembering that drainage represents serous fluid loss, and the doctor may wish to prescribe replacement intravenously, using clear fluid or blood or other blood products. Keep medical staff informed.
- If the drain is a pleural drain, look for the fluid level swinging within the tubing, as the pressures change when the child breathes. Positive pressure ventilation will cause a reverse swing to the negative pressure of spontaneous ventilation. If the fluid is no longer swinging, the air may have completely drained, or the chest drain may have become blocked. This should be reported and discussed with the medical staff (Carroll 1995).
- If the water is bubbling, this may indicate air draining. If the bubbling is continuous, and the child is not receiving positive pressure ventilation, this may indicate an air leak in the drainage system. The system will need to be checked by briefly clamping the chest tube near the patient; if the bubbling continues, there is an air leak. If suction has been applied, the water will bubble gently, but excessive bubbling may indicate too high suction. This will not affect the lungs, but may cause increased water evaporation and disturbing noise for other children and parents (Carroll 1995).
- Check the bottle. It should be well secured, at least 1 foot below the child's chest. Check the different chambers, and whether there is sufficient water.
- Check the suction level.
- The system will need changing if the chambers are two-thirds full. Daily change is not necessary as long as the system remains closed and drainage is small. (See also Control of Infection, p. 13.)

Do and do not

Chest drain 'milking', when the tubes are stripped with a roller or clamp, has been widely practised in many units. It was believed to encourage drainage and prevent clots. Its practice is now discouraged, as the negative pressure created can be exceedingly high, up to $-400 \text{ cmH}_2\text{O}$, and cause trauma to the mediastinum or pleural space. It has also been shown that milking has no effect on clot formation, as the pleura have a defibrinating effect on blood (Carroll 1993, 1995).

Clamping chest drains when transferring or moving the child is another traditional nursing practice that has been shown to be potentially dangerous. If air is draining, clamping the chest drains can cause a build-up of pressure in the pleural space, leading to tension pneumothorax and sudden lung and circulatory collapse. The only indications now accepted for clamping underwater seal drains are:

- following pneumonectomy, to maintain the central mediastinal position (Williams 1992)
- when changing chest drainage bottles (Williams 1992)
- in children with pneumothorax, when reinflation of the lung is confirmed by chest X-ray, allowing for observation of a recurring pneumothorax before the drain is removed (Williams 1992)
- on accidental disconnection of the chest drain, though it has been argued that a more appropriate response if this has occurred is to submerge the disconnected chest drain under water, while quickly reconnecting the drainage tubes, or reassembling a new drainage system if the previous one has been contaminated (Carroll 1995).

If the bottle is accidentally tipped over or raised above the child's head, it should be immediately returned to its proper position. It should not normally need replacing, as long as the contents of one chamber have not spilled into another. Modern devices have systems that prevent this happening.

Removing the tube

The doctor will decide to remove the drain on the basis of clinical signs and/or chest X-ray, which will indicate whether the original problem has resolved. Removing the drain can be distressing and uncomfortable. Only the older child will be able to cooperate, so sedation and analgesia may be required.

The tube is removed using an aseptic technique. Any tape holding the tube in position is removed. The tubing is clamped, and any suction discontinued. If the timing can be coordinated, the drain is removed on expiration.

If a purse-string suture has been used, the suture is pulled tight to occlude the wound, while the drain is gently and firmly withdrawn. This prevents air being sucked into the pleural space on inspiration. An impermeable dressing is applied to the skin till the wound has healed, so that air cannot enter the pleura through the open drain wound.

The child is made comfortable and observed for recurrence of the problem.

References

Carroll P 1993 Technical update brief: the child with a chest tube. Pediatric Nursing 19(4): 370–371

Carroll P 1995 Chest tubes made easy. Registered Nurse 58(12): 46–56

O'Hanlon Nicholls 1996 Commonly asked questions about chest tubes. American Journal of Nursing 96(5): 60–64

Smith R N, Fallentine J, Kessel S 1995 Underwater chest drainage; bringing the facts to the surface. Nursing 25(2): 60–63

Williams T 1992 To clamp or not to clamp? Nursing Times 88(18): 33

Wyatt T 1995 Pneumothorax in the neonate. Journal of Obstetrics, Gynaecology and Neonatal Nursing 24(3): 211–216

10

Ear Care

Introduction

Caring for the ear should be part of routine hygiene care for all children. Occasionally the child will require clinical care of the external or middle ear; it is important that this is performed knowledgeably.

Learning outcomes

After reading this section the nurse will understand:

- signs and symptoms associated with common childhood conditions of the ear
- nursing care associated with common childhood conditions of the ear.

Factors to note

The ear comprises three connecting areas (Fig. 10.1):

- The outer ear (pinna).
- The middle ear. The eardrum acts like a drum skin, vibrating and conducting sound through to the

inner ear. Pressure between middle and inner ear is balanced by the auditory tube.

- The inner ear contains the cochlear bones and the organ of Corti through which the vibration is converted into nerve impulses and transmitted to the brain. The inner ear also contains cells controlling equilibrium.

Problems of the ear experienced by children include:

- deafness
- otitis media or externa
- foreign bodies
- wax or 'glue'
- perforated eardrum
- conditions requiring surgery.

Guidelines

The ear has two important functions: hearing and balance. If either of these functions is disturbed, the child's

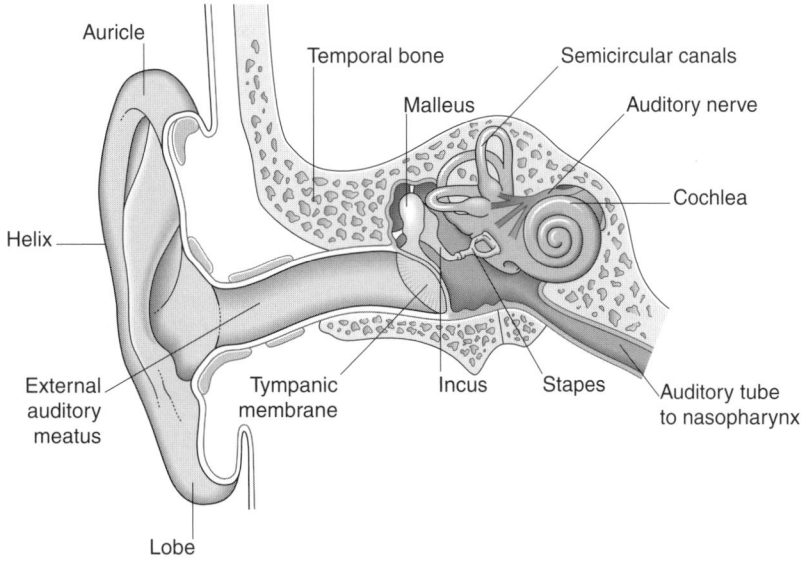

Figure 10.1
The structure of the ear.

Auricle · Temporal bone · Semicircular canals · Malleus · Auditory nerve · Cochlea · Helix · External auditory meatus · Tympanic membrane · Incus · Stapes · Auditory tube to nasopharynx · Lobe

normal sensations and perceptions can be altered, causing anxiety and confusion. Ear infections can also cause severe pain in children and attention should be paid to pain-relieving methods.

General hygiene and ear care

The external ear is covered by skin, and just like the rest of the body, skin needs daily care. Children often forget to clean behind their ears; something if they cannot see it, it does not exist. Daily ear cleansing should, however, form part of the child's hygiene routines. Just like other areas of skin, the ear can become itchy, dry or eczematous, and if this is the case, skin creams may be needed (Martin 1994) (see also Hygiene, p. 131).

Never insert anything into the ear canal other than an auroscope or tympanic thermometer (and even in these cases, care must be taken). Cotton buds, hairgrips, fingers, all have been known to cause inner ear damage (Martin 1994).

Observation and examination of the ear

The nurse or parent should observe the outer ear during general hygiene care of the child.

If the nurse observes inflammation, this may indicate infection. Because ear infections can be so painful, they may also be observed by the child's behaviour. Small children especially may be distressed, clearly in pain, and some may be able to locate the pain to the ear; others may try to rub their ear, or rub it against something to gain relief.

It is quite normal for a small amount of wax (cerumen) to be seen at the entrance to the ear canal. Cerumen is normally honey coloured, becoming darker as it is exposed to air. However if the exudate is clear, this could indicate cerebrospinal fluid leakage, which may indicate a serious condition, for example head injury. If the exudate is green and/or offensive, this could indicate infection. The presence of blood may indicate haemorrhage, for example after surgery or trauma.

Equipment and method

More detailed examination of the middle ear and eardrum will be facilitated by an auroscope. Aural examination is usually performed by a doctor, as part of the general assessment of any unwell child. If the child is small, she is usually held sideways on a parent's lap, with the side of the head firmly held to the parent's chest. Explain to the child and parent what is about to happen, and allow the child to explore the auroscope before use.

Assessment of hearing

Hearing loss may be caused by congenital structural or conductive disorders. Examination of a child's hearing forms a routine part of developmental assessment. In older children, deafness can be acquired through chronic ear infections, or damage to the structure of the ear (for example perforated eardrum). In this instance, tell-tale signs might include being easily distracted, speech difficulties, or learning difficulties. For further reading on hearing assessment, see Hall 1991 and McQuaid et al 1996.

Foreign bodies (Surkitt Parr 1989)

Foreign bodies, such as buttons, small toys, ends of cotton buds, even batteries, are not uncommon reasons for children to attend accident and emergency departments. The under-fours are particularly prone to putting foreign bodies into their ears. The presence of a foreign body will sometimes go unnoticed for some time, but may be indicated by signs of infection, hearing loss, bleeding, otorrhoea (discharge) or pain.

Removal of the foreign body will sometimes be attempted by the accident and emergency doctor using a speculum or aural hook, but a successful first attempt is important, so as not to push the item further into the ear canal. The item may also be syringed out (see below) as long as it is not absorbent, in which case it will absorb the water and swell, becoming even more difficult to remove. The ENT surgeon may decide that a general anaesthetic is the safest course of action, as there is no danger of the child struggling. It is important to check that there is no underlying pathology; in some cases a child may have pushed something into the ear to relieve pain, say from an ear infection.

In rare instances, an insect will enter the ear canal, and may still be alive, causing an incessant buzzing and tickling of the ear. If a light is shone into the ear, the insect may be drawn out. Alternatively, a small amount of oil is inserted into the ear to drown the insect, which is then syringed away.

Ear syringing (Thurgood & Thurgood 1995)

Equipment
- Receiving dish
- Protective clothing or apron

- Ear syringe pump (Propulse)

Ear syringe pumps have replaced the traditional syringe. Water is warmed in a bath and can then be pumped into the ear via a probe at low pressure.

Method

Ear syringing, or irrigation, is a common procedure for removing excessive ear wax or foreign bodies in adults. It can be a dangerous enterprise if the patient is uncooperative, and therefore is not undertaken routinely in children. The anatomy of the ear also differs in children, whose external auditory meatus is shorter and straighter than in adults, and therefore requires a different technique. The pinna, instead of being pulled up and back, is pulled down and forward in children. Recognised complications include tympanic membrane perforation and external auditory meatus damage. It is a skilled task which should only be undertaken by those who have received appropriate training. In children, this will most frequently be a trained ENT doctor. Contraindications to the procedure include previous ear surgery or hearing loss.

Administration of ear drops

Equipment

The doctor may prescribe ear drops. There are many preparations recommended for removing wax; olive or almond oil ear drops may be prescribed, as well as pharmaceutical preparations, such as Cerumol and Waxsol.

A swab should be available to catch drips.

Method

Ear drops should be checked according to local policies for administration of medicines. They should be stored safely and according to manufacturers' instructions. They often have a short shelf-life once opened, so expiry dates should be noted carefully. Labels should indicate the patient's name and the expiry date of the product. (See also Administration of Medicines, p. 29.)

Administering ear drops to children can be tricky because they often find the sensation uncomfortable and tickly, and are likely to wriggle or protest.

- Lay the child on her back (supine) and turn her head to the side. A younger child may need to be held.
- In children under 3 years, pull the pinna downwards to straighten the external ear canal.

- Instil the drops as prescribed.
- Keep the child lying still, and gently massage the area in front of the ear, to help the droplets descend.
- Some nurses recommend small cotton wool pledgets to be placed in the ear to prevent the fluid leaking out, but they must not be so small that they become lost, nor so large that they prevent the leakage of exudate. On balance it is safer to avoid them (Campbell & Glasper 1995).

Ear surgery

In severe, recurrent, or chronic cases of otitis media, and in some other conditions, surgery may be necessary (Maw & Bawden 1993). The main goals of postoperative ENT nursing care should be:

- to protect the airway
- to provide adequate pain relief
- to identify and treat haemorrhage
- to identify and treat infection.

(See also Postoperative Care, p. 225.)

If grommets are inserted, the child should normally be able to go swimming, but should not jump or dive into the water. The grommets may fall out at any time postoperatively, which is quite normal and need not cause concern.

Do and do not

- Do not attempt to insert anything into a child's ear.
- Do not attempt to undertake any task for which you have not received training.

References

Campbell S, Glasper E A (eds) 1995 Whaley and Wong's children's nursing. Mosby, London

Hall D M B (ed) 1991 Health for all children, 2nd edn. Oxford University Press, Oxford

McQuaid L, Huband S, Parker E 1996 Children's nursing. Churchill Livingstone, Edinburgh

Martin R L 1994 Nuts and bolts: how to care for the external ear. Hearing Journal 47(2): 43–44

Maw R, Bawden R 1993 Spontaneous resolution of severe chronic glue ear in children and effect of adenoidectomy, tonsillectomy, and insertion of ventilation tubes (grommets). BMJ 306(6880): 756–760

Surkitt Parr D 1989 The removal of foreign bodies. Nursing 3(35): 11–13

Thurgood K, Thurgood G 1995 Ear syringing: a clinical skill. British Journal of Nursing 4(12): 682–687

11

Eye Care

Introduction and rationale

Vision is a sense most of us take for granted. Vision problems for children range from the minor to the profound. We should make certain that any nursing care ensures the child's comfort and does not cause problems that may worsen the child's eyesight.

Ensuring that the eyes are clean is part of the general care of any child. Equally, the nurse may see serious eye conditions where good eye care is part of the essential treatment. These may include common infections of the newborn, including for example chlamydia infection, tear duct abnormalities, and postoperative care. Traditional practice, as taught on many paediatric wards, has not always been based on up-to-date research.

Learning outcomes

After reading this section the nurse should know the theory, and be able to describe:

- general eye care for the well child (see Hygiene, p. 131)
- eye care for the vulnerable child
- instillation of eye drops/ointment
- management of the infant/child with an eye infection.

Factors to note

Eye problems in children (McQuaid et al 1996)

- Infection: may be caused by a variety of organisms, including some of the sexually transmitted diseases in neonates (*Chlamydia trachomatis, Neisseria gonorrhoeae*), as well as the commonly found *Staphylococcus aureus* and streptococci.
- Cataract: opacity of the lens, causing loss of vision. This may occur as a result of rubella infection in the first trimester of pregnancy. Corneal transplants are now used to treat this condition.
- Squint: this refers to an inaccurate alignment of the axis of the eye. It may be congenital or acquired. Treatment includes corrective exercises, spectacles, and surgery.

- Retrolental fibroplasia: the retina detaches, and the area behind the lens becomes opaque, causing blindness. It is caused by raised blood oxygen levels in premature infants.
- Retinoblastoma: congenital tumour seen in babies and young children.
- Ptosis: the eyelid loses muscular control and droops over the eye. This can be characteristic of the neurological disease myasthenia gravis.
- Congenital glaucoma: fluid does not drain from the eye normally, causing increasing intraocular pressures. Treatment is by drops, or surgery.

The following groups of children will be particularly at risk of complications, which may include corneal damage, and infection:

- unconscious children, especially those receiving muscle-relaxing drugs
- children whose eyes are not properly shut; note that incomplete eye closure of 1–2 mm can go undetected, but may still result in exposure keratitis (Winceck et al 1989)
- immunosuppressed children
- low birthweight infants, in whom visual problems are common (Shrader 1991)
- newborn babies under 6 weeks old, who do not produce tears, which contain a natural antibiotic agent, lysozyme (McQuaid et al 1996)
- children undergoing eye surgery
- children who cannot blink.

Guidelines

As with all nursing procedures, assessment is the vital first step. Early detection of eye problems can prevent further damage.

Eye care is a distressing experience for any child. Explaining what will happen and building it into games, for example with dolls, may help the child to cooperate. Eye care may be performed by the parent or carer, or the children themselves, if they are happy to do so and have been taught any special techniques.

As eye care can require specialist knowledge, links with specialist ophthalmology colleagues should be developed by any paediatric unit.

Frequency of eye care

This will be variable. Healthy children may only have their eyes cleaned once or twice a day as part of their general hygiene routine (see Hygiene, p. 131); a sick or vulnerable child may need more frequent specific care. Lloyd (1990) recommends 6-hourly care for the unconscious child, where the eyes are dry. In other circumstances, for example if a child's eyes are discharging, they may require hourly treatment.

Purpose of eye care

- To maintain cleanliness of the eyes, thereby promoting comfort and preventing cross-infection
- To keep mucosa moist
- To treat existing infection
- To administer medication

Equipment

- Warm water and bowl. If a child is prone to infection, sterile water should be used. Saline solution is not recommended, as it increases evaporation of tear fluid and can sting (Lloyd 1990, Tree & Tomlinson 1990).
- Clean face flannel or wipes.
- If the eye is infected, or the child is particularly vulnerable to infection, use sterile swabs. Fluffy cotton wool balls or material should not be used, as wisps of cotton may scratch the cornea (Laight 1996).
- Eye swab if infection is suspected and cause unknown. Remember swabs for chlamydia need to be transported in special viral transport medium.
- Disposal bag.

The following may be required, depending on circumstances.

- If the eyes are being cleaned normally as part of everyday hygiene care for a well child, gloves need not be worn. Non-sterile latex gloves should be used if the eye is infected.
- Eye dressing.
- Gelatine-based eye occlusion for the unconscious child, e.g. Geliperm.
- Eye drops/ointment as prescribed.

Preparation

- Explain to the child and parents what will occur, and why the eye care is needed.

- Collect all equipment.
- Position the child in a comfortable position, where his eyes are easily accessible. A child who is very young may need holding by a parent or carer, and an assistant may be needed.
- Wash your hands carefully.

Method

- Observe the condition of the eyes for redness, inflammation, swelling, presence of any discharge, foreign body, or eyelash defect. Each eye should be assessed independently.
- Wash your hands, and put on gloves if necessary.
- If there is any concern that the eye is infected, swab the eye using an appropriate swab.
- In the well child, a clean face flannel or wash wipe can be used, and the eyes cleaned first with a different section of the flannel. Wipe from the inside to the outside of the eye. Do not use soap, which is unpleasant if it gets into the child's eyes.
- If the eye is infected, or the child particularly vulnerable to infection, use sterile swabs and sterile water. To avoid cross-infection, clean the non-infected eye first, then the infected eye. Always wipe from inside to outside, and use a different swab for each eye.
- In a child who is at risk of corneal drying and ulceration, eyes should be kept moist using approved, prescribed artificial tear drops, for example Hypromellose.
- Eye protection may be useful in such children if they are unconscious. This may be a simple eye dressing, or a gelatine-based product such as Geliperm. Geliperm should never be re-used, or resoaked, because of the risk of contamination. Each pack of Geliperm is for single patient use only. The Geliperm should be cut with a sterile cutter to a size sufficient to ensure that both eyelids are generously covered. Geliperm should not be allowed to dry out; the frequency of change will depend on environmental conditions, but may need to be reviewed 2-hourly. Unused Geliperm should be discarded after 48 hours (see manufacturer's instructions).

Administration of eye drops/ointment

Equipment

Eye drops and ointment should be checked according to local policies on administration of medicines. Separate bottles or tubes should be kept for each eye. They should be stored safely and according to manufacturers' instructions. They often have a short shelf-life once opened, so expiry dates should be noted carefully. Labels should indicate the patient's name, left or right eye, and the expiry date of the product. (See also Administration of Medicines, p. 29.)

Method
- If the child will cooperate, lay him flat and ask him to look up at the ceiling.
- Wash your hands, and put on gloves if needed.
- With one hand, pull down the eyelid. Rest the other hand on the child's forehead so that it moves with the child and is thus less likely to cause trauma (Campbell & Glasper 1995).
- Drops:
  - administer each drop separately
  - instil the correct amount of drops, as prescribed, into the lower inner corner of each eye, not directly onto the eyeball.
- Ointment: squeeze the ointment along the inside of the lower eyelid.
- Do not touch the eye with the bottle or tube, or your fingers.
- Ask the child to gently close his eyes and then roll them around to spread the fluid.
- Wipe away any excess fluid from around the eye.
- Record on a drug chart.

Administration of eye drops can be particularly difficult in young children and toddlers, who may struggle and close their eyes protectively. Play, patience, and asking the parent to hold the child firmly on her lap, will help.

Do and do not
- Do assess the child's eyes carefully, especially if they fall into one of the risk groups.
- Do not confuse eye care as part of general hygiene with clinical eye care. This can over-hospitalise the child. Most children will just need a clean wet flannel.

References
Campbell S, Glasper E A (eds) 1995 Whaley and Wong's children's nursing. Mosby, London

Laight S 1996 The efficacy of eye care for ventilated patients: outline of an experimental research pilot study. Intensive and Critical Care Nursing 12(1): 16–26

Lloyd F 1990 Making sense of eye care for ventilated and unconscious patients. Nursing Times 86(19): 36–37

McQuaid L, Huband S, Parker E 1996 Children's nursing. Churchill Livingstone, Edinburgh

Shrader B 1991 Visual problems and very low birthweight. Nursing Times 87(4): 55

Tree G R, Tomlinson A 1990 Effect of artificial tear solutions and saline on tear film evaporation. Option-vis-Science 67(12): 886–890

Winceck J et al 1989 Exposure keratitis in comatose children. Journal of Neuroscience Nursing 21(4): 241–244

Further reading
Farrell M F, Wray F 1993 Eye care for ventilated patients. Intensive and Critical Care Nursing 9(2): 137–141

Laight S 1995 A vision for eye care: a brief study of the change process. Intensive and Critical Care Nursing 11(4): 217–222

Feeding

Part 1: Breast, Bottle and Weaning

Introduction

An adequate diet is vital to promote a child's growth and development. Children are dependent upon adults to feed them safely and appropriately when young and, later, to teach them how and what to provide for themselves when able.

Learning outcomes

By the end of this section you should:

- be able to explain how feeding impacts on a child's development
- be able to describe how to feed a baby/toddler
- be able to list the benefits of breastfeeding
- be able to describe how to calculate a baby's feed requirements.

Rationale

Feeding supplies the baby with food and fluids to aid growth and to promote recovery when he is ill. It also plays a vital role in his development. A children's nurse must be fully aware of how, what and when to feed a child and be able to teach families how to feed their child.

Factors to note

The children's nurse should be familiar with how to assess the child's nutritional status. Being able to plot height and weight on a percentile chart and then interpret those results is an important skill (see Assessment, p. 45).

Hands should always be washed thoroughly prior to handling a child's food or feed and before feeding a child. Feeding always presents the risk of cross-infection by introducing bacteria into the body via the intestine. Babies are particularly at risk because of their immature immune system.

Sick infants

Fasting times for procedures. Fasting time is an important consideration, especially for small babies who can dehydrate rapidly and experience hypoglycaemia (Bates 1994). In his article, Bates describes how, further to a research study, fasting times for children have been reduced to 4 hours for solids or milk and 2 hours for clear fluids.

Guidelines

Parental involvement in feeding is not just desirable, but essential. Feeding is one of the basic, vital life functions which parents undertake for their child and is an important part of the bonding process. Parents should always be included.

Breastfeeding

The first choice of feed for a healthy baby is breast milk. Breastfeeding secures for the baby optimum health, growth and development, and immunity against illness (DoH 1994, 1996). There is now significant evidence to support the existence of a variety of advantages of breastfeeding both to the infant and mother (BPA Standing Committee on Nutrition 1994), which are summarised in Box 12.1.

However, in the UK breastfeeding rates are still low. By the baby's sixth week of life, only 40% of mothers are still breastfeeding (DoH 1996), yet it is recommended that babies are breastfed until at least 4 months of age (DoH 1994).

The reasons why a mother stops feeding vary, but a recurrent issue is the lack of help and support to continue when difficulties are encountered (DoH 1996, Hambridge et al 1995). Social and cultural factors, e.g. early return to work, can also influence a mother's decision to cease breastfeeding. Lack of knowledgeable support can be a particular issue if the baby is admitted to a children's ward, as education about breastfeeding for children's nurses has been sketchy or non-existent in the past.

Box 12.1   **Advantages of breastfeeding (DoH 1996)**

Advantages to the baby
Reduced risk of developing:

- gastrointestinal illness and gastroenteritis in particular
- middle ear infection
- respiratory system infection
- urinary tract infection
- insulin-dependent diabetes mellitus
- allergies, e.g. eczema

and for the preterm baby:

- optimum neurological development
- reduced risk of necrotising enterocolitis

Advantages to the mother
Reduced risk of:

- premenopausal breast cancer
- some forms of ovarian cancer

Social gains:

- ready availability for feeding baby
- unique contact between mother and baby
- may help mother to lose weight naturally

Breast milk

There are three types of breast milk produced. The first is colostrum, produced in the first 3 days after the baby's birth. This is not as rich as mature breast milk but is well suited to the newborn baby's nutritional requirements and contains many maternal antibodies. After about the third day, the mother's milk is 'let down' and mature breast milk is produced. Foremilk is the milk released at the beginning of a feed and is high in lactose but low in fat; later in the feed, hindmilk is produced which is four to five times higher in fat, providing more calories and being more satisfying to the baby.

Frequency and length of breastfeeds

Baby-led feeding is important for a plentiful milk supply (Chadderton et al 1997). 10–15 times in 24 hours is not an unusual frequency, particularly at first, and in the first few days after birth, babies may want to feed for long periods, sometimes up to an hour. Remember that the baby must be allowed to suckle for long enough in order to receive both high-lactose foremilk and high-fat hindmilk, i.e. not just for a brief 3–5 minutes.

Night feeding is important in a breastfed baby. Maternal prolactin secretion is greater at night and prolactin is the hormone which promotes lactation.

Expressing breast milk

A mother may need to express milk:

- to relieve her breasts if they are full or uncomfortable
- if her baby is unable to feed because of illness (e.g. he is too small or sick, or is being starved in preparation for an operation)
- if she is going to be away from her baby for more than an hour or two, or going back to work
- to help the baby attach to a full breast.

There are three ways to express breast milk: by hand, hand pump or electric pump. Any equipment used for expressing milk must be sterilised before use and the mother's hands must be washed and carefully dried. In hospital, kits for electric breast pumps can be re-used after autoclaving if recommended for multiple use by the manufacturer, e.g. Egnell Breast Pump kits. Nurses should familiarise themselves with the type of pump their department offers to mothers to use.

If a mother is expressing milk to maintain a supply whilst her baby is unable to suckle, she should aim to express six to eight times in each 24 hours, including once at night.

Breast milk can be stored for up to 24 hours in a refrigerator (which must maintain a temperature of 2–4°C) or up to 3 months in a freezer. However, from an infection control viewpoint, breast milk is a body fluid and therefore should be stored in a refrigerator or freezer containing nothing but breast milk. It must not be stored with any other type of artificial baby milk or any food.

Breast milk that has previously been frozen then thawed must be stored in the refrigerator and used within 24 hours. If not used, thawed milk must be thrown away.

Equipment to breastfeed
- The only 'equipment' necessary for breastfeeding will be a drink for the mother, close to hand.
- Breast pads or tissues may be required to mop any leakage from the breast from which the baby is not feeding.
- The mother must feel comfortable if she is to breastfeed well, so she may require a special chair or pillow in order to find her optimum position.

- Nipple shields should be avoided as they can reduce the mother's milk supply (Chadderton et al 1997).

Method

This method is based on Chadderton et al 1997.

1. Ensure that the mother is comfortable with a drink close at hand.
2. If the baby is calm and relaxed, feeding is likely to progress better.
3. Position the baby so that he is lying comfortably close to his mother with his head and body in line and not twisted. His head should be slightly higher than his bottom, well supported, but free to move. His nose and mouth should be in line with the nipple.
4. Depending on its size and shape, the mother's breast may need support from her hand. Place her hand with fingers flat against her rib cage so that the breast is supported by the angle of thumb and forefinger. The breast can also be supported with the hand underneath and thumb lightly on top well back from the areola so she can form her breast into a good shape for the baby to latch on.
5. Allow the baby to root for the breast letting tongue and lips touch the nipple. Moving him slightly away now will encourage him to open his mouth wide. Then bring him back to the breast quickly, but smoothly, aiming the lower jaw at the base of the areola. This brings his tongue over his lower lip to scoop up the areola, nipple and as much breast tissue as possible, ensuring that the tongue can reach the lactiferous ducts within the tissue behind the areola. The lactiferous ducts are small reservoirs of milk from which the milk is released.
6. Allow the baby to empty the first breast before moving on to the second, to ensure that both fore- and hindmilks are released.

Observations and complications for breastfeeding

Observations (Chadderton et al 1997)

- Observe that the mother and baby are comfortable and relaxed, with baby close to mother with his head and body straight, his chin touching her breast (and in the young infant < 6 months, with his bottom supported).
- Observe the baby's responses. Does he reach (root in the newborn) for the breast, explore it with his tongue, stay attached? Are there signs of milk ejection (afterpains, milk leakage)?

- Is there evidence of emotional bonding (mother has a secure, confident hold, watches and touches her baby), does he watch her?
- Anatomy – are the breasts soft and full, the nipples protractile, skin healthy and breasts round during feeding?
- How does the baby suckle? Is his mouth wide, lower lip turned outward, tongue cupped around the breast? Are his cheeks round? Does he produce slow, deep sucks in bursts followed by short pauses? Can you see or hear him swallow?
- Note how long the baby feeds and record if required.
- Observe for signs of possible difficulty – see below.

Complications/difficulties

There are no complications of breastfeeding as such, but there may be some difficulties in establishing effective breastfeeding.

- Mother is tense and not relaxed – give the mother time to talk through worries and fears, and provide emotional and practical support.
- Baby is uninterested, sleepy or lazy – try switch feeding. Allow the baby to suckle at one breast until he loses interest, then switch to the other breast and back again when he has lost interest in this breast. Switch two or three times in all until the baby has been feeding long enough to receive hindmilk.
- If the baby is uninterested at the start, try cuddling him well into the breast, skin, to skin between feeds. This will help him to become used to the smell, feel and appearance of the breast (Chadderton et al 1997). Do not give dummies, bottles or pacifiers which can confuse a baby trying to learn how to breastfeed (Shore 1998).
- Mother's nipples become cracked and sore. Avoidance is the best treatment. Encourage the mother to maintain good personal hygiene, ensuring that the breasts are dried carefully, and do not allow the baby to suck at just the end of the nipple which can lead to soreness and cracked skin.
- Be aware that many drugs can be excreted in breast milk and therefore ingested by the baby. The British National Formulary provides information on drugs known to be excreted, but the list is not exhaustive.

Do and do not

- Do promote breastfeeding; provide encouragement, help and support to mothers trying to breastfeed.
- Do ensure that a breastfeeding mother has access to a well-balanced diet and sufficient fluids.

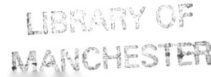

- Do be aware of where to obtain expert help for the breastfeeding mother, if unable to provide it from available staff.
- Do ensure that a breastfeeding mother has access to facilities to enable her to express milk when necessary.
- Do not give a breastfed baby a dummy or pacifier.
- Do not give a breastfed baby artificial milk, water or juice unless absolutely necessary.
- Do not give a breastfed baby a bottle. If a breastfed baby has to be given anything by mouth, it should be fed to him using a cup or cup and spoon.

Artificial feeding

Not all mothers will choose or be able to breastfeed their babies. Hull & Johnston (1993) list some contra-indications to breastfeeding:

- the very premature infant's inability to suck
- some severe abnormalities of an infant's mouth, e.g. severe cleft palate
- severe maternal ill health may contraindicate breastfeeding, e.g. active tuberculosis and HIV infection can both be transmitted to the infant via breast milk
- the mother who is severely undernourished or has poor renal function may find breastfeeding an unacceptable drain on her own nutritional reserves
- the child has a condition, e.g. phenylketonuria, which necessitates a special diet that precludes feeding with breast milk.

A children's nurse must be able to undertake and advise on artificial methods of feeding as well as calculate if a baby is taking appropriate amounts of feed to sustain expected growth and development. This is calculated by multiplying the child's body weight by a figure which is determined by his age (see Table 12.1).

On the basis of the figures in Table 12.1, a 3-month-old baby weighing 5.2 kg should receive: $5.2 \times 150 = 780$ ml in 24 hours.

Exceptions to this calculation are determined by a children's dietitian (if available) or a paediatrician. Exceptional circumstances might include a baby failing to thrive, who requires 200 ml/kg/day, or a child in renal failure or with cerebral oedema, who requires restricted fluids, e.g. 75 ml/kg/day.

It is a matter of parental choice as to which artificial feed their healthy baby is given. They may require guidance from health care staff as to the most suitable breast

Table 12.1   **Average fluid requirements of a healthy baby**

Age of baby	Average total fluid requirement in 24 hours in ml/kg
Newborn	30
2 days	60
3 days	90
4 days	120
5 days	150
1 week to 8 months	150
9–12 months	120

milk substitute, infant formula or follow-on milk, but it should be made clear to all parents that cow's milk is not suitable for children under 12 months of age (Shore 1995). Formula milks are mostly some form of modified cow's milk, containing protein in the form of casein (the protein in cow's milk). Hull & Johnston (1995) summarise the four basic types of formula milk as:

- a whey-based formula with a whey : casein ratio of 60 : 40 like human milk, e.g. SMA Gold Cap
- a casein-based formula with a whey : casein ratio of 20 : 80 like cow's milk, e.g. SMA White Cap
- a soya protein-based formula with no milk constituents, e.g. Wysoy
- a follow-on formula for infants who have been weaned; these are iron enriched, with a higher protein content, e.g. Progress.

Vitamin and iron supplements for infants

The DoH (1994) recommends that vitamin supplements are not necessary for breastfed babies under 6 months, provided that the mother's vitamin intake is adequate, or for formula-fed infants taking more than 500 ml daily. An infant taking less than 500 ml/day or an infant over 6 months whose main source of nutrition is breast milk should receive vitamin A and D supplements.

Preparing artificial feeds

Larger children's units and children's hospitals will usually have a special feed unit or milk kitchen where baby feeds are made under sterile conditions. If feeds are to be made on the wards, very careful attention must be paid to the risk of cross-infection. A separate area should be set aside for feed preparation, away from any other food.

Equipment

- Documentation listing type and quantity of feed to be made
- Washed and sterilised bottles with fluid measure on side
- Washed and sterilised manufacturer-supplied milk powder scoop
- Boiled, cooled water (that has only been boiled once and has not been artificially softened)
- Milk powder of the same brand as the scoop; check that the milk powder is within its expiry date
- Washed and sterilised plastic knife with straight-edged back
- 70% isopropyl alcohol spray or impregnated swab
- Patient identification labels

Method

1. Wash and dry hands thoroughly; put on disposable plastic apron.
2. Ensure that the work surface is clean and dry; spray or wipe the surface with 70% isopropyl alcohol.
3. Pour the required amount of boiled, cooled water into each of the bottles. The amount required is the total amount of feed per bottle. For example, if the baby requires 125 ml at each feed, put 125 ml water in each bottle.
4. Using the correct brand of scoop for the type of milk powder being used, scoop up the milk powder. Do not pack the milk tightly into the scoop. Using the flat edge of the back of the knife, level off the top of the powder with the top of the scoop. Add the powder to the water. One scoop of powder is added to each fluid ounce (28.4 ml) of water. Any less powder than this and the baby will be underfed; any more powder than this and the too concentrated feed can lead to diarrhoea and even hypernatraemia.
5. Once all the powder has been added to the feed, put the lid on each bottle and shake well to mix the milk powder and water thoroughly.
6. Label the bottle with the baby's identification label, the type and quantity of feed and the expiry date (24 hours later). All the feeds should then be autoclaved/pasteurised and stored in a refrigerator specifically for milk feeds only.

Bottle feeding a baby

Equipment

- Plastic apron
- Sterile bottle of milk of correct formula type and quantity

- Sterile teat
- Jug of hot water with sealable lid or bottle warmer to heat bottle
- Bib
- Comfortable chair with support for arm
- Sterilising unit containing 125 parts per million of hypochlorite in solution
- Documentation to record feed given

Method

1. Prior to feeding, ensure that the baby's nose is clean and that he has a clean, dry nappy. He is less likely to feed well if his nose is blocked with mucus or he is uncomfortable from a wet or soiled nappy.
2. Wash hands thoroughly and put on an apron (to prevent cross-infection).
3. If using a proprietary preprepared formula milk, first check the cap according to the manufacturer's instructions to ensure that the seal has not been broken.
4. Check that the expiry date of the feed has not passed and check again that the feed is of the correct make and the quantity to be given.
5. If the feed is to be heated (some babies prefer milk at room temperature), place the bottle in a jug of hot water. If the feed has been refrigerated prior to use, this will need to be nearly boiling water. Care must be taken if very hot water is to be carried through the ward. Ideally it should be carried in a sealed container and be placed on a tray to reduce the risk of accidental spillage which could harm a child or adult.
6. After approximately 2 minutes, check the feed to see if it feels warm enough to test whether it is ready to feed to the baby.
7. If it feels warm enough, put the teat onto the bottle and test the temperature of the milk by squirting a small amount onto the back of the hand or onto the skin on the underside of the forearm. Ideally the milk should be at approximately blood temperature (37°C), as breast milk would be, therefore it should feel just warm and not hot on contact with the skin. Too hot milk can easily burn the baby's mouth. If it feels hot, it must not be given to the baby until it has cooled down; the temperature must be tested again after cooling, before giving it to the baby.
8. Put the bib around the baby to protect his clothing.
9. The baby should be held well supported for feeding, with his head above his stomach. This reduces the risk of accidental aspiration of stomach contents. A baby should never be bottle-fed whilst he is lying flat because of the increased risk of vomiting and aspiration of feed and vomit into the lungs.

10. Offer the bottle by placing it gently to the lips. Never force a bottle into a baby's mouth. If he is reluctant to accept the bottle, it may help to gently stroke his skin just to the side of his mouth. This can stimulate the sucking reflex, as can stroking him gently under the chin.

11. Hold the bottle at a sufficiently steep angle to keep the teat filled with milk, to help prevent the baby sucking in too much air which can cause discomfort and vomiting (Hull & Johnston 1993). Most babies can take approximately half of the total amount of feed before requiring to be winded. Winding the baby helps to bring up any air swallowed during feeding (Hull & Johnston 1993) and therefore promotes comfort and helps reduce the incidence of vomiting after feeding.

12. Gently remove the bottle and sit baby up, supporting his head if he is unable to do so for himself. Gently rubbing his back can help to bring up the wind. Some babies like to be put up onto the shoulder to be winded, but take care to protect the shoulder and back in case he regurgitates some milk with the wind. Regurgitating a small amount of milk with wind is normal and is known as posseting (Hull & Johnston 1993).

13. Remember that feeding is a time to promote physical contact, eye contact and verbal stimulation for the baby.

14. After the feed is completed, wind the baby again and then make him comfortable. Ideally (and particularly if the baby is prone to vomiting), he should be allowed to sit up for 20–30 minutes after a feed to prevent aspiration and vomiting.

15. Record what feed was given, how much feed was taken and note if there was any vomiting. If vomiting has occurred, describe the consistency and quantity.

16. Clear away. If the bottle and/or teat (if not a single-use teat) are to be used again, the bottle should be washed thoroughly clean in warm, soapy water then rinsed carefully. The teat should be washed thoroughly and salt may be rubbed inside it to remove all traces of milk. It should then be rinsed thoroughly to remove all salt. The clean bottle and teat are then submerged completely in the sterilising solution, ensuring that there are no air bubbles, and left in the sterilising unit for at least 30 minutes. The presence of any organic matter, e.g. milk, saliva, in a hypochlorite solution will destabilise it and render it incapable of sterilising. Hypochlorite solutions should be discarded every 24 hours or if there is evidence of contamination of the solution. It is not necessary to rinse the hypochlorite solution off the teat prior to offering it to the baby.

Observations and complications

Observations

Feeding is a good time to assess whether the baby is developing as expected for his age. Be aware of how he is on handling. Is his head control appropriate for his age? Is he abnormally stiff or floppy or does he handle as would be expected of a child of his age? Observe the baby's face, his expressions, eye movements, eye contact. Check that he is achieving developmental milestones, e.g. fixing and following by 4 weeks. Observe how he feeds, noting if he has a good, strong suck or if he is slow to feed and sleepy or unusually drowsy. If there is vomiting, observe the physical nature of the vomiting and the vomit itself, e.g. is it effortless, or is it projectile, is the vomit milky or bile-stained? Report any unusual findings.

Complications of bottle feeding

As with any calculation, there is the risk of human error resulting in too much or too little being given. Parents unaware of how much feed they should give their baby could overfeed, leading to excessive weight gain over a prolonged period, or underfeed, resulting in weight loss and dehydration. In addition, a child with medical problems such as congenital heart disease or renal disease may not cope with a feed calculated at the normal quantities. The incorrect feed could be given which could be a problem if special additives are omitted or given accidentally. A feed that has been reconstituted incorrectly may cause hypernatraemia (salt overload) if it is too concentrated, or provide insufficient calories if too dilute.

Do and do not

- Do calculate the feed correctly.
- Do ensure that, if making up feeds, the correct brand of milk scoop is used for the correct type of milk powder.
- Do ensure that exactly one level scoop of milk powder is added to each fluid ounce (28.4 ml) of cooled, boiled water.
- Do ensure that the correct type of formula and amount of feed is given to the right child.
- Do remember to test the temperature of a feed before it is given to a baby.
- Do not bottle feed a baby lying flat on his back.
- Do not reconstitute baby milk powder with water that has been boiled more than once.
- Do not reheat bottle feeds more than once.

Toddler feeding

Weaning

Shore (1995) summarises the COMA report (DoH 1994) and its recommendations for weaning. The main points include:

- Solid food should not be introduced before the age of 4 months.
- Suitable first weaning foods to be given by spoon are: non-wheat cereals, fruit, vegetables, potatoes.
- Diet should include good sources of vitamin C to aid iron absorption.
- Non-breastfed babies should only receive infant formula milk for the first year (they may be given follow-on, iron-rich formula milks from 6 months onwards).
- By 6 months the child should be receiving a mixed diet, totally free from added salt and, wherever possible, free from added sugar.
- Drinking from a cup is to be encouraged from 6 months.
- If there is doubt that dietary iron is adequate, consider the continued use of iron-enriched formula/follow-on milk.
- Cow's, goat's or sheep's milk must not be introduced before 12 months of age.
- Discourage bottle feeds from 12 months.
- Water should be the drink of choice when milk is not required.
- 1–5 years: vitamin A and D supplements should be given unless there is certainty that the child is receiving adequate quantities in the diet and moderate exposure to sunlight.
- Prevent dental caries: promote healthy dentition by avoiding sugared or fizzy drinks and fruit juices. Give only at meal times via cup, not bottle or pacifier.

Note. However adequate the dietary iron intake, it is useless without intake of substances such as vitamin C which enables the iron actually to be absorbed (Palmer 1993). In addition, other dietary substances (tea, egg yolk) can inhibit the absorption of iron (Palmer 1993).

Factors to note

Feeding is important to several areas of the toddler's development. Social, fine motor and perceptual development is demonstrated by a 10-month-old attempting to grasp and manipulate the spoon with which he is being fed and his determination to try to feed himself (Bee 1997). Whilst it can be frustrating for child and carer to see him continually drop food just before he gets it to his mouth, it should not be discouraged. Neither should he be discouraged from handling his food, as exploring texture teaches him about the surrounding world. However, it is important to distinguish between acceptable learning behaviour in comparison to what would constitute unacceptable social behaviour if allowed to become established.

Feeding a toddler (approximately 9–24 months)

Equipment
- High chair
- Food of appropriate consistency according to his age and level of development, e.g. will he require finger foods, can he tolerate lumpy foods?
- Bib
- Feeder beaker of water or diluted fruit juice; avoid fizzy drinks and sugary squashes.
- Spoons for feeding (the toddler will often want one to himself, even if he is unable to feed independently)
- Documentation to record food given if required

Method
1. Wash the child's hands and utilise the opportunity to teach him about washing his own hands prior to meals.
2. Wash hands thoroughly and put on an apron (to prevent cross-infection).
3. Ensure that the toddler is strapped safely and securely into the high chair.
4. Allow him to hold a spoon of his own. He may accept help to put food onto his spoon.
5. Put a small amount of food onto the spoon. If he is managing well with his own spoon, let him carry on. Do not try to get him to take food from your spoon.
6. If he is having difficulty, intersperse his own efforts at feeding by placing your spoon just into the front of his mouth. Never force the spoon into his mouth.
7. Constantly encourage him and praise him when he manages to put food into his mouth himself and when he accepts food from you.
8. As children learn to manipulate their mouth and tongue muscles, inevitably some food gets spat out accidentally. However, it will become clear if there is a particular food which he does not like. He will try to spit it out and may well purse his lips and

refuse to take another mouthful. Offer that particular food once more. If he still refuses or spits it out again, try another item of food from the plate instead.

9. Encourage him to feed himself finger foods, e.g. carrot, bread, fruit. This teaches him independence, different textures of food (not purée) and enables him to experience the achievement of feeding himself.

10. Offer him a drink from his feeder cup once or twice during the meal and at the end of the savoury course and at the end of the meal. The last drink of the meal would ideally be water to help rinse his mouth and prevent dental caries.

11. Allow him to feel his food if he so wishes, but discourage him from throwing his plate or utensils. Be firm and consistent in what behaviour is allowed and what is not tolerated.

12. At the end of his meal, clear away the remains and clean his face and hands.

Observations and complications

Observations

Observe how the toddler reacts to being fed. Does he help himself, or is he very passive? This can tell you something about his level of development.

Establish the toddler's likes and dislikes in different foods and textures.

Relate your observations of how he feeds and what he does and does not like to the information given to you by his parents.

Observe how he behaves when fed by his parents. Useful information about how he and his parents interact can be gained from observing them during a meal time.

Complications

There are few complications associated with feeding a toddler. There could be a risk of him choking on a piece of food, in which case he should be given emergency treatment for choking, following resuscitation guidelines.

If the food he is given is too hot, there is a risk of him burning his mouth.

Do and do not

- Do check the temperature of his food before feeding him.
- Do praise and encourage him when he succeeds in feeding himself.
- Do allow him to help feed himself.
- Do let him touch and feel his food.
- Do be prepared for a messy meal time.
- Do not give him a lot to drink prior to a meal that would fill his stomach and make him less hungry.
- Do not ever force him to take food.

References

Bates J 1994 Reducing fasting times in paediatric day surgery. Child Health 90(48): 38–39

Bee H 1997 The developing child, 8th edn. Addison-Wesley, New York, ch 5, pp 128–129

British Paediatric Association Standing Committee on Nutrition 1994 Is breastfeeding beneficial in the UK? Archives of Disease in Childhood 71: 376–380

Chadderton M, MacDonald A, Munn J et al 1997 A healthy start – infant feeding policy. South Birmingham Community Health Trust, Birmingham Children's Hospital NHS Trust, Birmingham

Department of Health (DoH) 1994 Report of working group on weaning diet of the committee of medical aspects of food policy. Weaning and the weaning diet. HMSO, London

Department of Health (DoH) 1996 Breastfeeding: good practice guidance to the NHS. HMSO, London

Hambridge K M, Krebs N F, Sokol R J 1995 Infant feeding. In: Roy C, Silverman A, Alagille D (eds) Pediatric clinical gastroenterology, 4th edn. Mosby, St Louis, ch 36, pp 1020–1021

Hull D, Johnston D I 1993 Essential paediatrics, 3rd edn. Churchill Livingstone, Edinburgh, ch 5, pp 75–89

Palmer G 1993 Any old iron. Health Visitor 66(7): 248–249, 252

Shore C 1995 The COMA report: nursing implications. Paediatric Nursing 7(3): 14–17

Shore C 1998 Good practice guidelines for breastfeeding in paediatric units. Paediatric Nursing 10(1): 29–24

Further reading

Agnew T 1996 Battle of the breast in the classroom. Nursing Times 92(2): 15

Coldicutt P 1994 Children's options. Nursing Times 90(13): 54–56

Elia I 1994 Adoptive breastfeeding. Nursing Standard 8(43): 20–21

Henshel D, Inch S 1996 Breastfeeding: a guide for midwives. Books for Midwives Press, Hale

Payne D 1995 A lot of bottle. Nursing Times 91(17): 20–21

Royal College of Midwives 1991 Successful breastfeeding. Churchill Livingstone, Edinburgh

Part 2: Enteral Feeding

Introduction

Enteral feeding is an artificial method of supplying the child with nutrition via a nasogastric tube or gastrostomy.

Learning outcomes

By the end of this section you should:

- be able to identify some typical situations in which a child may require enteral feeding
- be able to describe the techniques of providing enteral nutrition and hydration to the child who is unable to feed orally
- understand the possible risks and side-effects associated with some feeding techniques.

Rationale for enteral feeding

A children's nurse should be able to undertake enteral feeding, teach children and their families the different techniques and be aware of possible positive and negative effects of enteral feeding.

Factors to note

See Factors to note in Part 1 of this section, page 107.

Hambridge et al (1995a) give reasons why some children are unable to feed orally:

- The child has cancer and the treatment causes anorexia and vomiting.
- The child is unable to take in sufficient nutrition for growth and development in an acute or chronic illness, e.g. severe bronchiolitis, gross reflux, renal failure or liver disease, particularly when she has increased calorific and nutrient requirements.
- The child is unable to absorb her food, e.g. short bowel syndrome and severe, acute diarrhoea.
- The premature infant may not yet have developed a swallowing reflex.

These children can be fed enterally via nasogastric (NG) tube or gastrostomy (Hambridge et al 1995a).

The multidisciplinary team is essential when a sick child has special dietary requirements:

- A children's dietitian and/or paediatrician may be required to prescribe a feed or extra calories (Maxijul) or additives, e.g. a thickening agent (Nestargel).
- A doctor may need to prescribe drugs, e.g. antireflux treatment, electrolyte supplements or intestinal motility regulators (cisapride, loperamide).
- Nutritional care nurse specialists may be available in some hospitals to help advise on practical aspects of feeding children.
- A speech therapist may conduct an assessment of the child's oral motor function, and is a source of valuable advice with regard to the child's developmental needs associated with feeding (Langley 1994).

Nasogastric tubes

There are two main types commonly used. A polyvinylchloride (PVC) tube, e.g. Portex, and polyurethane tubes, sometimes known as 'silk' tubes. They are single-use only and the PVC tube is primarily for short-term feeding. The polyurethane tubes for longer-term feeding can remain in situ for up to a month. The tubes are sized according to the width of their internal lumen; 6, 8 and 10 French gauge (Fg) are most commonly used in children. If a thickening agent has been added to the child's feed, the small 6 Fg diameter tube may be too narrow to facilitate instillation of the feed. Tubes commonly come in two lengths, 50 and 100 cm. The length used will depend on how big the child is. The tube must be long enough to cover the length from the outer edge of the child's face, through her nasopharynx and down into her stomach (see Fig. 12.1).

The PVC tubes should be changed every 5–7 days and polyurethane tubes monthly to prevent increased risk of bacterial contamination and the material of the tube being eroded by gastric juices (Taylor & Goodison-McLaren 1992).

Gastrostomy tubes

Gastrostomy tubes are made of silicone. There are three main types: skin-level 'button' or 'key' devices;

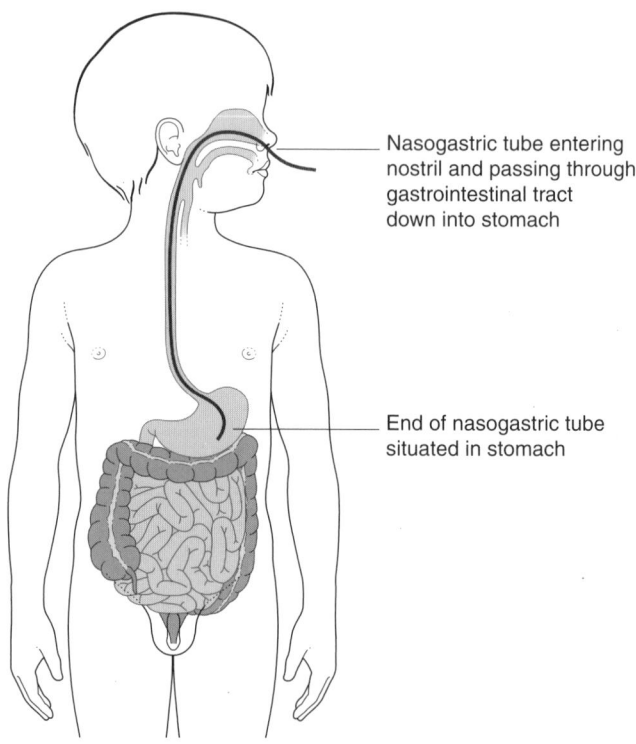

Nasogastric tube entering nostril and passing through gastrointestinal tract down into stomach

End of nasogastric tube situated in stomach

Figure 12.1
*The length and position
of an NG tube in situ.*

percutaneous endoscopic tubes; and surgically placed tubes, e.g. Foley catheter (Fig. 12.2).

Once healed, the skin around a gastrostomy site should be washed daily with soap and water to prevent the skin around the site becoming sore (Coldicutt 1994). Frequency and timing of tube changes varies according to the device used and the child's condition. The gastrostomy button is a device in which the exterior of the tube sits flush with the skin and when not in use, resembles a button on the surface of the skin (see Fig. 12.2A). It is usually changed once every 3–6 months but must not be used until the tract from the initial gastrostomy has formed – at least 3 months after insertion of the original tube (Gauderer et al 1988). However, in some areas, when the gastrostomy tract has been formed via a Stamm procedure (full surgical procedure), tubes are placed directly.

The percutaneous endoscopic tube (PEG) is a gastrostomy tube that is inserted through the skin into the stomach under endoscopic control, therefore avoiding the need for a full, laparoscopic surgical procedure (Booth 1991). It can stay in situ for some months.

A surgically placed tube such as a Foley catheter is usually much shorter-term in use and should only be changed by a surgeon or nurse who has received training in the procedure. If it becomes displaced in the first 2 weeks postoperatively, before the tract has properly formed, it must be re-inserted as a matter of urgency or the skin and tissues will close over. Gastrostomy tubes are most commonly sized between 8 and 15 Fg, although smaller or larger tubes may be used in small babies or older children.

Research-based practice relating to the risks of enteral feeding

Research has highlighted the risks of nasogastric feeding, in particular the risk of aspiration of feed because of misplaced tubes, blocked tubes, infection transmission and the excessive vacuum pressure caused by using smaller-volume syringes.

Maintaining patency of nasogastric and gastrostomy tubes. NG and gastrostomy tubes must be flushed before and after a feed. During continuous feeding or when not in use, NG tubes should be flushed regularly to maintain patency, e.g. every 4 hours during the day-time (Lifshitz et al 1991, Paul et al 1993). Gastrostomy tubes must also be flushed regularly to maintain patency (Lifshitz et al 1991, Paul et al 1994).

Preventing infection transmission via enteral feeding. Whenever an NG or gastrostomy tube is flushed, it should be done with boiled, cooled or sterile water (not tap water), whatever the age of the child (Anderton 1995, Coldicutt 1994, Paul et al 1993, 1994).

In addition, feeds should only be prepared on surfaces which have been cleaned thoroughly with soap and water, dried and then wiped with 70% isopropyl alcohol-impregnated wipes. Any feed delivery systems should be single-use only, and feed containers, NG and gastrostomy tubes should also be cleaned with the alcohol-impregnated wipes prior to use (Anderton 1995, Paul et al 1993, 1994).

Size of syringe used when administering feed/flush via NG or gastrostomy tube. A polyurethane tube (e.g. silk tube or gastrostomy tube) is softer and more prone to damage. The smaller the syringe, the smaller is the bore (the hole in the middle) and the greater the pressure created when injecting with it. 1–5 ml syringes produce the highest pressure for a given force. Using a larger-sized syringe reduces the pressure on the tube,

thus minimising the risk of damage (Paul et al 1993, Sidey 1995, Taylor & Goodison-McLaren 1992). This is also mentioned in the manufacturers' guidelines, e.g. for a Merck tube.

Guidelines

Parents and older children should be encouraged to be involved with enteral feeding. This can include being involved in or even trained to pass the nasogastric or gastrostomy tube if they so wish. Involvement can help them to feel in control of the procedure and help their acceptance of the problem (Holden et al 1997).

Passing a nasogastric (NG) tube

Equipment

- Plastic apron
- Disposable latex gloves
- Boiled, cooled sterile water for flushing tube
- 2 sterile gallipots
- pH paper that is capable of indicating an acid range of pH 0–3
- 2 syringes – 5/10 ml for PVC tube or 50/60 ml for polyurethane tube

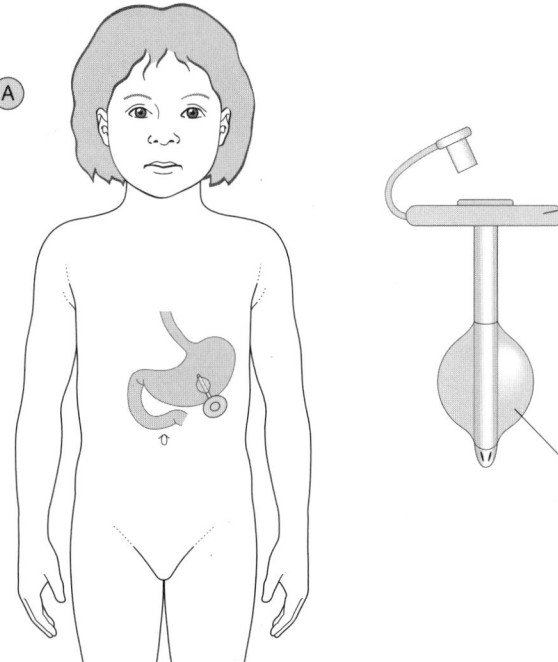

Sits flush with skin

Balloon or mushroom-shaped end to sit inside and prevent device falling out

Figure 12.2
Types of gastrostomy tube: (A) skin-level 'button' or 'key' device.

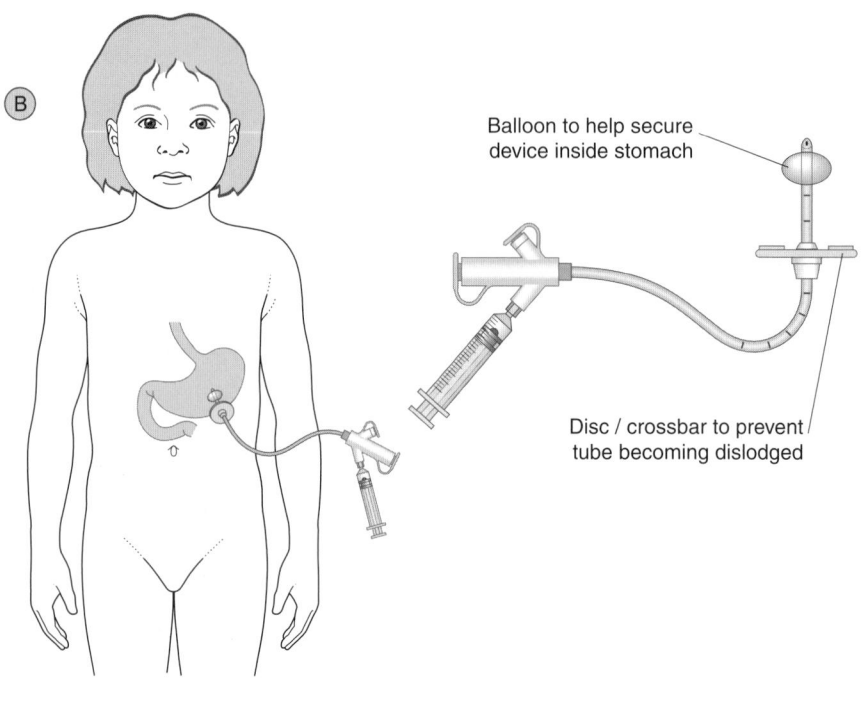

Balloon to help secure
device inside stomach

Disc / crossbar to prevent
tube becoming dislodged

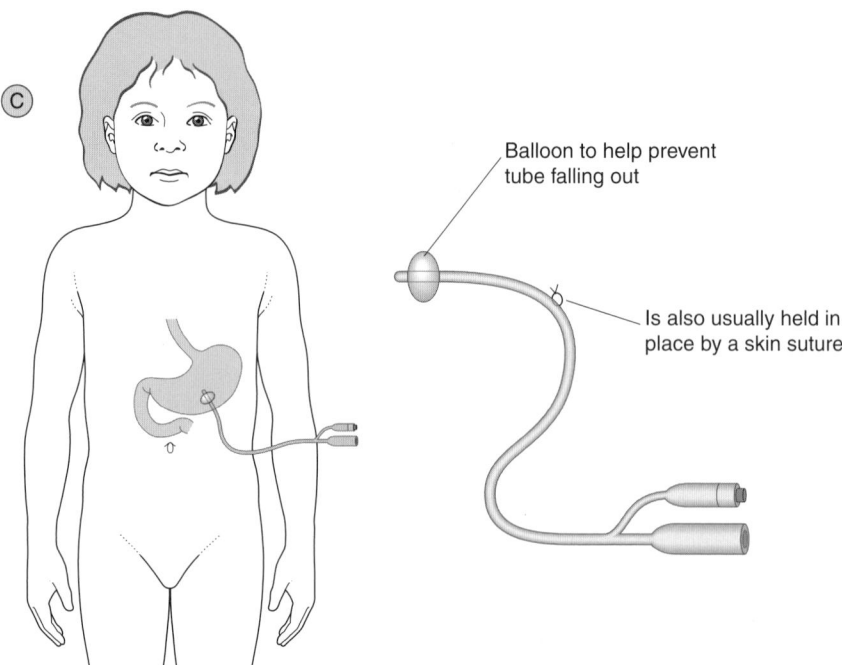

Balloon to help prevent
tube falling out

Is also usually held in
place by a skin suture

Figure 12.2
*Types of gastrostomy
tube: (B) percutaneous
endoscopic tube; (C)
surgically placed tube,
e.g. Foley catheter.*

- 70% isopropyl alcohol-impregnated wipes
- Tape to secure the tube to the child's cheek (check that she is not allergic to the tape)
- Scissors
- If the child has especially sensitive skin, you may need a hydrocolloid dressing such as extra-thin Granuflex to provide a protective layer between the child's skin and the adhesive tape holding the tube in place
- Dummy if child uses it
- Drink of water if the child is older

Method

Note. Generally two people are needed to pass an NG tube, one to comfort and support the child and one to pass the tube.

1. Wherever possible, the child and family should have had psychological preparation to reduce the distress caused by the procedure (Holden et al 1997).
2. Wash hands thoroughly, dry them and put on a plastic apron to prevent cross-infection (Anderton 1995).
3. Clean the work surface/trolley on which equipment is to be placed, and spray or wipe with alcohol (Anderton 1995). Allow alcohol to dry (it sterilises as it dries).
4. If using hydrocolloid dressing, cut a piece and place it within easy reach. It should be wide enough to be at least three times the diameter of the NG tube and long enough to cover at least two-thirds of the child's cheek from the side of her nostril towards her ear (see Fig. 12.3). Normally, a piece 1.5 cm × 5 cm would be adequate for most children except a very tiny neonate who would need less.
5. Cut a piece of adhesive tape and place it in easy reach. It should be wide enough to cover the NG tube with overlap at each side sufficient to hold it securely in place, and long enough to secure at least 3 cm of tube. If hydrocolloid dressing is used, the adhesive tape should not extend beyond the boundary of the hydrocolloid.
6. Draw up 2–5 ml of the water into one of the syringes. Place on one side, in easy reach.
7. Put approximately 10 ml water into a gallipot in easy reach.
8. Open up the second syringe and place it in easy reach.
9. Take a strip of litmus paper and place it in the second gallipot.
10. Wash hands thoroughly, dry them and put on disposable gloves to prevent bacterial contamination of the tube (Anderton 1995).
11. Take the NG tube out of its sterile packaging. Ensure that it is not damaged in any way. If the tube has a guide wire, check that the wire is not bent and is correctly inserted down the middle of the tube. Measure what length of tube is to be passed. With the fingers of your dominant hand, hold the distal end of the tube (the one which will sit in the stomach) by the child's nostril. Measure the first length of tubing from the nostril to the edge of the cheek, by the ear (Fig. 12.4A). Then measure the second length of tubing from the edge of the ear down to the child's stomach – just past the xiphoid process (Fig. 12.4B). Mark this point

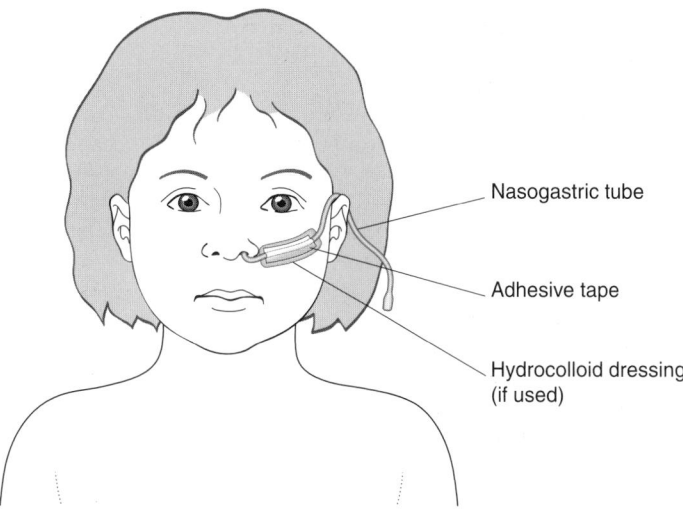

Figure 12.3

Size and position of tape securing nasogastric tube to cheek.

Nasogastric tube

Adhesive tape

Hydrocolloid dressing (if used)

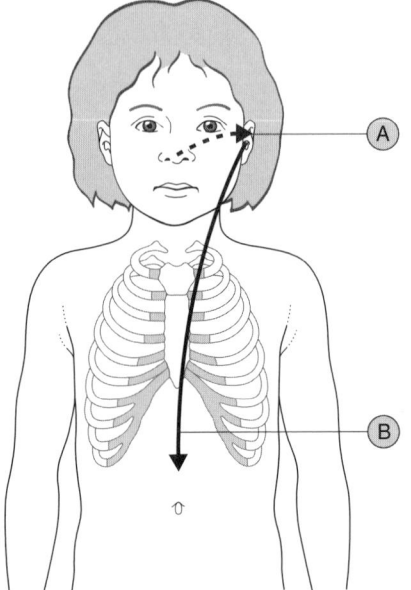

Figure 12.4
Measuring the length of NG tube to be passed: (A) holding the tip of the tube, measure from nose to ear: (B) then measure from ear to stomach, aiming for the space in the middle below the ribs.

on the tube by holding it in the fingers of your non-dominant hand. Some tubes have black markings on the tubing at 10 cm intervals to give you a visual guide as to what length of tubing needs to be passed.

12. Ask the person holding the child to position her so that you can access her nostril. A baby is best held wrapped in a sheet and in position as if for bottle feeding. An older child should be encouraged to sit upright.

13. Maintain your hold on the proximal end of the tube (the one which will remain on the exterior) at the end of the pre-measured length. Lubricate the distal end of the NG tube by dipping it in the gallipot containing water.

14. Gently pass the distal end of the tube into the child's nostril. Angle it slightly upwards and gently guide it over the back of the nose and into the nasopharynx.

15. Continue to feed the tube downwards. As it gets to the back of the child's throat, she will gag. To try to ease the passage of the tube encourage a baby to suck on her dummy and try to persuade the older child to have a sip of water. Advance the tube as the child swallows. This will help ease her discomfort and reduce the risk of the tube passing into the trachea as her epiglottis will cover her trachea as she swallows.

16. Continue to advance the tube. You may have to

pause in order for the tube to pass through the cardiac sphincter into the stomach. When the place you have marked on the tube is at the opening of the child's nostril, the distal end should now be in her stomach.

17. Ask the person holding the child, or the child herself, to place her fingers against the tube to prevent it slipping.

18. Check that the NG tube is in the correct position.

19. Connect a syringe (5/10 ml or 50/60 ml depending on type of tube) to the end of the NG tube and withdraw the plunger until fluid appears in the syringe – only a very small amount ($\frac{1}{2}$–1 ml) of fluid is required. Disconnect the syringe and close off the end of the tube.

20. Put the contents of the syringe onto the blue litmus paper and observe for an acid reaction (the aspirate must be in the pH range 0–3) indicating that the fluid originates from the stomach and the tube is correctly positioned.

    If no fluid was obtained, try changing the child's position and then aspirating the tube again. If still no fluid can be withdrawn and it is safe to do so, give the child a few millilitres (5 ml) of water, juice or milk orally and then aspirate the tube again.

    If it is still not possible to be sure that the tube is correctly placed, it may need to be withdrawn a little or passed further, in order to obtain acidic aspirate. In exceptional circumstances it may be necessary to obtain an X-ray picture to determine whether the tube is correctly positioned.

21. Having established that the tube is correctly placed, gently flush the tube with 2–5 ml of water to ensure that it is patent. Remove the guide wire if one has been used. Disconnect and close off the end of the tube.

22. Secure the tube to the child's cheek using the adhesive tape (and hydrocolloid if necessary).

Feeding via an NG or gastrostomy tube

Equipment
- Plastic apron
- Disposable latex gloves
- Boiled, cooled sterile water for flushing tube
- 2 sterile gallipots
- Blue litmus paper
- 2 syringes – 5/10 ml for PVC NG tube or 50/60 ml for polyurethane NG tube
- 70% isopropyl alcohol spray or impregnated wipes
- Sterile feed – correct type and quantity at room temperature
- Bottle opener if required
- Documentation to record feed given

For bolus feed
- Gravity feed delivery system with plunger if feed thickened or narrow bore (6 or 8 Fg)
- Separate clamp for gravity feed tube if roller clamp not integral to the system
- Dummy if appropriate (and breastfeeding is not to be established in the future)
- Toys related to feeding – plastic dishes, utensils, etc.

For continuous feed
- Enteral feeding pump with fully charged battery and lead to connect it to a mains electrical supply
- Continuous enteral feeding administration set and label to indicate when set changed

Method
1. Clean the work surface/trolley on which feed is to be prepared and wipe it with alcohol (Anderton 1995). Allow alcohol to dry (it sterilises as it dries).
2. Check that the expiry date of the feed has not passed.
3. Wash and dry the bottle opener and separate clamp if used. Clean bottle opener and clamp (if used) and top of feed container by spraying or wiping with alcohol to prevent cross-infection (Anderton 1995).
4. Open the feed administration system and put all equipment on the work surface.
5. Wash hands thoroughly and put on disposable latex gloves to prevent bacterial contamination of feed (Anderton 1995).
6. Reassure the child and parent; explain what you are about to do.
7. Ensure that the patient is comfortable and is positioned with her head above the level of her stomach to prevent aspiration, preferably sitting or nursed at an angle of about 30 degrees (Lifshitz et al 1991). The neonate should be placed prone or on her right side (Taylor & Goodison-McLaren 1992).
8. Draw up 5–10 ml of sterile water (for flushing tube) into the appropriate size of syringe for the type of tube.
9. Check that the NG/gastrostomy tube is in the correct position and patent. See steps 19–21 for passing an NG tube. A gastrostomy tube should be allowed to free drain a small amount of fluid onto litmus paper placed in one of the gallipots.
10. Prime the feed administration system. Apply a clamp to the tubing, fill the barrel/bag/burette with feed and then fill the tubing by gradually releasing the clamp. If necessary, run excess feed into the second sterile gallipot. When the tubing is primed and all air removed, apply the clamp again.

Bolus feeding
11. Connect the feed administration set to the tube (Anderton 1995).
12. Slowly release the clamp and raise the barrel of the feed system to allow feed to flow into the tube by gravity. The higher the tube is raised, the faster the flow rate. Administration of the feed should take the same length of time as it would take the child to have the same amount orally – usually 15–30 minutes.

    If the feed is too thick or the bore of the NG tube too narrow to allow feed to drip in by gravity, then the feed must be instilled using the plunger. *Gently* depress the plunger to deliver the feed at the same rate as if feeding by gravity. Never use force; this will make the child vomit.
13. Top up the barrel with the remaining feed as it begins to empty. Do not allow it to empty as far as the tubing until the feed is complete (to prevent instilling air into the tube, leading to discomfort and wind).

14. Whilst the feed is being given, encourage the child to suck (on a dummy) so that she associates sucking with the sensation of feeding. The older child can be tube fed at the dinner table to encourage normal socialisation associated with feeding. Similarly, the older child should be encouraged to play with feeding utensils whilst being tube fed.
15. When the feed is complete, remove the empty gravity feed system and close off the feeding tube before air can get into the tube.
16. Gently flush the feeding tube with the remaining 2–5 ml of sterile water in the appropriate size of syringe. Cap off the feeding tube.
17. Make the child comfortable and clear away equipment.
18. A gravity feed system may be re-used over a 24-hour period as long as it is sterilised in between feeds. It must be discarded and a new system used after 24 hours to reduce the risk of bacterial contamination (Anderton 1995).

Continuous feeding

11. If the feed has preservatives and is sterile (e.g. a proprietary brand such as Cow and Gate formula), the full amount of feed (up to 24 hours' worth) should be primed in the administration set to prevent the set being accessed frequently and therefore reduce the risk of bacterial contamination (Anderton 1995). If the feed does not have preservatives (e.g. it is made daily by a special feed kitchen), the set should be primed with enough feed for 4 hours at a time (Anderton 1995).
12. Plug in and switch on the enteral pump. Test the alarm system on the pump. Load the administration set into the pump.
13. Set the pump to the correct rate (in ml/hour) to deliver the desired quantity in the required time period. If it is important that a limited, specific quantity of feed is to be delivered, use the appropriate function on the pump and set a total volume for delivery.
14. Connect the feed administration set to the tube.
15. Set the pump to run. The nurse should check the pump hourly and document the amount of feed that the pump has administered.
16. Aspirate the patient's tube every 4 hours to test that the tube remains correctly in situ in the stomach.
17. If the set is to be topped up with feed 4-hourly, then a cleaned work surface/trolley should be used

and apron and disposable gloves worn. The top of the feed container and the opening of the administration set are both wiped with alcohol before feed is put into the system (Anderton 1995).
18. Change the feed administration set every 24 hours (Anderton 1995).

Observations and complications of enteral feeding

Observations
- Check when the tube was last changed.
- Check the skin around a gastrostomy site for any signs of soreness caused by leakage from the stoma.
- Always check the position of the tube before using it. Be aware that blue litmus paper will not be sufficiently accurate to indicate an acid reaction if the child is on antireflux treatment. An acid reaction of 0–3 using pH paper is the safest way to indicate an acidic aspirate, therefore indicating that the tube is correctly placed.
- Whilst feeding, check that the child appears comfortable and is not showing signs of discomfort such as heaving or retching.
- Check the child's breathing and colour whilst administering the feed.

Complications
- Incorrect feed calculation could lead to too much or too little feed being given.
- The wrong feed or wrongly constituted feed could be given.
- The biggest risk of NG feeding is the tube being or becoming misplaced. This can cause feed to be delivered into the lungs or feed to be aspirated. If at any time during an NG feed the child becomes blue or has difficulty breathing, the feed must be stopped immediately, the tube aspirated and the child may require suction. It used to be common practice to check the position of an NG tube by listening with a stethoscope for the sound of air injected into the stomach via the NG tube. Research has shown this to be an inaccurate and dangerous practice (Hendry et al 1986, Metheny et al 1990).
- NG and gastrostomy tubes can also be misplaced in the wrong part of the gut. If either tube is in the small intestine rather than the stomach, aspirate will be obtained, but will not be acidic. In this case, the tube should be repositioned and re-checked for correct position before use.

- Vomiting can occur if the feed is given too fast.
- Tubes may become blocked, but force should never be applied to try to unblock them as this could damage the tube and increase the risk of feed being instilled in the wrong place. If a tube remains blocked, it must be removed.
- Rarely, a gastrostomy tube can migrate into the small intestine with the peristaltic action of the intestine. This can cause diarrhoea, vomiting and even intestinal obstruction and/or perforation, causing the child great discomfort and distress (Coldicutt 1994). Prevention is better than cure and the importance of correctly fitting and securing the tubes must be stressed.
- Bacterial contamination can lead to gastroenteritis.
- Prolonged absence of oral feeding can lead to developmental delay. Oral stimulation, sucking and swallowing can disappear and speech development can be affected (Evans Morris & Dunn Klein 1987, Taylor & Goodison-McLaren 1992). Manipulating food – chewing, swallowing, etc. – enables the child to learn the control of tongue and mouth muscles that is necessary to produce intelligible speech.

Without oral feeding, pleasant associations with oral stimulation such as gratification of hunger are lost and the child can become hypersensitised to touch and taste (Evans Morris & Dunn Klein 1987). This makes it increasingly difficult to reintroduce oral feeding after prolonged NG/gastrostomy feeding when the only associations with oral feeding are unpleasant sensations, e.g. vomiting and suction (Langley 1994). This can then lead to problems with social development as the child may not learn appropriate social behaviour associated with meal times.

All these aspects of development must be considered and action taken to try to mitigate the negative side-effects in children who are unable to feed orally.

COMMUNITY PERSPECTIVE

Many children who require enteral feeding are cared for by their families at home. It is therefore imperative that the carers are aware of all aspects of this care, including potential pitfalls.

Organisation of equipment is essential prior to discharge. This may include a feed pump and an ongoing supply of disposable equipment, nasogastric tubes, syringes, feed bags, gastrostomy button extension tubes, litmus paper, etc. It can be frustrating if a child's discharge from hospital is delayed because of lack of supplies. Parents also need to know who to contact for further supplies, whether this is a company supplying the entire package, e.g. Caremark, or a local chemist, a community dietitian or the CCN. They must also be aware of local policy regarding the servicing of feed pumps. In smaller houses, the sheer volume of supplies needing to be stored can be a problem.

The role of the CCN is to support the carers, ensuring that they are not only competent in the techniques required but are also happy to undertake them. Whereas enteral feeding is a routine procedure in hospital, it is a major commitment for families at home, both physically and emotionally.

Concerns about altered body image may be problematic for parents, siblings and the sick child herself. The CCN will have the opportunity to recognise and address any such problems in the safe environment of the home. If necessary she may refer the family for further psychological support.

Nasogastric feeding

Some parents are happy to undertake not only the technique of feeding but also that of replacing the tube. This is advantageous for carers and nursing staff, as tubes are frequently pulled up at most inconvenient times, resulting either in parents having to trek back to hospital at short notice or community nurses having to reorganise their schedules to ensure that a child does not miss a feed.

Passing a nasogastric tube can be a frightening experience on the first few occasions and support for the carer at this time is vital. The opportunity to undertake the procedure in hospital prior to discharge is therefore most helpful and, on the first few occasions at home, the presence of a member of the CCN team is reassuring. There is the added advantage that the CCN can observe the carer's technique and check her level of knowledge. Discussion can take place at this time on how to modify infection control measures, as the risk of cross-infection in the home is smaller. Sensible hygiene precautions with emphasis on hand-washing techniques are more appropriate as it is important that the home does not become an extension of hospital. The importance of including the tube-fed child at family meal times should not be overlooked, the emphasis being on the maintenance of as normal an environment as possible. Parents should not be pressurised into taking on the responsibility of repassing the nasogastric tube if they are reluctant. Often when they have gained confidence in managing feeds at home, they will feel ready to take on this skill.

It is important to remember mouth care (see Oral Hygiene, p. 179). Twice daily brushing of the teeth and the use of mouth washes will improve the feel of the mouth as well as being good health promotion.

A useful tip to stop the skin on the cheeks becoming sore is to apply a strip of Stomahesive or Granuflex wafer to the cheek (see above, p. 119). The tape securing the tube is thus stuck to the wafer, rather than directly to the skin.

Gastrostomy feeding

Gastrostomy feeding is likely to be long term and therefore the child or the family will undertake the majority, if not all, of the care. The procedure should therefore fit in with the family's normal lifestyle and not dictate it. They should therefore be in a position to make decisions, in conjunction with medical, nursing and dietetic staff, relating to the type of device and the administration of the feed.

In addition to the points related to nasogastric feeding, the family need to be aware of the following:

- The stoma site should be cleaned with mild soap and warm water every day, care being taken to dry the area well.
- As part of this routine, the device must be turned daily. This helps form a healthy stoma and prevents the formation of adhesions.
- The use of Sofradex eye ointment around the entry site is often helpful if the area around the stoma appears inflamed, or granulation tissue is forming.
- Once a stoma site is fully healed, after 2–3 weeks, bathing and swimming are allowed.
- Balloon devices should be deflated and reinflated weekly to ensure that the correct amount of fluid remains in the balloon.
- When and how to change a balloon device.
- Methods of unblocking tubes, using carbonated water, pineapple juice, coca cola or Pancrex.
- Manufacturers' recommended life of button extension sets, as these vary considerably.
- How to use a decompression tube if applicable.

The aim of the CCN is to ensure that families are empowered to give the recommended nutritional support to their child, whilst maintaining as relaxed a home environment as possible. This is best achieved by ensuring a smooth transition from hospital to home and providing ongoing support from the appropriate members of the multidisciplinary team without overwhelming families with professional input. Respite care should if possible be offered, either by nursing staff or by carers especially trained to undertake this care.

Do and do not

- Do always check that NG and gastrostomy tubes are correctly positioned before instilling anything into the tube.
- Do stop an NG feed immediately if the child experiences difficulty in breathing or develops cyanosis.
- Do aspirate and flush NG tubes 4-hourly to check position and maintain patency.
- Do secure a gastrostomy tube carefully to prevent peristalsis causing the tube to migrate into the wrong part of the intestine.
- Do encourage the child who is not fed orally to use her mouth in play – blowing, kissing, touching her mouth and putting fingers into her mouth.
- Do take all measures to prevent bacterial contamination of feed.
- Do not ever use an NG or gastrostomy tube if there is any doubt that it is correctly placed in the stomach.

References

Anderton A 1995 Reducing bacterial contamination in enteral tube feeds. British Journal of Nursing 4(7): 368–376

Booth I W 1991 Enteral nutrition in childhood. British Journal of Hospital Medicine 46: 111–113

Coldicutt P 1994 Children's options. Nursing Times 90(13): 54–56

Evans Morris S, Dunn Klein M 1987 Pre-feeding skills. A comprehensive resource for feeding development. Therapy Skill Builders, USA, pp 320, 352

Gauderer M W L, Olsen M M, Stellato T A et al 1988 Feeding gastrostomy button: experience and recommendations. Journal of Pediatric Surgery 23: 24–28

Hambridge K M, Sokol R J, Krebs N F 1995 Enteral and parenteral alimentation. In: Roy C, Silverman A, Alagille D (eds) Paediatric clinical gastroenterology, 4th edn. Mosby, St Louis, ch 37, p 1030

Hendry P J, Akyurekli M D, McIntyre R, Quarrington A, Keon W J 1986 Bronchopulmonary complications of nasogastric feeding tubes. Critical Care Medicine 14(10): 892–894

Holden C E, McDonald A, Ward M et al 1997 Psychological preparation for nasogastric feeding in children. British Journal of Nursing 6(7): 376–381, 384–385

Langley P 1994 From tube to table. Nursing Times 90(48): 43–46

Lifshitz F, Finch N M, Lifshitz J Z 1991 Children's nutrition. Jones & Bartlett, Boston, ch 27, p 518

Merck Tube Manufacturer's Guidelines. Bio Material, Lenten House, Lenten Street Alton, Hampshire G034 18G

Metheny N, McSweeney M, Wehrle M A, Liersema L 1990 Nursing Research 39(5): 14

Paul L, Holden C, Smith A et al 1993 Tube feeding and you. Birmingham Children's Hospital NHS Trust, Birmingham

Paul L A, Holden C, Smith A et al 1994 Gastrostomy feeding and you. Birmingham Children's Hospital NHS Trust, Birmingham

Sidey A 1995 Enteral feeding in community settings. Paediatric Nursing 7(6): 21–24

Taylor S, Goodison-McLaren 1992 Nutritional support – a team approach. Wolfe Publishing, London, ch 15, pp 258, 273

Further reading

Booklets produced by the manufacturers of the devices

Holden C E, Pontis J W L, Charlton C P L, Booth I W 1990 Naso-gastric feeding at home, acceptability and safety. Archives of Disease in Childhood 66: 148–154

Holden C, McDonald A, Ward M et al 1987 Feeding time with Roo and Joe. Sherwood Medical Industries, Crawley

Patchell C J, Anderton A, MacDonald A, George R H, Booth I W 1994 Bacterial contamination of enteral feeds. Archives of Disease in Childhood 70: 327–330

Sidey A, Torbet S 1995 Enteral feeding in community settings. Paediatric Nursing 7(6): 21–23

13

Gastric Lavage

Introduction

Improperly stored household products, such as bleach, cleaning materials and medications like paracetamol, pose the greatest danger to the curious child.

There are a variety of treatments used to minimise the effects of these ingestions, including the use of syrup of ipecacuanha, activated charcoal and gastric lavage.

Although gastric emptying remains a controversial method of treatment for toxic ingestions (Emergency Medicine 1991, Proudfoot 1993), this method of treatment is still routinely used in emergency departments of children's hospitals.

Although gastric lavage is mainly associated with poisoning, there are other therapeutic uses for lavage. Gastrointestinal tract haemorrhage is rare in children; however, upper gastrointestinal bleeding, as a result of oesophageal varices, can be controlled by gastric lavage using chilled fluid (Abernathy et al 1994).

Gastric aspirate may be obtained to help in the diagnosis of tuberculosis (Campbell & McIntosh 1992, Summitt 1990).

In cases of pyloric stenosis where there is persistent excessive vomiting preoperatively, gastric lavage may be performed.

Learning outcomes

On completion of this section the nurse should be able to:

- explain the reasons for performing gastric lavage in children
- identify the child requiring gastric lavage
- perform gastric lavage safely.

Rationale

The stomach of the child who has ingested a toxic substance can be emptied by inducing vomiting or by passing a gastric lavage tube and manually evacuating the contents. Whether induction of vomiting is more efficient than gastric lavage, or vice versa, in recovering ingested substances is doubtful, as neither will empty the stomach completely (Proudfoot 1993).

The decision on which method to adopt depends on age, degree of cooperation and conscious level. Although induction of vomiting is the preferred method used for emptying the stomach in children, there are circumstances which necessitate the use of gastric lavage. Gastric lavage has a diagnostic purpose as well as being therapeutic.

Factors to note

In children over 6 months old the first-line management of ingestion of a toxic substance, where gastric emptying is advised, is the use of syrup of ipecacuanha.

Recommended doses of syrup of ipecacuanha are related to the age of the child.

Gastric lavage is not indicated in cases of caustic substance ingestion.

Children seen within 1–2 hours following a known large ingestion of a toxic substance benefit from gastric lavage (Barkin & Rosen 1994, Deason 1995).

Children who are convulsing, comatosed or uncooperative should be considered for lavage.

Loss of the gag reflex will result in aspiration if vomiting is induced. In these cases gastric lavage is indicated.

For the aforementioned, the airway should be protected using a cuffed endotracheal tube, which is inserted by the anaesthetist prior to performing gastric lavage.

The use of gastric lavage in treating hydrocarbon ingestions, e.g. turpentine substitute or white spirit, is controversial.

Chilled fluid should be used if lavage is being performed to control an upper gastrointestinal bleed.

Obtaining a gastric aspirate to help in the diagnosis of tuberculosis is normally performed in the morning once the child has been fasted (Summitt 1990).

Always refer to the local or national poison information centre for advice regarding gastric emptying. Most casualty units now have Toxbase computers for direct access and immediate information.

Equipment
- Large-bore gastric tube
- Funnel/catheter tip syringe
- Beaker or calibrated jug to measure fluid.
- Appropriately sized cuffed endotracheal tube
- Water-soluble lubricant
- Warmed lavage fluid; chilled fluid should be used if being used to control bleeding
- Collecting receptacle
- Specimen container (if required)
- Gloves, goggles and gown or plastic apron
- Blanket to swaddle child (if required)

Method
- Explain the procedure to the child and parent.
- Protect the child's airway. This may involve endotracheal intubation by the anaesthetist.
- Position the child on his left side and elevate the foot of the bed/trolley (Trendelenburg position). This will help to prevent aspiration in the unintubated child, and aid drainage by syphonage.
- Select a large-bore orogastric tube. The size of the tube will depend on the substance that has been ingested or the reason for performing the lavage, i.e. a smaller tube may be used for controlling a gastrointestinal bleed or obtaining an aspirate for analysis. A smaller-bore tube may be used if a fluid has been ingested.
- Lubricate the tube using water-based lubricant and slowly insert the tube into the mouth, down the oesophagus and into the stomach.
- Ensure that the tube is in the correct position by aspirating the stomach contents.
- Attach the funnel/catheter tip syringe to the end of the tube and instil the warmed lavage solution into the child's stomach. The amount of fluid is based on 15 ml/kg of body weight (Wojner 1993).
- Once the fluid has been instilled into the stomach, the upper abdomen may be gently massaged to enhance distribution of the lavage fluid within the stomach and hence removal of toxin (Wojner 1993).
- Aspirate the fluid or allow it to drain from the stomach by syphonage, depending on local policy.
- Repeat the procedure until the effluent is clear.
- Once the effluent is clear, activated charcoal, an agent to reduce absorption of toxins, or an antidote to the toxin may be prescribed by the medical staff

for instillation, in order to limit the effects of the toxins.
- Pinch the tube and remove it gently.
- Leave the child comfortable.

Observations and complications
- Ensure that the child's airway is protected as there is the danger of aspiration of gastric contents.
- Measure the appropriate amount of warmed/chilled fluid accurately.
- Maintain accurate records of the fluid used and the fluid obtained.
- Observe the effluent for signs of toxic substance. Retain a sample, occasionally all, of the effluent for laboratory analysis.
- Oesophageal perforation may occur during insertion of the tube. If blood is noted in the aspirated fluid, stop the procedure immediately and inform the medical staff.

Do and do not
- Do ensure that the child's airway is protected.
- Do ensure that the child's head is lower than his abdomen throughout the procedure. This aids gastric emptying.
- Do have oxygen, suction and resuscitation equipment available at hand.
- Do not use excessive force when inserting the tube.

References
Abernathy T L, Beck M L, Becker S I et al 1994 Handbook of therapeutic interventions. Springhouse, Pennsylvania

Barkin R M, Rosen P 1994 Emergency pediatrics. A guide to ambulatory care, 4th edn. Mosby, St. Louis

Campbell A G M, McIntosh N 1992 Forfar and Arneil's textbook of paediatrics, 4th edn. Churchill Livingstone, Edinburgh

Deason J G 1995 Acute iron ingestion in a 2 year old child. Journal of Emergency Nursing 21(1): 9–11

Emergency Medicine 1991 Is gastric emptying harmful? Emergency Medicine 23(10): 83–84

Proudfoot A T 1993 Acute poisoning, 2nd edn. Butterworth-Heinemann, Oxford

Summitt R L 1990 Comprehensive pediatrics. Mosby, St. Louis

Wojner A W 1993 Seconds count when a child is poisoned. Registered Nurse 56(10): 46–52

Further reading
Barkin R M, Rosen P 1994 Emergency pediatrics. A guide to ambulatory care, 4th edn. Mosby, St. Louis

Paynter M 1993 Gastric lavage in accident and emergency.
    Nursing Standard 7(18): 32–33

14

Hygiene

Introduction and rationale

Meeting the child's hygiene needs is an essential element of nursing care; it will enhance comfort, promote self-esteem and prevent infection. As the child grows physically and becomes more independent, these needs change.

This section describes hygiene practices for normal children, at home or in hospital. More specific care of problems common in sick children can be found in other sections.

Learning outcomes

After reading this section, the nurse should be able to explain:

- essential hygiene practices for the healthy child
- prevention of cross-infection through good hygiene practice
- adaptation of techniques to suit the sick child.

Factors to note

Observation

Performing hygiene tasks for a baby or child gives the nurse a privileged opportunity to observe and monitor the health or general well-being of a child. As each element of hygiene care is performed, there is an opportunity for detailed assessment of the condition of a particular area (for example ears or eyes). The nurse may observe, for example, signs of malnutrition; chest recession in a child with respiratory distress; bruises or bite marks on a child who has been abused; skin infections such as impetigo or ringworm. Assisting a child with hygiene tasks also gives the nurse an opportunity for health education.

Privacy

The nurse should respect the differing need for privacy at different stages of development. In the older child or adolescent, a need for privacy emerges as sexual awareness develops. Illness and disability require that intimate tasks, that would normally be performed by the child or

teenager herself, may need to be performed by nurses and parents. The nurse should involve parents where appropriate, allocating same-sex nurses and carers if requested and feasible given staffing resources, and encourage independence and self-care where possible.

Routine

Hygiene tasks form an important element of the child's daily routine in many households, sometimes developing into ritualistic behaviour. The admitting nurse should ask about these routines, and they should be maintained as much as possible while the child is in hospital or sick at home. Keeping to established routine provides comfort and reassurance to the child, especially during periods of stress.

Cross-infection

Good hygiene represents an important defence against infection. A child's ability to fight infection will depend on her age, health and immunological status. If we over-protect children from normal contact with micro-organisms, we can render them unable to develop a natural immunity, but allowing children to develop preventable illness because of sloppy hygiene practices is unacceptable.

Guidelines

Before commencing any hygiene task, consider:

- Is the task really necessary? Children who are sick, or babies who are premature, should be left in peace with minimal disturbance unless there is a good reason to do otherwise.
- Have you collected all necessary equipment together?
- Could any other aspect of care be combined with hygiene needs? Examples include: observations of vital signs, topical drug administration, specimen collection.
- Could the parents be involved in performing the task, or would they prefer the nurse to do it?

- What can the child do independently? Or what can the child begin to learn to do on her own? If a child is able to learn a basic skill, for example hairbrushing or getting dressed, in hospital, this will give her a personal sense of achievement and a feeling that something positive has occurred.
- How can you make the experience fun? Can you introduce play or toys into the experience?

Infection control: good practice

Universal precautions to prevent infection should be taken (see Control of Infection, p. 13). Hands should be washed thoroughly before and after handling any baby or child, in the home or in hospital, and especially before any procedure requiring intimate contact, such as feeding or bathing. If dealing with body fluids, the nurse should wear gloves.

Newborn baby care

The newborn infant is covered with a protective substance called vernix caseosa and with blood from the mother. Birth is a traumatic, exhausting experience for mother, father, and baby. Midwives now resist the impulse to bath the baby immediately after birth; instead, excess moisture is wiped away and the infant is placed naked on the mother's abdomen or breast, covered perhaps by a clean towel to maintain warmth. Bathing can wait till parents and baby have recovered from the birth and can participate fully in the event.

The timing of hygiene activities should be planned for when the baby will enjoy them, when she is awake and content. For example, nappies should be changed regularly, as the acidity of urine and faeces can cause nappy rash and cause discomfort (Scowen 1995). The timing will depend on circumstances. On balance, changing a nappy immediately before a feed is preferable, though it can be frustrating for the baby, who will cry from hunger. Changing the nappy immediately after a feed may make the baby sick, or interrupt the progression to a postprandial snooze. However, if the baby has defecated during feeding, the nappy should be changed after the feed.

Hygiene activities can form a useful way for mother and baby to bond. They give an opportunity for face-to-face contact, touch and 'talking'. For example, if the newborn baby is in a neonatal intensive care unit, inviting the mother to help with these activities can encourage bonding when she can no longer fulfil other caring functions.

Bathing very newborn babies daily is unnecessary, and may be unwise if the cord is still in situ (Skale 1992). Newborn babies do not get especially dirty, as older babies and toddlers do. Many newborn babies are distressed if undressed; being naked leaves them insecure and exposed. Their body temperature may be lowered unnecessarily when undressed. Newborn babies' skin should be slightly dry and flaky (though not cracked); the instinct to apply moisturising creams is inappropriate (Brennan 1996).

Topping and tailing is a useful alternative to bathing.

Top and tailing

Equipment

- A small dish of warm clean sterile water for the baby's eyes and face
- A bowl of warm water for the nappy area
- Non-sterile swabs for eye care (or at home a clean soft cloth) (*Note:* Cotton wool balls should not be used, as, if small cotton strands enter underneath the eyelid, they can damage the cornea; see also Eye Care, p. 103.)
- Cotton wool balls/wash wipes/clean soft flannel for the rest of the baby's body
- Soap or baby bath solution is not necessary unless the baby's nappy area is very soiled (Brennan 1996)
- A clean nappy
- Disposal bag or bucket for soiled nappy and clothes
- Nappy creams are not necessary under normal circumstances, if the baby is changed regularly (Brennan 1996); however, if a baby is prone to nappy rash, a protective barrier cream can be useful
- Soft baby hairbrush
- Clean clothes
- Clean towel
  (*Note:* Many parents use talcum powder, but the hygiene benefits of this are unclear. Powder tends to cling and cake to moist areas, can cause skin irritation, and can be inhaled by the baby (Skale 1992, Campbell & Glasper 1995).)

Method

- Ensure that the room is warm and comfortable, with no cool draughts.
- Place the baby, dressed, on the towel.
- Clean the baby's eyes. (Clean the corners and outside the eye; do not attempt to clean under the lids.) Use a different swab for each eye, to prevent cross-infection. Gently wash the rest of the face and around the mouth before commencing, with a clean cloth or swabs. Pat dry gently.

- Do not attempt to clean inside any orifice, be it nose, eye, ear or mouth. All body orifices clean themselves naturally by production and secretion of mucus or fluid.
- Wash baby's hands with a wet washcloth, and dry. If nails are long, snip very carefully with blunt-ended baby scissors.
- Undress the baby so that the nappy area is accessible. With most baby clothing this is possible without undressing the baby fully.
- Take off the nappy. If the baby is wet, just clean with warm water. If the baby is soiled, wipe excess faeces away with cotton wool balls, the nappy or wipes. Observe for nappy rash. Always clean from front to back, thus avoiding contaminating the urethra with faeces. Wash the baby's bottom with a washcloth and dry.
- Only the visible surface of genitalia should be cleaned: do not retract the foreskin (which often will not retract till the boy is much older anyway) or clean inside the labia in a girl.
- Put on a clean nappy (underneath the umbilicus if the cord is still attached) and dress the baby in clean clothes.

Umbilical cord care

Umbilical sepsis is a cause of septicaemia and neonatal infection. However, the reduction in the incidence of staphylococcal infection, along with anxieties about the safety of traditional hexachlorophane treatment in the 1980s, led many units to opt for a non-interventionist policy, keeping the cord clean and dry but not using antiseptic treatments (Bourk 1989/1990). Practices in UK hospitals now vary widely, which is confusing to nurse and parent alike.

In 1993 a study by Verber & Pagan examined a variety of different regimes of cord care. The regimes examined included:

- hexachlorophane powder (Sterzac) to umbilicus, axilla and groin during routine morning care, and to umbilicus only at other nappy changes
- dry cord care (no intervention other than to keep clean and dry)
- chlorhexidine 4% detergent liquid (Hibiscrub), once daily, massaged into the cord for 2 minutes, then rinsed off in the bath (these infants were bathed daily from day 1, other infants were bathed from day 4)
- no intervention apart from daily bathing from day 1.

The results showed a clear reduction in colonisation of staphylococci for the babies treated with chlorhexidine,

and a slightly less, but still significant, reduction in colonisation for those treated with hexachlorophane. Cross-infection between infants and staff was reduced with either method. Chlorhexidine resulted in delayed cord separation, and the midwives found it difficult and unpleasant to use. Hexachlorophane powder has for some time now been shown to be safe (Plueckhahn & Collins 1976). The authors of this study therefore recommend treatment of all neonates with hexachlorophane powder.

The umbilical area must be observed for infection and swabbed for microbiological culture if any signs of infection are present (raised temperature, general unwellness, redness, inflammation, swelling of umbilicus or surrounding skin). If there is evidence of infection, systemic antibiotics will be required. If an umbilical catheter is in situ, care should be as for an intravenous or arterial line: the line must be secured carefully and the entry site kept clean and dry; a strict aseptic technique should be used if handling is necessary.

Baby bath

Newborn babies, as mentioned above, do not need bathing daily unless they are sick or have very dirty nappies. Babies who are crawling will get very dirty indeed and a daily bath becomes a necessity. A baby bath may be too stressful for a sick child, for example a child with breathing difficulties or neurological disturbance. If this is the case, a top and tail can be performed instead.

Equipment

As for top and tail.
The baby bath itself should be prepared, adding cold water first, then warm, to reduce the risk of the water not mixing properly and hotter water remaining at the base of the tub. The water temperature should be comfortable; 29–32°C is recommended by Leach (1989). It is essential that the temperature of the water is tested; a scald can occur if the water is too hot. The traditional method of assessing the temperature of the bath is to dip one's elbow into the water. It should feel comfortably warm. A water thermometer can be used by those who are inexperienced in this technique.

Method
- Make sure that the bath is placed at a comfortable height, preferably on a stand. Kneel or sit, whichever is easiest. Stooping while holding the baby can lead to back problems, and will mean that the person bathing the baby cannot relax and enjoy the occasion.

- Undress the baby. If the nappy area is very soiled, clean off the faeces with cotton wool balls or wipes. Wrap the baby securely in a towel.
- Clean the baby's eyes, face and mouth before commencing, with a clean cloth or swabs. Start with the eyes, and use a different swab or corner of a clean flannel for each eye, to prevent cross-infection.
- Whilst the baby is still wrapped in the towel, hold her head over the bath and gently wash water over the hair, avoiding the eyes. Mild shampoo or a small quantity of baby bath solution can be used, though they are not strictly necessary. Use a corner of the towel to dry the hair.
- Unwrap the towel. Hold the baby securely, with one hand grasping the farther upper arm, and the baby's neck and shoulders supported on the forearm (see Fig. 14.1). Place the baby gently in the water, allowing her a little time to get used to the sensation. If the baby is learning to sit, support her sitting in the water with a hand around her back, but *never* leave her unsupported. It can only take a moment for a baby to topple over. This may put the baby off baths for some time or, in the worst

scenario, the baby may drown. A non-slip mat or seat cradle should be used to prevent an accidental slip.
- If bathing an active baby in the 'big' bath, make sure she cannot accidentally touch the hot tap.
- Gently wash the baby with the free hand, under the arms, her back and the nappy area. Pay particular attention to skin creases. Allow the baby to kick and splash, exploring the weightless sensation. This should be fun for both carer and baby, but if the baby is clearly distressed, bring her out of the bath as soon as possible.
- Do not let the baby lose heat.
- Wrap the baby in the towel. When dry, dress her in clean dry clothes. The room should be warm enough for older babies to play naked for a while, to kick and wriggle, free from the constraints of a nappy.

Oral care

As soon as teeth erupt, a toothbrushing routine should commence. A small soft toothbrush can be used with a pea-sized amount of toothpaste. Advice from local

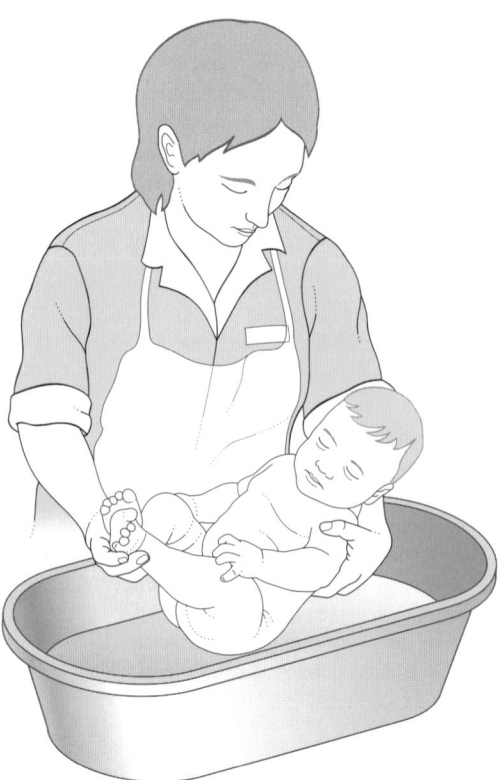

Figure 14.1
Holding baby safely for a bath.

health visitors should be sought about whether additional fluoride is necessary (Bowsher 1997). (See also Oral Hygiene, p. 179.)

Other aspects of baby hygiene

Good hygiene practice also involves keeping the baby's environment, and anything she is likely to come into contact with, clean. Newborn babies have very little defence against microorganisms; once the placental transference of immunity has worn off at 3 months, or breastfeeding has stopped, babies must develop their own defences.

The most likely sources of contaminants are feeds, feeding bottles or pacifiers. If formula feeds are to be used, they must be made up under sterile conditions. Feeding bottles and pacifiers should be sterilised. Weaning foods must be prepared using strict food hygiene practice. (See also Feeding, Part 1, p. 107.)

Once the child is older and can reach for toys and put them in her mouth (usually at about 3 months), toys should be kept 'socially' clean, though sterilising them is not necessary.

Handwashing is important for all carers and siblings. Older children should be told to wash their own hands after using the toilet and before and after meals, especially if they want to hold or touch the baby, or share toys.

The environment around a baby, at home or within a hospital cubicle or ward, should be clean and as free as possible from excessive build-up of dust and dirt. Once a child is crawling, the floor and other surfaces should be kept socially clean.

Visitors, including staff, who have coughs or colds or other infections should not have intimate care of a baby.

The toddler and preschool child

A healthy normal toddler will probably spend a lot of time on the floor, in the dirt outdoors, or exploring the content of the rubbish bin or dog faeces in the park. A preschool child will be a little more discriminatory about what she explores, but will still get very dirty through play. A daily bath or shower will become essential. Frequent washes of face and hands before, after and in between meals will also be necessary. Nappies should be changed every few hours. Preschool children who are toilet trained are unlikely to be able to wipe themselves clean after defecating, and help should be

given. Hands should always be washed after using the toilet.

Toddlers are learning and developing fast through play and experience, but can also become immensely frustrated, especially when they cannot understand *why* they must have a clean face, change clothes or get in the bath.

Preschool children are developing independence, as well as gross and fine motor skills. They will be learning how to make choices within certain limits, for example deciding between baby or adult toothpaste, soap or bubble bath.

Even if a child is ill, make hygiene activities fun, develop a comforting routine, encourage the child's independence and learning.

Most toddlers and preschool children enjoy a bath, and will happily play in the water; either a soapy bath solution or soap can be used, though soap in the eyes can sting badly. If the child has eczema, special bath solutions and creams may be necessary. Some children will dislike baths, and prefer spraying themselves with the shower head, or having a sponge bath.

Safety is paramount and small children must not be left alone in the bath even for a moment. They should be warned not to touch the hot tap, and the temperature of the hot water should be controlled so it cannot scald if turned on accidentally.

Attention will also need to be paid to hair, teeth and nails, continuing routines which should start as a baby. Children under 7 years of age will need to have their teeth brushed for them, as it is unlikely that they have developed sufficient dexterity. A good idea is to get the child to start brushing her own teeth, and for the parent to finish the task (Bowsher 1997). (See also Oral Hygiene, p. 179.)

Hairwashing can become a battleground unless it is handled sensitively. Children hate getting shampoo into their eyes, and great ingenuity is used by most parents to make hairwashing fun and painless. Hair should be examined periodically for head lice, a common infestation once the child has started mixing at toddlers' groups or playschool.

Children learn by imitation. By watching their parents or older siblings wash their hair, have showers, or brush their teeth, they will want to copy them (Cadoff 1995). All children need praise and reward for good behaviour, and approval from their parents.

At this age, toys, eating utensils, carpets, etc. should be kept socially clean, but do not need to be sterilised.

Older school children and adolescents

As school children grow older they become more independent. Hygiene needs change as the body changes in adolescence: problems with acne, greasy hair or body odour may emerge; the menarche will occur and other sexual changes of puberty. Such changes can be disturbing even for the best-prepared teenager, especially when they manifest themselves outside the safety and reassurance of home or school. Teenagers can be very embarrassed if they cannot manage their own hygiene needs independently (Atmarow et al 1993). Sensitivity is needed if the adolescent requires assistance with hygiene activities in hospital.

The bed bath

A bed bath is usually given when a child is too sick or disabled to get into a proper bath, and when a 'top and tail' wash is insufficient. Critically ill or unconscious children, children who have fevers and are sweating profusely, or children in traction after orthopaedic surgery may all need bed baths.

Parents and children should be asked whether they would like the nurse to give the bed bath, or whether they would prefer the parent to do it. To some parents of chronically ill children it can be a welcome relief to have someone take over this aspect of care, whereas to parents of children who are acutely ill, continuing to care for their child's hygiene needs can be a way of maintaining control and feeling useful. The children may much prefer the parents to give the care, and their preferences should be respected.

The basic principles of a bed bath are:

- being well organised
- privacy
- comfort
- total body care.

Equipment
- Wash bowl with warm water
- Flannels or washcloths: at least two, one for the face and one for the genital area
- Soap or bath solution
- Disposal bag
- Linen skip
- Hairbrush or comb
- Toothbrush

- Nail scissors
- Clean towel
- Clean clothes or night clothes
- Clean bedlinen

Make sure that there is sufficient of everything. Ensure that the water remains hot enough; it may need changing several times, if it becomes cool or particularly soapy or dirty.

Method
- Discuss the need for a bed bath with the child and parents. Explain what will occur.
- Ensure that the child is given privacy, for example curtains around the bed.
- Raise the bed to a comfortable working height. Ensure that you are comfortable and safe; you may need assistance from colleagues or parents with turning or lifting. Use manual handling aids where possible. Do not stretch over the bed, but walk around to the other side if necessary.
- Strip the bed and bed area of any non-essential items or bedclothes. Clear a surface, either a trolley or bedside table, for washing equipment.
- Undress the patient and leave covered with a flannelette sheet and/or gown.
- Wash the patient's eyes, using a different corner of the washcloth for each eye. Use more specific eye care if indicated (see Eye Care, p. 103).
- Wash the child's face, paying special attention to mouth and ears (see Oral Hygiene, p. 179; Ear Care, p. 99). Help the child to clean her teeth.
- Before washing each body part, place a dry towel beneath it to prevent water dripping onto the sheets.
- Cover the upper body with a sheet or towel, but leave the arms exposed. Using soap and water, or bath solution or special lotion, wash the child's hands, and trim and clean the nails if necessary. Wash each arm, paying particular attention to hands and nails, and the underarm area. Rinse the flannel and rinse off the soap. Rinsing may need to be repeated.
- Gently remove the cover from the upper body, leaving genitalia covered, and wash and rinse the chest and abdomen.
- Cover the upper body again, and wash the front of the legs and feet. Check for pressure sores on heels or ankles (see Pressure Area Care, p. 235).
- With a different washcloth or flannel, wash the 'front' genitalia and rinse. Children or adolescents may prefer to do this for themselves, if possible. (*Note:* For boys post-puberty, the foreskin should be pulled back and the penis washed underneath (Campbell & Glasper 1995)).

- With assistance, turn the patient onto one side.
- Wash back, legs and finally buttocks, and dry.
- Position the patient comfortably.
- Brush or comb the hair, and check behind the head for skin lesions or sores. If hairwashing is necessary and the child can tolerate the procedure, wash the hair by holding the child's head over the end of the bed (help will be needed) over a washbowl, using a jug to rinse.
- Dress the patient in clean clothes as appropriate.
- Tidy away the bowl of water and wash things.

At the same time as doing a bed bath there may be an opportunity to:

- Slide in a clean sheet to replace the old bottom sheet; top sheet and pillow slips may also need replacing.
- Change the position of leads from monitoring equipment, or of catheters or tubes taped to the skin, to avoid skin irritation or damage due to prolonged adhesion or pressure. Some units will have their own local policies on frequency of repositioning. Clean off any remaining adhesive with a gentle adhesive remover.
- Perform passive limb exercises if indicated.
- Perform other nursing care, for example observations, topical skin treatments.
- Talk with the child. This may be an opportunity for the child to express her fears and thoughts about her illness, or just to have a good chat.
- Use play and make the bed bath fun. The more alert child will enjoy toys and games appropriate for her age; if the child has learning or sensory disabilities she may enjoy the touch, smell, feel of the experience.

'Bag baths'. Carruth et al (1995) describe an alternative technique, a 'bag bath', in which eight washcloths are placed in a polythene bag, together with a measured amount of dilute moisturising wash solution, and heated in a microwave. One washcloth is used for each limb or body area. The skin is left to air dry. They reported a significant improvement in comfort, reduction in cross-infection, and savings in laundry and linen costs and in nursing time.

> ## COMMUNITY PERSPECTIVE
> The hygiene of the sick child who is at home will, as a general rule, be undertaken by the family. There may be occasions when they require help with this care and this gives the CCN the opportunity to assess the child in an informal but effective manner. It is important not to be judgemental about the family's standards of hygiene unless they pose a threat to the child's well-being.

References

Atmarow G, Blomfield J, Brady S 1993 The clean gang: the health education teaching package designed for schoolchildren. Nursing Times 89(45): 30–32

Bourk E 1989/1990 Cord care: too much or too little? Australian Journal of Advanced Nursing 7(2): 19–22

Bowsher J 1997 Paediatric dental care: oral care in the early years. Professional Care of Mother and Child 7(2): 47–49

Brennan G 1996 Opinion: care of the new born baby's skin. Midwives 109(1303): 240

Cadoff J 1995 Just like mommy! Your child learns how to wash, comb, and brush from watching you. Parents Magazine 70(2): 70, 77

Campbell S, Glasper E A (eds) 1995 Whaley and Wong's children's nursing. Mosby, London

Carruth A K, Ricks D, Pullen P 1995 Bag baths, an alternative to the bed bath. Nursing Management 26(9): 75–78

Leach P 1989 Baby and child: from birth to five years, 2nd edn. Penguin, London

Plueckhahn V D, Collins R B 1976 Hexachlorophane emulsions and antiseptic skin care of newborn infants. Medical Journal of Australia 1(22): 815–819

Scowen P 1995 Skin care and nappy rash. Professional Care Of Mother and Child 5(5): 138

Skale N 1992 Manual of paediatric nursing procedures. J B Lippincott, Pennsylvania

Verber I G, Pagan F S 1993 What cord care; if any? Archives of Disease in Childhood 68(5): 594–596

15

Incubator Care

Introduction

The maintenance of a neutral thermal environment is of the utmost importance when nursing the preterm, ill or cold infant. A neutral thermal environment is one which balances heat production and heat conservation and dissipation, thus enabling the infant to maintain a normal core temperature with minimal oxygen requirements and calorie expenditure (Campbell & Glasper 1995, Marshall 1997).

The neutral thermal environment can be maintained in three main ways:

- by the use of an open crib with blankets and clothing: the dressed infant covered with blankets has the ability to maintain body temperature within a wide range of environmental temperatures; however, observation is greatly diminished
- by using radiant heaters, e.g. Baby Therms: infants can be nursed naked allowing for improved observation of the ill infant
- by using an incubator, where infants can be nursed naked (Fig. 15.1); however, the environment is enclosed.

This section discusses the care of the infant nursed in an incubator.

Learning outcomes

By the end of this section the nurse should:

- develop an understanding of thermoregulation in the term and preterm infant
- be able to identify the infant who requires to be nursed in an incubator
- be able to prepare an incubator to receive an ill infant
- demonstrate an understanding of temperature regulation devices used in the incubator

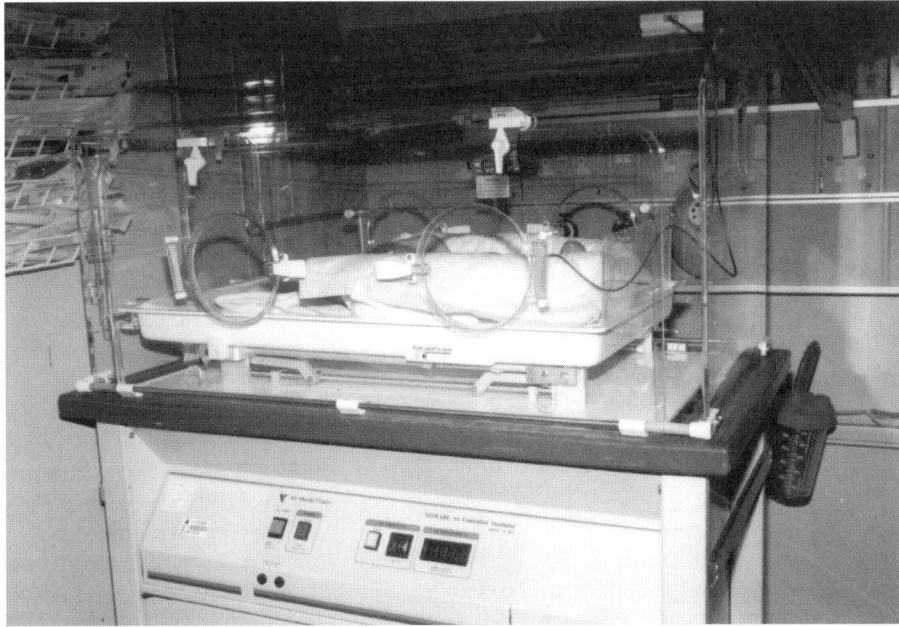

Figure 15.1
Infant being nursed in an incubator.

- provide safe and effective care to the infant nursed in the incubator.

Rationale

Both term and preterm infants have difficulty in maintaining body temperature owing to an inability to control their heat loss. Prevention of heat loss in ill and distressed infants is crucial to their survival; thus the provision of a neutral thermal environment when nursing the infant is of the utmost importance (Campbell & Glasper 1995). Environmental temperature which maintains the infant's skin temperature between 36.5 and 37.5°C (rectal 37°C) is known to promote minimal metabolic rate and oxygen consumption (Hazinski 1992, Merenstein & Gardiner 1993). This is defined as the neutral thermal environment.

Factors to note

Infants are at risk of poor temperature control caused by an immature hypothalamus resulting in poor control of heat loss and heat production (see Temperature Control, p. 277). This is more marked in the preterm infant.

Preterm infants lack glycogen and stored fats, particularly brown fat which is important both as an energy source and for heat production (Sheeran 1996). It is laid down in a variety of locations in the body between 26 and 28 weeks of gestation; hence infants born before this time may lack the ability to generate their own heat. Infants who do have brown fat have the ability to generate heat from birth. Brown fat in infants differs from that in adults in that it has a higher number of mitochondria and an abundant sympathetic nerve supply. Brown fat accounts for 10% of the term infant's total adipose tissue (Flaherty 1996, Hughes & Griffith 1984, Sheeran 1996).

Infants have a thin subcutaneous fat layer resulting in poor insulation (Bennett & Brown 1993).

Term and preterm infants do not have the ability to shiver to produce heat in response to cold, and their metabolic response is limited. Changes in peripheral vascular tone, with constriction of skin vessels, occur in an attempt to reduce heat loss, thus keeping the blood in the central circulation. Non-shivering thermogenesis may occur where heat production is achieved from brown fat (Mitchell 1996, Sheeran 1996).

Heat loss in the infant is nearly four times greater, per unit of body weight, than that in adults. This is primarily due to the higher ratio of surface area to body weight in infants (Hughes & Griffith 1984).

Infants lose heat in four ways:

- by conduction – occurring when the infant comes into direct contact with a cooler surface, thus losing heat to that surface
- by convection – when warmth is lost to the surrounding air or water; this necessitates the maintenance of room temperature between 24 and 26°C (Sheeran 1996)
- by radiation – heat loss from the infant to a surface nearby without direct contact; this may occur if the infant is placed near cold external walls
- by evaporation – caused by the evaporation of surface body water; this water is converted into vapour and is of particular significance in the newborn (Sheeran 1996).

Exposed to extremes of temperature, infants will suffer from decreased lung surfactant, hypoglycaemia, increased oxygen consumption and decreased blood coagulability in cold conditions, and increased fluid loss, hypernatraemia and recurrent apnoea in heat. Both extremes of temperature may result in death (Roberton 1993).

Equipment

- Incubator
- Temperature monitor
- Servo control skin probe (if required)
- Sterile water (if required)

Method

Incubators can be used to maintain a neutral thermal environment in two ways: skin servo control and air (nonservo) control. Skin servo control involves attaching a skin probe to the abdomen of the infant, normally over the liver. Thus, the temperature of the infant's skin will then control the environmental temperature within the incubator by regulation of the heater, turning it on and off as required (Boyd & Lenhart 1996).

In the air (nonservo) control mode the heater is manually adjusted by the nursing staff to predetermined air temperature levels (Boyd & Lenhart 1996).

For detailed guidance on the use of individual incubators the nurse should refer to the manufacturers' operating guidelines.

- Position the incubator in an area of the ward away from direct sunlight and draughts. Direct sunlight will cause the incubator to overheat.
- Fill the water reservoir with sterile water if additional humidity is required. Ensure that the temperature of the incubator is maintained at a constant level, not in excess of the humidity, to prevent additional heat loss caused by evaporation.

- The room temperature should be maintained between 24 and 26°C (Sheeran 1996). This helps prevent heat loss through the incubator wall.
- The incubator heater should be switched on and temperature limits set (see Table 15.1). The incubator should be warmed to between these temperature limits before the infant is transferred into it.
- Attach the servo control probe to the infant's abdomen, if required, and adjust temperature limits for skin temperature (as per local policy).
- Prevent heat loss from the incubator by keeping the portholes closed when the infant is not being attended to.
- Minimal handling and coordination of care to prevent constant disruption (clustered care) will not only allow the infant to rest but will also reduce heat loss.
- Warm your hands before touching the child.
- Warm additional equipment before putting it into the incubator.
- Ensure that the infant is kept as dry as possible to reduce evaporative heat loss.
- Radiant and convective heat loss can be further reduced by the use of heat shields. Perspex heat shields should be placed over the infant's body, with his head being outside of the shield (Bennett & Brown 1993). Care should be taken to ensure that the foot end of the shield is closed to prevent the continued circulation of air through the shield.
- Significant heat loss from the infant's head can be reduced by the use of a hat (Roberton 1993).
- Clean the incubator in accordance with the manufacturer's instructions.
- Change the incubator as per local policy.

Observations and complications

- The infant's temperature should be checked on a regular basis, if not continuously monitored.

- Routine care should be clustered to reduce heat loss from the incubator.
- The incubator temperature limits should be set to ensure that the infant does not overheat or become hypothermic.
- Incubator temperature should be monitored continually and maintained within set limits.
- Replace the water in the reservoir fully every 24 hours to reduce infection risk.
- Porthole access may be problematic if the infant is unstable. Under these conditions the infant should be transferred to a radiant warmer.

Transition from incubator to open cot

Weaning from an incubator to an open cot is an important step in the discharge preparation of an infant. Practice will differ between units, with some units having detailed policies. These policies may be based on a combination of the following:

- The infant's condition should be stable.
- The weight of the infant.
- Steady weight gain demonstrated by the infant.
- The temperature of the incubator being gradually reduced. This may be reduced over a 24-hour period; however, the incubator should never be turned off as this will result in air not being circulated.
- Monitoring of the infant's temperature is important to ensure that he is maintaining his temperature.
- The infant should be placed in a cot, in a draught-free position in the ward.
- The infant should be clothed and wrapped. Special attention should be paid to the wearing of hats because of the increased heat loss from the head. Clothing and wrapping may be commenced when the infant is in the incubator, with suggestions

Table 15.1 **Neutral thermal environmental temperatures determined by age and weight (Hazinski 1992, Blumer 1990)**

Age	Under 1200 g	Over 2500 g (and > 36 weeks gestation)
0–24 hours	34.0–35.4°C	31.0–33.8°C
24–48 hours	34.0–35.0°C	30.5–33.5°C
48–96 hours	34.0–35.0°C	29.8–33.2°C
4–14 days	32.6–34.0°C	29.0–32.6°C
2–6 weeks	30.6–34.0°C	29.0–33.0°C

regarding clothing being the first stage of incubator weaning rather than decreasing incubator temperature (Medoff-Cooper 1994).

Do and do not

- Do ensure that the care is clustered to decrease disturbance of the infant.
- Do encourage parents in the care of their infant. This will help enhance the parent–child relationship.
- Do ensure that the infant is wrapped well and has his head covered if he is being removed from the incubator for feeding or cuddling.
- Do ensure that sheets etc. are warmed before putting them into the incubator.
- Do ensure that the sterile water in the reservoir, if used, is fully changed every 24 hours.
- Do not leave the incubator in direct sunlight or draughts.
- Do not leave portholes or incubator doors open unnecessarily.
- Do not allow the baby's head to be covered by the Perspex heat shield as this may cause hypoxia (Bennett & Brown 1993).
- Do not turn off the incubator while the infant is inside.

References

Bennett V R, Brown L K 1993 Myles textbook for midwives, 12th edn. Churchill Livingstone, Edinburgh, ch 36

Blumer J L (ed) 1990 A practical guide to pediatric intensive care, 3rd edn. Mosby, St Louis

Boyd H, Lenhart P 1996 Temperature control: servo versus nonservo – which is best? Neonatal Network 15(2): 75–76

Campbell S, Glasper E A (eds) 1995 Whaley and Wong's children's nursing. Mosby, London, ch 13

Flaherty L 1996 Neonates and premature infants: overview of differences and ED management. Journal of Emergency Nursing 22(2): 120–124

Hazinski M F 1992 Nursing care of the critically ill child, 2nd edn. Mosby, St Louis, ch 14

Hughes J G, Griffith J F 1984 Synopsis of pediatrics, 6th edn. Mosby, USA

Marshall A 1997 Humidifying the environment for the premature neonate: maintenance of the thermoneutral environment. Journal of Neonatal Nursing 3(1): 32–36

Medoff-Cooper B 1994 Transition of the preterm infant to an open crib. Journal of Obstetric, Gynaecological and Neonatal Nursing 23(4): 329–335

Merenstein G B, Gardiner S L 1993 Handbook of neonatal intensive care, 3rd edn. Mosby, St Louis

Mitchell A 1996 Step by step guide. Thermal monitoring of patients in NICU. Journal of Neonatal Nursing 2(2): 4-page insert

Roberton N R C 1993 A manual of neonatal intensive care. Edward Arnold, London

Sheeran M S 1996 Thermoregulation in neonates: obtaining an accurate axillary temperature measurement. Journal of Neonatal Nursing 2(4): 6–9

Further reading

Cusson R M, Madonia J A, Tackman J B 1997 The effect of environment on body site temperatures in full term neonates. Nursing Research 26(4): 202–207

Short M A 1998 A comparison of temperature in VLBW infants swaddled versus unswaddled in a double – walled incubator in skin control mode. Neonatal Network 17(3): 25–31

16

Inhalational Devices

Introduction and rationale

The use of inhalers is so common that most paediatric nurses will be required to administer medication in this way, and should therefore have an understanding of the techniques required. While asthma will be the most common illness seen by paediatric nurses where this treatment will be required, children suffering other conditions, such as cystic fibrosis, will also use this technique.

Inhalational drugs are used because this route proves a particularly quick and effective way of reaching the lung tissues, without causing systemic side-effects.

The range of inhalational devices is now huge and can confuse anyone who is not in constant touch with developments. It has been shown that many nurses do not understand the mechanisms sufficiently well to teach children and parents how to use them, and that the devices are often poorly used by those they are intended to help (Hall 1996, Howell 1996).

Learning outcomes

After reading this section, the nurse should be able to:

- understand the suitability of different devices for different age groups
- describe good practice in administering medication.

Nurses should develop a good understanding of respiratory physiology to complement this practice (see Further reading, p. 149).

Please note that there is not space here to include details of the pharmacology of drugs used via the inhalational route; the section concentrates on the technique of administering medications in this way.

Factors to note

Children are much more likely to comply with their medication if they understand why they need it, what the drugs do to help, and how to take their medication. There are many good picture books available both from drug manufacturers and from the National Asthma Campaign.

Children should have immediate access to their inhalers. Whilst many schools now have effective inhaler policies, unfortunately even as recently as 1992 many schools still did not allow small children immediate access to their inhalers (Warner et al 1992). Access is defined differently in different schools; an inhaler locked in the head's office is in fact not easily accessible to most children. If a problem is identified with access to inhalers at school, the school nurse should be informed.

Guidelines

Correct diagnosis and assessment of the child's respiratory function are important. It is helpful to teach parents and other carers, for example teachers, how to recognise if an asthmatic child's symptoms are not well controlled.

Assessment should include observation of respiratory rate and effort (see Assessment, p. 45). Skin colour and general well-being should be noted. Signs of increasing effort may include intercostal recession, or using accessory muscles to aid breathing. The child may seek a position with her chest upright and head forward to increase lung expansion. Peak flow measurement (see below) is a useful test of lung function. Oxygen saturation measurement may give an early indication of any hypoxia. X-rays and other more detailed lung function tests can be performed. The history of the illness should be noted, especially as classic signs of chronic respiratory distress, chronic night-time coughing and shortness of breath after exercise (Caldwell 1997) are still often ignored by parents and GPs.

Peak flow measurement

Peak flow measures peak expiratory flow – the fastest rate at which air can come out of the lungs – and is measured in litres per second or minute. To predict the normal peak flow for a child, the child's height must be measured and then plotted against a nomogram, which details height on one axis and predicted peak flow on the other axis of the graph (Godfrey et al 1970).

There are several brands of peak flow meter, but most paediatric wards will need meters suitable for children with low lung capacity. Some children's meters come with little toy fans: the faster you blow, the faster the fan rotates. If the child is very distressed, it may be unwise to undertake a peak flow reading, as this may encourage bronchospasm or tire the child unnecessarily. Under normal circumstances, however, most children enjoy the challenge of bettering their last score.

The child should be taught to follow the following steps:

1. Move the measurement bar on the meter to zero.
2. Stand up.
3. Hold the meter horizontally.
4. Open mouth, and slowly inhale as large a breath as possible.
5. Put mouthpiece on the tongue and seal with the lips.
6. Blow out: a short, hard and fast breath.
7. Relax and rest for several seconds.
8. Repeat steps 1–7 three times.
9. Record the best reading.

The reading should be compared to the child's own baseline measurement and the normal values for a child of her height. One would hope to see a gradual improvement as the child's condition improves.

Older children who are being taught self-management of their asthma may benefit from peak flow guidelines, which set levels above and below which certain medication should be taken or increased. While it is quite normal for morning readings to dip, variation above 15% may be significant.

Inhalers

Hall in 1996 showed that in 80% of people with poorly controlled asthma, poor inhaler technique is a factor. Hall recommends that inhaler technique needs to be taught consistently and repetitively, and technique checked at least every year by an experienced nurse.

Equipment

Different devices have different features, which make them amenable to different age groups, lifestyles and medication regimes (Logan 1992). New devices are being developed all the time, hence devices change in popularity from year to year. The child's understanding, the complexity of treatment, her gross and fine motor skills, and her respiratory function will all affect which device should be chosen. Tables 16.1 and 16.2 summarise the different features of common devices. As can be seen from these tables, children should be assessed individually to determine which device would be most suitable.

Aerosol inhalers used to contain chlorofluorocarbons (CFCs), gases which contribute to the depletion of the ozone layer. Some inhalers are now CFC-free, but there may be some adjustment in switching from the older inhalers to the new CFC-free inhalers; they may look, feel, smell and taste different, and for this reason compliance may be affected (National Asthma Campaign 1995, Partridge 1994, DoH 1998).

Table 16.1   **Summary of features of dry powder inhalers (positive attributes in bold)**

Device features	Capsule inhalers	Diskhalers	Multidose dry powder inhalers
Preloading required	Yes	Yes	No
Multiple doses available	No	**Yes 8/4 doses**	**Yes 50, 100, 200 doses**
Indicator of doses taken/remaining	N/A	**Yes**	**Yes (last 20 only)**
Inspiratory flow rate (1/min)	60	60	30 (60 = optimum)
Lactose carrier	Yes	Yes	Varies with manufacturer

None of these devices is suitable for children under 5 years old.
All the devices have the following attributes:

- discreet and portable
- do not contain CFCs
- do not need shaking before use
- do not require hand–lung coordination
- no time lapse between actuations required.

Adapted from Warner & Gregson 1995.

Table 16.2 **Summary of features of aerosol inhalers (positive attributes in bold)**

Device features	Metered-dose inhaler (MDI)	Large spacer and MDI	Breath-actuated MDI	Spinhaler
Discreet and portable	**Yes**	No	**Yes**	**Yes**
Require hand–lung synchronisation	Yes	**No**	**No**	Yes
Time lapse between actuations	Yes (30 s)	Yes (30 s)	Yes (60 s)	Yes (60 s)
Oropharyngeal impaction leading to inhibition of inhalation	Yes	**No**	Yes	Yes
Minimum age for use	7 years	**Infant**	7 years	No studies
Inspiratory flow rate (1/min)	30	22 (tidal volume breathing)	28–30	30
Medications available	**All**	Product specific	6	3

In addition, these devices have the following characteristics:

- no preloading required
- multiple doses available
- number of doses remaining/taken indicated
- require shaking before use.

Adapted from Warner & Gregson 1995.

Rees & Price (1995) suggest the devices listed in Table 16.3 as being appropriate for administering different medications to different age groups.

Method

With any device, only a small proportion of the inhaled drug reaches the child's lungs. A study by Jackson & Lipworth (1995) showed that the percentage of dose actually inhaled into the lungs ranged from 9% (using a metered-dose inhaler) to 21% with a spacer, and 28% with a Turbohaler. Much of the drug will remain in the oropharynx, and will then be absorbed systemically. It is important, especially with steroids which can cause side-effects if absorbed in this way, to teach children to wash their mouths out after inhaling (Barnes 1995). It is also important to know that different devices will have different therapeutic effects, and dosages may need to be adjusted accordingly when devices are changed.

The following common principles apply to all devices:

- Drugs should be checked and administered according to local policy and UKCC guidelines (see

Administration of Medicines, p. 29).
- Always remove the protective mouthpiece before use.
- Always check expiry date of drug canister and inhaler.

However, each type of device requires a different technique (see Figs 16.1 and 16.2). Pharmaceutical companies provide full instructions with their products, and these should be explained to children and their families.

Spacer for baby

Spacers enable drugs to be given to babies which would otherwise need to be given via the oral route, thus avoiding systemic effects.

Method
- Invert the spacer in such a way that the valve falls open.

Table 16.3   **Inhalational devices appropriate for different age groups**

Age group	Device
0–2 years	Large volume spacer + face mask + metered-dose inhaler
	Nebuliser
3–4 years	Large volume spacer + metered-dose inhaler
5 years up	Breath-actuated metered-dose inhaler
	Diskhaler/Rotahaler
	Spinhaler
	Multidose dry powder inhaler
10 years up	Metered-dose inhaler,
	Other devices as per 5 years old and over

- Attach a mask to the mouthpiece.
- Position the baby so that the mask can be placed comfortably over her face.
- Actuate the drug canister once.
- Hold the mask to the baby's face while she takes approximately five breaths. If the baby cries, the inhalation can continue as she will be taking nice big breaths.
- Repeat the dose if prescribed (Hubbard 1995).

Spacers, if washed too frequently, can develop a build-up of static. To avoid this, manufacturers' instructions should be followed and the spacer should be left to dry, not dried with towels or a cloth.

Nebulisers

Nebulisers are used commonly in hospital when asthma is acute, or to treat respiratory infections, for example in cystic fibrosis. They have the advantage that oxygen can be administered simultaneously, important if the child is hypoxic. The humidification can also be beneficial.

Nebulisers can also be misused, particularly in the community, where compressors can be bought without prescription. If home nebulisers are used, parents and child should be advised that they must only be used under regular medical supervision (Rees & Price 1995). They should not continue increasing the dose if the child's condition deteriorates, but must seek medical advice. Compressors should be regularly maintained.

Equipment
Nebuliser pot and mask or mouthpiece; different sizes are available to suit all ages. Some nebuliser types are better for specific drugs than others. If the child is venti-

lated, special connectors are available to connect the nebuliser to the ventilator tubing. The gas can be administered via a compressor, or via a bottled or piped gas supply. Oxygen should be used in acute asthma, as the child is likely to be hypoxic.

Method
- The medication should be checked against the prescription as per policy for administration of medications.
- To ensure adequate droplet formation, the nebuliser solution should be diluted to volume as recommended by the nebuliser manufacturer (2.5 ml for Medic Aid nebulisers (Medic Aid 1995)). Even though some medications come in prepacked nebules, they may need further dilution if the volume is too small, for example when a small baby receives only a small proportion of the nebule, as a small volume of the fluid always remains in the pot. Rees & Price (1995) recommend 4 ml minimum volume. The oxygen or air flow should reach 8–10 litres per minute (Rees & Price 1995).
- The child should be sitting comfortably, either in bed, on a chair, or on a parent's or nurse's lap.
- Tap the nebuliser during nebulisation, to ensure that large droplets are shaken down (Caldwell & Milroy 1995).
- Observe the child's condition during and after using the nebuliser.
- After the nebuliser has finished, dry tubing using driven gas, and wash and dry nebuliser pot and mask. Store for that patient only.

Summary of possible complications
The number of medications that may be given by inhaler precludes a comprehensive list of side-effects

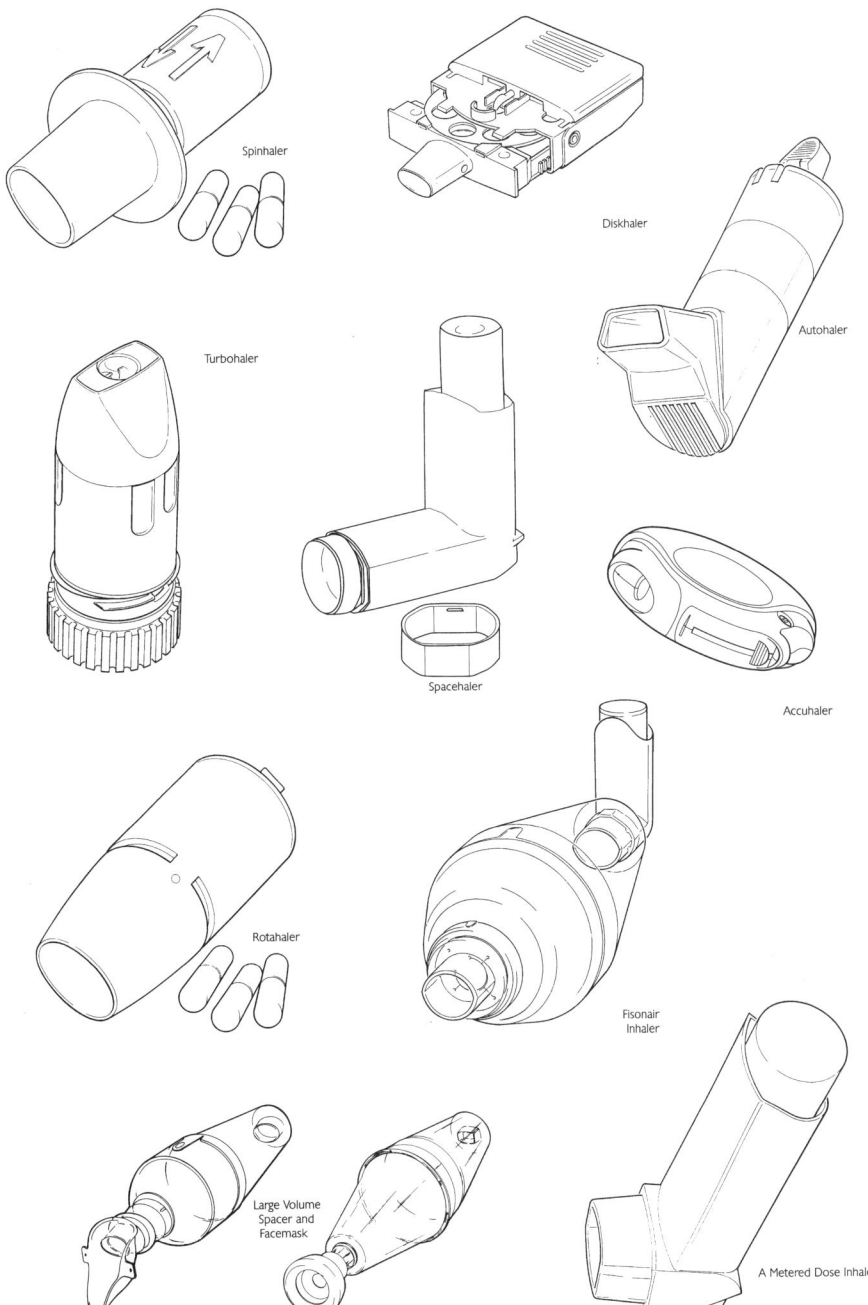

Figure 16.1

A selection of devices which require different techniques (reproduced by kind permission of the National Asthma and Respiratory Training Centre, © NARTC, Warwick).

being given here. A thorough knowledge of pharmacology is, however, necessary to understand and identify these side-effects. Rees & Price (1995) offer a good description of drugs used in asthma. It must be remembered that complications may occur, due both to the side-effects of the therapy and the natural history of the respiratory condition.

The possibility of side-effects of treatment can cause

HOW TO USE THE AEROCHAMBER

Method for patient who can use the device without help

1. Remove the cap.
2. Shake the inhaler and insert in the back of the Aerochamber.
3. Place the mouthpiece in the mouth (or the mask over mouth and nose).
4. Press the canister once to release a dose of the drug.
5. Take a deep, slow breath in. (If you hear a whistling sound, you are breathing in too quickly).
6. Hold the breath for about ten seconds, then breathe out through the mouthpiece.
7. Breathe in again but do not press the canister.
8. Remove the mouthpiece from the mouth and breathe out.
9. Wait a few seconds before a second dose is taken, and repeat steps 2 - 8.

Method particularly useful for young children

1. Remove the cap.
2. Shake the inhaler and insert in the back of the Aerochamber.
3. Place the mouthpiece in the mouth (or the mask over mouth and nose).
4. Encourage the child to breathe in and out slowly and gently. (If you hear a whistling sound the child is breathing in too quickly*).
5. Once the breathing pattern is well established, depress the canister with the free hand and leave the canister in the same position as the child continues to breathe in and out slowly (tidal breathing) five more times.
6. Remove the Aerochamber from the child's mouth.
7. For a second dose wait a few seconds and repeat steps 2 - 6.

* NB. The child Aerochamber device with mask & infant Aerochamber device with mask do not whistle.

Aerochamber

ALWAYS DEMONSTRATE TO THE PATIENT HOW TO USE THE SPACER DEVICE

HOW TO USE A SPACER DEVICE e.g. NEBUHALER
Method particularly useful for young children

1. Remove the cap, shake the inhaler and insert into the device.

2. Place the mouthpiece in the child's mouth, (if using the Nebuhaler be careful the child's lips are <u>behind</u> the ring).

3. Seal the child's lips round the mouthpiece by gently placing the fingers of one hand round the lips.

4. Encourage the child to breathe in and out slowly and gently. (This will make a 'clicking' sound as the valve opens and closes).

5. Once the breathing pattern is well established, depress the canister with the free hand and leave the device in the same position as the child continues to breathe (tidal breathing) several more times.

6. Remove the device from the child's mouth.

7. For a second dose wait 30 seconds and repeat sections 1-6.

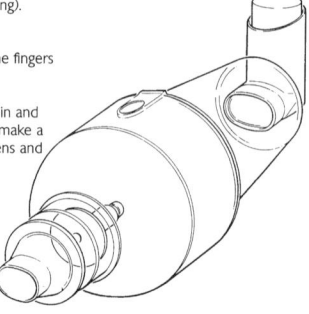

Nebuhaler

Figure 16.2
Two examples of devices with instructions for young children (reproduced by kind permission of the National Asthma and Respiratory Training Centre, © NARTC, Warwick).

ALWAYS DEMONSTRATE TO THE PATIENT HOW TO USE THE SPACER DEVICE

great anxiety for parents. The inhaler route is preferred, because less of the drug is absorbed systemically. Evidence suggests that mouth rinsing after inhalation may further lessen systemic side-effects (Jackson & Lipworth 1995).

COMMUNITY PERSPECTIVE

Many primary health care teams have asthma clinics, run by practice nurses who have undertaken an Asthma Training Centre course, and many children have their asthma managed in these clinics.

There will be instances where it will be more appropriate for CCNs to become involved with asthma management, for example as a follow-up after hospital admission. However, lines of communication should be maintained to ensure that no conflicting advice is given to families.

The role of the nurse involved in management of the child's asthma is:

- to ensure that the drug-delivery system is appropriate for the age and ability of the child
- to check that the child's inhaler technique is correct
- to check the family's level of understanding of the medication and to reinforce good practice, especially the benefits in terms of optimum drug deposition in the lungs when a large-volume spacer device is used
- to teach families ways in which to encourage the child to comply with treatment
- to act as liaison with the school nursing service should the child be experiencing difficulties in using the inhaler in school
- to encourage appropriate use of a home nebuliser where necessary, discouraging overdependence on the machine and ensuring that the family are aware of when to seek medical advice during an attack
- to ensure that local policy for servicing nebulisers is maintained.

Do and do not

- Children with asthma should carry their relievers at all times.

- Do offer regular and repeated teaching and follow-up checks of technique to all patients using inhalational devices.
- Do become familiar with features of different devices, in order to advise on the most suitable.
- Do encourage mouthwashing in patients who use inhalers, especially if inhaled steroids are prescribed.
- Do check that the school nurse is aware of a newly diagnosed child, and the school has a policy which will allow the child to use her inhaler when needed.

References

Barnes B 1995 Inflammation is the key to asthma. Supplement to MIMS Weekly (March): 2–3

Caldwell C 1997 Management of acute asthma in children. Paediatric Nursing 9(6): 29–32

Caldwell N A, Milroy R 1995 Optimising nebuliser practice within a large teaching hospital; easier said than done. Respiratory Medicine 89: 58–59

Department of Health 1998 Why your aerosol inhaler is being changed to CFC Free, DoH, London

Godfrey S et al 1970 Peak flow nomogram redrawn from original data. British Journal of Diseases of the Chest 64(15)

Hall J 1996 Evaluating asthma patient inhaler technique. Professional Nurse 11(11): 725–729

Howell M 1996 Staff knowledge of inhaler technique improved by survey. Nursing Times 92(13): 30–31

Hubbard J 1995 The correct use of inhalers for asthma in children. Maternal and Child Health (May): 168–175

Jackson C, Lipworth B 1995 Optimising inhaled drug delivery in patients with asthma. British Journal of General Practice 45(Dec): 683–687

Logan J 1992 Matching inhaler choice to patients' needs. The Asthma Training Centre, Colwood House Medical Publications, Stratford-upon-Avon

Medic Aid 1995 Information pack on nebulisers. Medic Aid

National Asthma Campaign 1995 New CFC free inhalers. National Asthma Campaign, London

Partridge M R 1994 Metered dose inhalers and CFC's: what respiratory physicians need to know. Respiratory Medicine 88: 645–647

Rees J, Price J 1995 Asthma in children: treatment. BMJ 310(June 10): 1522–1527

Warner J O, Gregson R K 1995 Asthma inhalers; developments or distractions? Maternal and Child Health (Dec): 383

Warner J O, Neijens H J, Landau et al 1992 Archives of Disease in Childhood

Further reading

Wooler E 1994 On course for knowledge. Nursing Times 90(15): 42–44

17

Intravenous Therapy

Introduction

Intravenous infusions for fluid replacement and drug administration are commonplace in the paediatric ward, whereas blood transfusion and platelet administration are seen more commonly in haematology units, with total parenteral nutrition often being seen in paediatric intensive care and neonatal units. Maintaining optimal function of intravenous infusions is of primary importance in children's nursing as fluid overload and electrolyte imbalance are potentially life-threatening and the frequent resiting of intravenous cannulae is stressful to the child and family (Smith & Wilkinson-Faulk 1994).

Learning outcomes

By the end of this section and following additional reading and practice the nurse should be able to:

- understand the differences between a child's and an adult's body fluids distribution
- recognise the need for intravenous fluid therapy
- ensure the safe administration of intravenous fluid therapy
- identify children who may require blood or blood products
- safely administer blood and blood products
- act appropriately should the child have a reaction to the treatment
- understand the need for total parenteral nutrition
- identify children who may require total parenteral nutrition
- safely administer total parenteral nutrition.

Factors to note

- Body surface area differs in children and adults, with the child and infant having a proportionally greater body surface area than the adult. There is also a different distribution, e.g. the head constitutes 20% of the infant's body surface area compared with 7–9% of the adult's (Davenport 1996).
- The proportion of body weight that consists of water is greater in the child and infant; 75–80% of the newborn's body weight is attributed to fluid compared with approximately 60–70% in adolescents. This reduces to between 50 and 60% in the adult, with females having slightly more body fluid (Hazinski 1988, Livesley 1996, Hiu Lam 1998).

- Body fluids are distributed between the intracellular and extracellular compartments. In adults, intracellular body fluid normally constitutes around two-thirds (67%) of total body fluid. The extracellular compartment constitutes the remaining third (33%). The extracellular fluid consists of plasma, lymph, interstitial fluid, bone water and connective tissue water. In infants and children the majority of body fluid is found in the extracellular compartment, with approximately one-half of this being exchanged daily to maintain homeostasis (Hazinski 1992, Livesley 1996).
- As a result of this distribution, dehydration will occur more quickly in the infant/child.
- Care should be taken when siting an intravenous cannula to be used for infusion of fluids that the child's dominant hand is not used.
- A suitable size of intravenous cannula should be selected that not only reflects the size of the child's vascular access but also the intended use.
- Intravenous administration sets may or may not have an 'in-line' burette. It is preferential to use a set with an 'in-line' burette for both neonates and toddlers, as this will minimise the amount of fluid that the child receives should there be free flow of fluid (Hazinski 1992).

Intravenous infusions

The delivery of intravenous fluids is common within acute paediatric settings. Normally used to maintain hydrational status, intravenous infusions can also be used to administer drugs. Selection of the intravenous cannula site is important (see Venepuncture and Cannulation, p. 311); sites should be chosen that present the best calibre vein and that can also be suitably immobilised. Once the intravenous cannula is inserted and secured, the intravenous infusion can be commenced.

Equipment
- Intravenous fluid for administration
- Intravenous administration set
- In-line burette (if required)
- Air inlet (if required)
- Intravenous infusion pump
- Splint to immobilise limb
- Surgical tape and/or bandage to secure splint to limb and prevent intravenous line trailing

Method
- Explain the need for the infusion and the procedure to the child and parent/carer.
- Ensure that hands are clean and dry.
- Intravenous fluid should be checked by two members of the registered nursing staff (or as per local policy) against the medical prescription chart.
- The expiry date on the bag and the batch number on the bag should be recorded on an intravenous infusion recording sheet or as per local policy.
- Priming of the intravenous administration set is an aseptic procedure, and care must be taken to avoid touching the spike or contaminating the system.
- Remove the intravenous administration set from the sterile packaging.
- Remove the in-line burette (if required) from the sterile packaging.
- Insert the intravenous spike of the administration set into the exit line on the sterile burette.
- Close all roller clamps attached to the burette and administration set.
- Insert the spike of the burette into the appropriate port of the intravenous fluid bag. *Note:* If the intravenous fluid is in a bottle, the spike should be inserted into the appropriate place in the rubber stopper and an air inlet inserted. Clean the rubber stopper with 70% isopropyl alcohol (e.g. Mediwipes) and allow to dry prior to insertion of the spike and air inlet.
- Fill the burette (if used) with around 20–30 ml of fluid by opening the roller clamp; then close the clamp.
- Half fill the in-line bubble of the administration set with fluid by gently squeezing the bubble to expel air into the burette.
- Open the clamp and allow fluid to flow into the administration set, thus expelling the remaining air.

Once fluid has reached the end of the administration set, close the clamps and ensure that all air has been expelled.
- Place the administration set into the intravenous infusion pump as per manufacturer's instructions.
- Check patency of the child's intravenous cannula.
- Attach the administration set to the child's intravenous cannula and secure with surgical tape. *Note:* Non-sterile tape should not be placed directly over the insertion site (see Venepuncture and Cannulation, p. 311).
- Immobilise the child's limb if necessary with a splint, ensuring that the intravenous cannulation site can be easily observed.
- Set the rate of infusion, as prescribed, on the infusion pump. Open all clamps and commence the infusion.

Observations and complications
- Check the intravenous cannula insertion site, venous pressure (read from some computerised infusion pumps), volume infused and rate at which the fluid is infused hourly.
- Observe the intravenous cannula insertion site for signs of redness and swelling. The area approximately 2.5 cm (1 inch) above and below the insertion site should be easily observed.
- If the child complains of pain or there are signs of intravenous infiltration, stop the infusion immediately and report to medical staff. Infiltration can be graded, indicating the degree of possible damage to tissues (see Table 17.1).
- Record the volume infused and the rate on a fluid balance chart.
- A running total of fluid infused should be maintained. This provides an accurate hourly fluid intake.

Do and do not
- Do check the site on an hourly basis.
- Do ensure that the child's limb is immobilised.
- Do stop the infusion if the child complains of pain. Inform the medical staff/nurse practitioner.
- Do stop the infusion if there are any signs of extravasation.
- Do refer to local extravasation policy.
- Do not obscure the intravenous cannula insertion site.
- Do not bandage fully the arm on which a cannula is sited.
- Do not put the bandage on too tightly.

Table 17.1   **Grading for intravenous infiltration (Flemmer & Chan 1993)**

Grade	Manifestations
I	Painful intravenous site. No signs of swelling or redness
II	Painful site. Slight swelling. Good pulse and capillary refill below infiltration site. No blanching evident
III	Painful site. Marked swelling with blanching and skin cool to touch. Good pulse below infiltration site with brisk capillary refill
IV	Painful site. Very marked swelling with blanching of skin. Skin cool to touch, pulses absent below infiltration with slow capillary refill (> 4 seconds). Skin breakdown or necrosis may be present; however, this may be delayed

Infiltration may not traverse through all stages. Infiltration at Grade IV is possible on first detection.

Blood transfusions

Transfusion of blood or blood products is performed in children for a variety of reasons, including anaemia, acute haemorrhage, haematological disease, following surgery and in other acute and chronic conditions.

Advances in both surgery and medicine have been made possible partly through the availability of blood and blood products (Contreras 1990).

Factors to note

- Erythrocytes (red blood cells) are formed in the red bone marrow from haemocytoblasts. As the red blood cell matures it loses its nucleus and caves in on both sides giving the characteristic shape of the biconcave disc.
- The usual life span of the red blood cell is 120 days. Once the cells grow old, their membranes become fragile and rupture, the contents being phagocytosed by the macrophages in the spleen, liver and bone marrow.
- The balance of production and destruction is equal under normal homeostasis.
- The main function of red blood cells is to transport oxygen, bound to haemoglobin, to all cells of the body. Other functions include the transport of waste carbon dioxide and the maintenance of blood pH.
- Fetal haemoglobin has a greater affinity for oxygen than adult haemoglobin, which is suitable for the fetal environment. Towards the later stages of pregnancy, the fetus begins to develop adult haemoglobin. Neonatal haemoglobin level is higher than that of children.
- Whole blood transfusion will replenish the volume, red blood cells and oxygen-carrying capacity of the blood. Packed red blood cells, referred to as packed cells, consist of blood in which some 80% of plasma has been removed. A packed cell transfusion aims at replenishing red blood cell mass and thus the oxygen-carrying capacity of the blood; however, a packed cell transfusion will not replenish volume (Abernathy et al 1994, Place 1998, Fitzpatrick & Fitzpatrick 1997).
- Whole blood transfusion is normally reserved for exchange transfusion for rhesus incompatibility, severe haemorrhage with depletion of coagulation factors and situations where more appropriate blood products are not readily available (Hazinski 1992).
- Washed red cells have had the plasma proteins, leucocytes and platelets removed by rinsing with a special solution; this decreases the chance of transfusion reaction. This type of prepared blood may be used in children who have frequent blood transfusions (Abernathy et al 1994, Campbell & Glasper 1995).
- Following bone marrow transplant, children require to have blood products irradiated.
- Blood should be stored at 4°C; therefore it must be refrigerated in a specialised blood refrigerator. Blood can be stored for 36 days after which it will have to be discarded if not used (Contreras 1990).
- The blood transfusion should be commenced within 30 minutes following the arrival of blood from the blood bank (Campbell & Glasper 1995, McConnell 1997).
- The use of blood warmers is recommended in infants and young children. In this instance the blood is actively warmed during administration by using tubing coils in a water bath. This may be performed during exchange transfusions (Hazinski 1992).
- Blood should be transfused over 4 hours. Transfusions exceeding this time may become

contaminated with bacteria. If the volume of blood cannot be transfused within 4 hours, it should be divided into smaller volumes and stored accordingly in the blood bank until required (Abernathy et al 1994, Campbell and Glasper 1995).

- Blood is obtained from people who are between the ages of 18 and 65 years. Frequency of donations is normally two to three times per year.
- Since 1985, all donor blood has been tested for human immunodeficiency virus (HIV 1 and 2 antibody). Testing for hepatitis (A, B and C), syphilis and *Treponema pallidum* antibody are routine (Blood Transfusion Service 1996). Selective testing for specific agents may be considered when administering blood to susceptible recipients, e.g. the testing for cytomegalovirus in immunosuppressed children. All donated blood has serologic tests performed to determine blood group (A, B, AB and O) as well as rhesus factor (Rh D +ve or - ve) (Campbell & Glasper 1995, Contreras 1990).
- Children with blood group AB can be transfused with blood groups AB, A, B and O. Children with blood group A can be transfused with groups A and O, and those with blood group B can be transfused with groups B and O. Those children with blood group O can only be transfused with blood group O. However, the blood that a child is transfused with must be rhesus compatible, i.e. have the same rhesus status, +ve or - ve. Blood group O is regarded as the universal donor whereas blood group AB is the universal recipient (Contreras 1990, Wong 1996).
- Religious and cultural beliefs of the child and family must be taken into account when considering a blood transfusion. Families who are Jehovah's Witnesses may not agree to blood transfusions; therefore substitutes may have to be considered. In cases where volume expansion is necessary, colloidal fluids may be as effective; however, if blood is a necessity, a court order may have to be obtained if the family do not give consent.

Equipment
- 0.9% saline
- Blood administration set (this must be appropriate for the pump if one is being used)
- In-line burette (if required)
- Filter for blood products (if required)
- Leucocyte filter (if required)
- Infusion pump (e.g. Ivac pump)

Method
- Explain the procedure to the child and parent/carer.
- Wash and dry your hands.
- Assemble the equipment and prime the administration set with 0.9% saline (see Intravenous infusions, above). The blood filter should be placed between the blood administration set and fluid bag. Although all blood administration sets should have a filter within the chamber, an additional filter may be used.
- Check the blood for administration against the medical prescription and haematology/blood bank information. The child's name, date of birth, hospital identification number, blood group, rhesus factor status, blood bag number and expiry date should be checked using the identification label attached to the bag of blood, the haematology/blood bank information slip, the child's hospital notes and the child's identification band.
- Check the bag of blood for abnormal colour, gas bubbles, clumping or any extraneous material. This may give an indication of bacterial contamination (Abernathy et al 1994).
- Replace the 0.9% saline with the blood bag and prime the administration set with blood (if the child is not to receive the saline within the system, as may be the case if the child is fluid restricted) and attach to the child's cannula. Secure the child's limb as necessary (see Intravenous infusions, above).
- Monitor and record the transfusion as per intravenous infusions.
- Once the transfusion is complete, flush the administration set with 0.9% saline and proceed as per medical instruction.

Observations and complications
- The majority of blood transfusion reactions occur within the first 15–30 minutes of starting the transfusion. These reactions can be categorised as haemolytic reactions, febrile reactions, allergic reactions and circulatory overload (see Table 17.2).
- Monitor and record the child's temperature, pulse and respirations a minimum of every 15 minutes for the first hour of the transfusion, and then every 30 minutes until blood transfusion is complete (Carter & Dearmun 1995, Hazinski 1992).
- Monitor and record infusion as per intravenous infusions.
- If a reaction occurs, stop the transfusion and inform medical staff immediately (see Table 17.2).

Table 17.2 **Reactions to blood transfusions**

Reaction	Manifestations	Management
Haemolytic reaction (Cause: incompatible blood. Rare)	Chills, fever, shaking, pain at i.v. site and along venous tract, breathlessness, abnormal bleeding, haematuria, progress to shock and renal failure	Stop transfusion Inform medical staff Retain sample of donor blood Obtain sample of child's blood Medical treatment to reverse shock
Febrile reactions (Cause: leucocyte, platelet or plasma protein antibodies)	Fever or chills	Stop transfusion Inform medical staff Administer prescribed antipyretic
Allergic reactions (Cause: allergens in donor's blood)	Urticaric rash, wheeze, breathlessness, laryngeal oedema	Stop transfusion Inform medical staff Adrenaline/steroid therapy may be used to counteract reaction Prophylactic antihistamines may be used in children who have a known reaction
Circulatory overload (Cause: rapid infusion)	Chest pain, cyanosis, noisy respirations, dyspnoea, distended neck veins	Stop transfusion Inform medical staff Place child in upright position Use diuretics to diminish fluid overload in children who can pass urine

Do and do not

- Do reassure parents regarding the testing of blood and blood products.
- Do check with the parents whether the child has had a previous reaction to blood or blood products. Report promptly to medical staff.
- Do ensure that the blood is thoroughly checked prior to administration.
- Do stop the transfusion if there is any indication of a reaction.
- Do keep emergency equipment at hand in case of severe haemolytic or anaphylactic reactions.
- Do not, in the case of reaction, restart a transfusion until the child's condition has been fully medically evaluated.
- Do not administer any other medication

intravenously using the same cannula during the transfusion.

- Do not give intravenous dextrose immediately before or after transfusion as haemolysis and clotting may occur within the administration set (Brunner & Suddarth 1991).

Platelet transfusion

Platelets can be administered both prophylactically and therapeutically to children with thrombocytopenia, leukaemia or those undergoing chemotherapy (Abernathy et al 1994). These children are at risk of bleeding, which can be fatal in some instances.

Factors to note

- Platelets are formed from cells within the bone marrow. They are disc-shaped cells and there are between 50 000–400 000 per cubic millimetre of blood (Tortora & Grabowski 1996, Place 1998, Arnett 1998).
- The normal life span of platelets is approximately 5–7 days. The life span of transfused platelets is 4 days (Hazinski 1992).
- Platelets arrest bleeding through platelet plug formation, wherein the platelets adhere to the damaged blood vessel. This adhesion changes the characteristics of the platelets by activating a series of reactions within them. This reaction forms a platelet plug which prevents blood loss in small vessels. Although initially loose, the plug eventually becomes tight by being reinforced with fibrin threads during coagulation (Tortora & Grabowski 1996).
- Ideally, platelets are matched according to their ABO and rhesus factors; however, in emergency situations compatible (or even incompatible) platelet concentrates can be used (Contreras 1990).
- Platelet transfusion may not increase platelet count in children with idiopathic thrombocytopenic purpura, disseminated intravascular coagulation or antibody reactions, because such conditions destroy platelets. However, platelet transfusion is of use in the treatment of severe haemorrhage of such children (Abernathy et al 1994).

Equipment

- Platelets for infusion
- Platelet administration set
- Appropriate infusion pump (if used)

Method

- Explain the procedure to the child and parent/carer.
- Wash and dry your hands.
- Check the platelets for infusion using the same criteria as those for blood (see Blood transfusions, above).
- Prime the administration set (see Intravenous infusions, above).
- Place the administration set into the pump as per manufacturer's instructions.
- Attach the administration set to the child's intravenous cannula and secure.
- Administer the platelets as instructed by the medical staff. Platelets are normally administered rapidly in 20–40 minutes (Hazinski 1992).
- Once administration is complete, disconnect the platelet administration set and discard it according to hospital policy. Record the volume of platelets infused on the appropriate chart.

Observations and complications

- As the platelets are administered relatively rapidly, it is important that the child is constantly observed to monitor any adverse reactions and for the infusion being completed.
- Observe the child for signs of fever, chills or rash, as reaction to platelets can occur. Reactions to platelets are normally treated with antihistamine drug therapy. Report any reactions to the medical staff and stop infusion until the child has been evaluated.

Do and do not

- Do ensure that the platelets are agitated until they are to be transfused. This prevents them from clumping.
- Do administer the platelets rapidly.
- Do not administer platelets using a pump that is not designed for platelet infusion (refer to manufacturer's instructions).

Total parenteral nutrition

The development of total parenteral nutrition a quarter of a century ago has enabled children with a variety of congenital and acquired gastrointestinal conditions to survive (Bilodeau 1995). Parenteral feeding is considered when a child cannot tolerate or absorb adequate nutrition orally or enterally. Parenteral nutrition is administered intravenously and refers to a nutrient solution which comprises dextrose, amino acids, fat, electrolytes, vitamins, micronutrients and water (Abernathy et al 1994, Gaedeke Norris & Steinhorn 1994, Galica 1997).

Factors to note

- Total parenteral nutrition is used therapeutically for conditions such as short bowel syndrome, intestinal obstruction, bowel fistulae, chronic persistent severe diarrhoea, extensive burns or children receiving chemotherapy (Bilodeau 1995, Campbell & Glasper 1995).
- Total parenteral nutrition can be administered through a central venous catheter, e.g. a Hickman line, or a peripheral cannula. The route of administration will be determined by the length of time that the child is to receive parenteral nutrition and the concentration of dextrose that is to be used. A concentration of dextrose and amino acids of

20–30% may cause vein sclerosis or burns if extravasation occurs; hence for this concentration a central venous catheter is used. For dextrose concentrations of below 10% a peripheral cannula can be used. The use of peripheral veins in the acutely ill is becoming more common (Campbell & Glasper 1995, Carter and Dearmun 1995, Hazinski 1992).

- Parenteral nutrition can be administered continuously throughout the day, as is often the case in the acutely ill, or can be administered overnight. Overnight administration would be considered for the child who is to receive long-term parenteral nutrition as it allows for more freedom of movement during the day.
- Parenteral nutrition is prepared on a daily basis and stored in a temperature-controlled refrigerator. If the child is acutely ill, electrolytes are altered in accordance with the child's own biochemistry. Children who are to receive their nutrition for a longer period of time and who are stabilised may not require daily alterations to their nutrition (Bilodeau 1995, Carter and Dearmun 1995).
- Dextrose is primarily used as a source of calories; amino acids are a source of nitrogen for protein synthesis. Electrolytes, minerals, trace elements and vitamins are added to meet the child's known nutritional requirements. Fat emulsions provide a major source of calories as well as preventing essential fatty acid deficiency states (Hazinski 1992, Galica 1997).
- Fat solution, e.g. Intralipid, is administered separately, as mixing it with dextrose solution may cause denaturing of the fat solution (Poskitt 1988). However, the same cannula/central line can be used for administration. Fat and dextrose solution are infused into the same central line using a three-way tap or a Y extension.
- The dextrose constituent of the total parenteral nutrition renders the child more prone to infection. An aseptic technique must therefore be used when changing bags of solution, and handling or changing intravenous lines (Hazinski 1992).
- Bags of nutrition should be stored in the refrigerator and removed around 30 minutes prior to the commencement of administration. This allows the solution to warm to room temperature.

Equipment
- Dextrose solution with additives
- Fat emulsion solution
- Amino acid solution, e.g. Vamin

- Intravenous administration set
- Intravenous infusion pump, e.g. Ivac pump
- Sterile drapes or dressing pack
- Sterile gloves
- 70% isopropyl alcohol
- Three-way tap Y extension (if required)

Method
- Explain the procedure to the child and parent/carer.
- Wash and dry hands.
- Open all equipment and place on a sterile drape.
- Two registered nurses (or as per local policy) should check the parenteral nutrition solution against the medical prescription. Check the solution for clarity, turbidity and particles. Check the expiry date.
- Wearing sterile gloves, prime the intravenous administration set as described for intravenous infusions (p. 152); however, care should be taken to maintain asepsis.
- Clean the child's central line with alcohol solution 2.5 cm (1 inch) from the tip. If the child has an existing administration set attached, clean 2.5 cm (1 inch) on either side of the join. Allow the alcohol to dry.
- Attach the administration set and thread the line through the infusion pump.
- Commence the infusion.
- Monitor and record the infusion as per intravenous infusions (p. 152).

Observations and complications
- Monitor fluid and electrolyte balance closely.
- Protect the bag of dextrose solution from sunlight, if necessary. Some additives degrade in sunlight; hence the solution bag may have to be covered, e.g. with a bag made out of paper or dark plastic. Coloured infusion sets can also be used. Guidance should be sought from the pharmacy department.
- Monitor and record the child's temperature 4-hourly. Pyrexia (temperature > 38.5°C) may indicate sepsis, and blood cultures should be obtained (Hazinski 1992).
- Monitor and record capillary blood glucose 4-hourly. The frequency of monitoring can be gradually reduced in accordance with the child's condition, but the test should be performed at least daily. Urine may also be tested for glucose as per local policy.
- Monitor weight daily. Height should be measured, but the frequency of measurement need not be the same as for weight (Gaedeke Norris & Steinhorn 1994).
- Observe for any signs of oedema.

- Change the intravenous infusion set every 24 hours (or as per local policy).
- To prevent oral dryness, perform oral hygiene frequently.
- If a central line is used, change the dressing in accordance with local policy.
- Sepsis, abnormalities in liver function, hyperglycaemia and hypocalcaemia are some complications of this therapy (Abernathy et al 1994, Bilodeau 1995).

Do and do not

- Do ensure that asepsis is maintained and manipulation of the line is kept to a minimum.
- Do ensure that the intravenous administration infusion set is changed every 24 hours.
- Do ensure, where necessary, that the bag of solution is protected from sunlight.
- Do ensure that parents are involved in care.
- Do not change intravenous lines without using aseptic technique.
- Do not use a central line or peripheral cannula for other drug or fluid administration.

COMMUNITY PERSPECTIVE

There are many issues surrounding these procedures when undertaken in the home; however, providing these are addressed, with safety being paramount, home intravenous therapy may be implemented. The responsibility for instigating such treatment must be given due consideration and, should the CCN feel insufficiently experienced or trained, she must consider her accountability in practice (RCN 1990). Specialist team input may be required, for example for the administration of TPN and immunoglobulin infusions (RCN 1994).

There will be situations where the CCN administers the infusion, others where the carers undertake the role.

The suitability of the home environment should be assessed before any suggestion is made to the family. Not every environment will be suitable and the presence of boisterous siblings and pets, for example, must be taken into account. Even in the most motivated families, a moment's inattention to a toddler intent on grabbing an i.v. line could be disastrous. These issues need to be discussed with the family before any decision is made. It may be possible to recruit the help of a neighbour or friend in arranging a 'special outing' for the sibling to coincide with a crucial period in the treatment.

There are advantages for some families in that the child is likely to be more relaxed in the home environment and able to maintain a more normal lifestyle. The responsibility of undertaking this type of treatment, however, may be too overwhelming for some families even with a skilled teaching input and support from the CCN. This must be assessed, ensuring that carers are not left with feelings of guilt should they decide not to participate in this area of care. Other families may welcome the opportunity to be involved.

The carers will need an intensive teaching programme and issues such as cross-infection should be discussed. The CCN must feel confident in the ability of the carers to cope safely with the procedures – most will be meticulous in their care.

Telephone contact is imperative and the CCN must feel confident that the phone is not likely to be cut off because of non-payment of bills.

General principles

It is necessary to ascertain whether clinical responsibility rests with the hospital paediatrician or with the GP.

The CCN will be responsible for ensuring that carers are fully informed about the therapy to be given, including side-effects and possible complications. They will need to be competent in the use of any pumps or syringe drivers which may be required and be able to recognise signs of infection, local or systemic.

Where an i.v. pump is to be used, this should be capable of running on its own batteries for some hours, in case of power failure.

Anaphylaxis kits should be provided and carers given the guidelines and information concerning dosages and usage.

Whenever possible, home i.v. therapy should be checked by two people; this will include dose, drug, dilution and expiry date, and always with the prescription sheet which will be written in line with local policy (see Administration of Medicines, p. 29).

Carers must know who to contact at any time during the treatment and, if the CCN is unavailable, be given a link to the ward.

Consideration should be given as to which i.v. system will be simplest for the families to use. This may not be the cheapest, and the CCN may need to convince the budget holder of the importance of this.

Commercial sharps boxes must be provided for safe disposal of ampoules, needles and syringes and disposed of as local policy dictates. This may entail making an arrangement with the council refuse department.

Specific considerations

Blood and blood products are only likely to be given in the community to enable a terminally ill child to remain at home. Should a child have had previous severe reactions then transfusion should not take place in the community (RCN 1994).

The GP must be aware that the procedure is taking place and ensure that she or a member of the paediatric medical team is immediately contactable if necessary.

The CCN will need to remain in the home for the duration of the transfusion and for 30 minutes afterwards, monitoring vital signs throughout.

Kits for dealing with any spillage should be available (RCN 1994).

Home parenteral nutrition

Close links need to be developed between hospital and community-based staff, specialist pharmacists, dietitians and specialist commercial companies, e.g. Caremark.

A home TPN (total parenteral nutrition) information document containing procedures and troubleshooting guidelines should be provided.

It should always be remembered that parents are shouldering a tremendous responsibility and, however competent they become, will need ongoing support.

References

Abernathy T L, Beck M L, Becker S I et al 1994 Handbook of therapeutic interventions. Springhouse, Pennsylvania

Arnett C 1998 Thrombocytopenia in the newborn. Neonatal Network 17(8): 27–32

Bilodeau J A 1995 A home parenteral nutrition program for infants. Journal of Obstetrics, Gynaecology and Neonatal Nursing 24(1): 72–76

Blood Transfusion Service 1996 Handbook of transfusion medicine, 2nd edn. The Blood Transfusion Service of the United Kingdom. HMSO, London

Brunner L S, Suddarth D S 1991 The Lippincott manual of paediatric nursing, 3rd edn. Chapman and Hall, London

Campbell S, Glasper E A (eds) 1995 Whaley and Wong's children's nursing. Mosby, London

Carter B, Dearmun A K 1995 Child health care nursing. Blackwell Science, Oxford

Contreras M C 1990 ABC of transfusion. British Medical Journal, London

Davenport M 1996 Paediatric fluid balance. Care of the Critically Ill 12(1): 26–31

Fitzpatrick L, Fitzpatrick T 1997 Blood transfusion. Keeping your patient safe. Nursing 27(8): 34–42

Flemmer L, Chan J S L 1993 A pediatric protocol for management of extravasation injuries. Pediatric Nursing 19(4): 355–358

Gaedeke Norris M K, Steinhorn D M 1994 Nutritional management during critical illness in infants and children. AACN Clinical Issues 5(4): 485–492

Galica L A 1997 Parenteral nutrition. Nursing clinics of North America 32(4): 705–717

Hazinski M F 1988 Understanding fluid balance in the seriously ill child. Pediatric Nursing 14(3): 231–236

Hazinski M F 1992 Nursing care of the critically ill child, 2nd edn. Mosby, St Louis

Hiu Lam W 1998 Fluids in paediatric patients. Care of the critically ill 14(3): 93–96

Livesley J 1996 Peripheral IV therapy in children. Paediatric Nursing 8(6): 29–33

McConnell E A 1997 Clinical do's and dont's. Safely administering a blood transfusion. Nursing 27(6): 30

Place B 1998 The transfusion of blood and its products. Nursing Times 94(34): 48–50

Poskitt E M E 1988 Practical paediatric nutrition. Butterworths, London

Sidey A 1994 RCN PCN Forum. Administering IV therapy to children in the community, 2nd edn. RCN, London

Smith A B, Wilkinson-Faulk D 1994 Factors affecting the lifespan of peripheral intravenous lines in hospitalised infants. Pediatric Nursing 20(6): 543–547

Tortora G J, Grabowski S R 1996 Principles of anatomy and physiology, 8th edn. HarperCollins College Publishers, New York

Wong D 1996 Wong and Whaley's clinical manual of paediatric nursing, 4th edn. Mosby, St Louis

Further reading

Blood Transfusion Service 1996 Handbook of transfusion medicine, 2nd edn. The Blood Transfusion Service of the United Kingdom. HMSO, London

Davenport M 1996 Paediatric fluid balance. Care of the Critically Ill 12(1): 26–31

Dodsworth H 1995 Making sense of the use of blood and blood products. Nursing Times 91(1): 25–27

Glover G, Powell F 1995 Blood transfusions. Nursing Standard 9(33): 31–37

Hazinski M F 1992 Nursing care of the critically ill child, 2nd edn. Mosby, St Louis

18

Isolation Nursing

Introduction

The aim is to minimise the risk of infection to both the child and others by implementing appropriate precautions early. This will reduce the spread of pathogenic organisms by the exogenous route and avoid unnecessary isolation of the child.

Learning outcomes

By the end of this section the nurse should be able to:

- perform standard precautions and identify the need for additional transmission precautions (see Control of Infection, p. 13)
- prevent the spread of infection whilst caring for the child and family
- plan safe individualised care for the child and family
- alleviate any anxiety or stress felt by the child and/or family while the child is nursed apart from others
- protect the susceptible child from opportunistic infections from both staff and the environment
- protect susceptible health care workers from infection or colonisation by the organism.

Rationale

Adherence to basic hygiene principles, wearing appropriate protective clothing, a clean environment and segregation of the child where necessary, will minimise the risk of cross-infection or colonisation by pathogenic organisms by interrupting the chain of transmission (Professional Development Unit No. 21 1995).

Factors to note

- The duration of separation will vary. Microorganisms cause a variety of infections and the incubation period and mode of transmission will vary according to the site of the infection and the microorganism involved (Benenson 1995). Global and local epidemiological patterns of infection will vary and should be taken into account. For example multiple antibiotic-resistant organisms such as methicillin-resistant *Staphylococcus aureus* (MRSA),

vancomycin-resistant enterococcus (VRE) and aminoglycoside-resistant Gram-negative bacteria such as klebsiellae are an increasing problem worldwide (Goldmann & Huskins 1997). Seasonal viral diarrhoeal illnesses such as those caused by rotavirus may be more prevalent in the winter months and blood-borne viruses will be endemic in many countries as well as in specific high-risk behaviours such as intravenous drug misuse. The need for ongoing microbiological surveillance samples must be considered.

- If there is a history of communicable disease in the family (for example chickenpox or blood-borne viruses) or signs of infection such as diarrhoea and vomiting, rash, cough or pyrexia, initiate appropriate microbiological investigation (see Specimen Collection, p. 261) and precautions as soon as possible
- Assess the risk of infection to the family, siblings and other visitors. Consider the precautions they should take whilst visiting in hospital. For example have the family members had chickenpox or are they incubating it? If they have had the disease they can visit, but if not, do they pose a risk to others on the ward? Should visiting be restricted?
- Assess the risk of infection to the child and staff (Macqueen 1996) and implement the wearing of appropriate protective clothing such as gloves, aprons, masks, visors or goggles. A careful explanation to the child and family must be given to avoid feelings of alienation. The wearing of protective clothing by family members will depend on the type of infection. For example gloves should be worn where there is a risk of blood-borne viruses being transmitted through blood or bloodstained body fluid.
- Check the need for prophylactic antibiotics for the family with diseases such as *Neisseria meningitidis* – meningococcal disease (Begg 1992, PHLS Meningococcal Infections Working Party 1989). Check whether relevant exposure of health care workers to the disease warrants prophylaxis. Health

care workers should seek advice from the occupational health department or infection control team.

- Discuss with the medical staff the need to notify the infectious disease to the local consultant in communicable disease control (CCDC).
- If last offices are to be performed consider the requirements for protective body bags (see Bereavement Care, p. 55). Consider the cultural, legal and safety needs of the family and other health care workers (Health Service Advisory Committee 1991).

Equipment

- A notice on the door of the cubicle or area to indicate to staff and visitors:
  - the need for separation and the risk of cross-infection
  - the need to discuss entry to the area and visiting arrangements where individuals are non-immune to the infection, e.g. chickenpox
  - the necessity to comply with handwashing and the wearing of protective clothing
- Handwashing equipment – disposable hand towels, liquid soap or antiseptic solution, alcoholic hand-rub
- Protective clothing such as disposable gloves, plastic aprons, facial protection (mask, goggles, visor)
- Foot-operated pedal bin with appropriately coloured, labelled disposable clinical waste bag with ties
- Sharps bin, if necessary
- Individual examination equipment such as a stethoscope, auroscope with earpieces, tape measure, tongue depressors, ophthalmoscope, patella hammer, sphygmomanometer with disposable or washable cuff, disposable thermometer
- Suction and oxygen equipment; easy access to resuscitation equipment
- Weighing machine
- Scissors
- Pens, ruler, chart holder, calculator
- Disposable equipment according to the needs of the child such as suction catheters, sticky tape, sterile packs, syringes and disposable hypodermic needles, equipment for intravascular cannulation
- A clock with a second hand should be easily visible
- Equipment for summoning attention such as a call bell or intercommunication system

- Television, radio, reading material, play equipment, according to the needs of the child

Guidelines (see Control of Infection, p. 13)

General principles

- A careful explanation must be given to the child and parent as to why there is a need for segregation from others. Details of the mode of transmission, the need for protective clothing and appropriate precautions to take including handwashing should be given. Consider the cultural and social implications some infectious diseases may have for the individual and family, such as tuberculosis, measles or human immunodeficiency virus (Helman 1994).
- Assess the need for a single room or for cohortion (nursing children together who have the same infection) and to implement the appropriate transmission precautions. Consider whether the likely organism is transmitted via airborne, droplet or contact routes and whether the door of the room should be open or closed.
- Consider the environmental need for special high-efficiency particulate air filters (HEPA) for the child who is or may become severely immunosuppressed (a compromised host) and needs protection from opportunistic infections such as *Aspergillus*, a normal environmental fungus (Rogers & Barnes 1988).
- Respect the need for privacy for the child and family by providing curtains/blinds for the bed area and knocking on the door before entry.
- Alleviate stress and anxiety felt by the child whilst he is separated from others. Increase play activity, schooling, television/videos and where necessary plan visiting as appropriate. Consider the need for voluntary workers.
- Consider the precautions to be taken when visiting other departments such as the operating theatre or X-ray department. It may be advisable to place the child last on the operating list or to go to the X-ray department when the least number of children are there, such as at the end of the day.
- When conducting ward rounds minimise the number of health care workers entering the isolation area. To reduce the risk of cross-infection it is sensible to examine children who are most immunosuppressed first and those with a communicable disease last. It is important that all children who are segregated from others receive the same care and time allocation as others.

- To prevent cross-infection occurring in nursery or primary schools, follow good housekeeping and hygiene principles (Niffenegger 1997, Ross 1993).
- Local infection control guidelines should be easily available to both staff and parents.
- Know how to contact the local infection control nurse and infection control doctor for advice.

Hand hygiene

- Handwashing facilities with appropriate liquid soap, antiseptic solution, alcohol hand-rub and disposable paper towels (Gould 1994) must be available inside the room, immediately outside it or in the cohorting area.
- Hands must be washed and thoroughly dried:
  - when dirty
  - before entry to the cubicle or cohorting area
  - before and after caring for the child
  - before aseptic procedures
  - before handling food
  - after dirty tasks such as toileting
  - after removal of protective clothing including gloves
  - after handling specimens
  - on exit of the single room or cohorting area.
- When leaving the isolation area apply alcohol hand-rub solution to prevent cross-infection (Elliot 1992).

Protective clothing

- Have available outside the room or cohorting area disposable gloves, aprons and facial protection (visors, goggles and masks as per local policy). Gloves and aprons should be worn if caring for the child. Assess the risk of procedures which may contaminate the health care worker. If there is a risk of aerosols (fine sprays) or splattering of body fluid into the face or mucosal surfaces, protective facial wear must be worn. Additional protective clothing may be required if there is extensive bleeding or explosive diarrhoea or vomiting and the risk of contamination to the health care worker and the environment is high.
- Non-latex and/or powder-free gloves should be available for health care workers who are allergic to latex or starch powder (Booth 1995).
- The individual need for health care workers, parents, siblings or visitors to wear protective clothing should be assessed with each child and discussed with the parents.

Specimen collection (see Specimen Collection, p. 261)

- All specimens must be regarded as potentially infectious.

- Plan the need for appropriate specimens to be taken in consultation with the medical staff before explaining to the child and family. This aids better continuity of care and reduces the likelihood of unnecessary and repeated specimens. Document specimens taken.
- Wear protective clothing such as gloves when obtaining or handling specimens and remember to wash your hands before and after collection.
- Ensure that containers are adequately sealed and not leaking. Do not contaminate the outside of the container.
- Ensure that all specimens and laboratory forms are correctly labelled, safely packed and dispatched to the appropriate laboratory as soon as possible.
- Do not store specimens in food or drug refrigerators.

Clinical waste

- Ensure that waste is segregated at source, such as by the bedside, into clinical and non-clinical waste.
- Take the sharps bin to the source of the sharp. Sharps bins may be a source of infection and should be removed and disposed of frequently, or when two-thirds full, and on discharge of the child. Do not put your hand in the bin to retrieve articles or to push down sharps. This increases the risk of inoculation injury. Sharps bins must be kept out of reach of children but easily available to the health care worker.
- Use foot-operated pedal bins with lids for all clinical and non-clinical waste and laundry. Hands will become contaminated if used for opening lids.
- Sharps bins and clinical waste bags must not be overfull or contaminated on the outside. They must be tied securely and the hospital or health authority generating them must be identified. It is unnecessary to double bag clinical waste (Maki et al 1986).
- Ensure that the waste bins are cleaned regularly, and on discharge of the child, with hot water and detergent and dried to prevent the risk of cross-infection.
- Infected clinical waste, including sharps, generated in the home may be collected by special arrangement organised by the primary health care team.

Laundry

- Infected laundry should be placed into a red soluble bag or soluble stitched bag within an outer bag and secured with a tie. The bag should be identified as containing infected material before it is removed from the area. Local policies must be followed.

- Dispose of laundry bags when two-thirds full.
- Well-maintained domestic washing machines on a hot wash cycle may be used to decontaminate laundry in the home setting. This includes infections such as those causing diarrhoeal illness and blood-borne viruses.

Excreta

- If disposable potties, bedpans or urinals are used, they must be covered during transport to the dirty utility area and placed in a well-maintained macerator for disposal. The supporting frame should be washed in hot water and detergent and dried before storage.
- If non-disposable utensils are used, they must be covered during transport and placed in a heat disinfector/bedpan washer which reaches a temperature of at least 80°C for at least 1 minute (Ayliffe et al 1992).
- Where the above equipment is not available, the excreta should be disposed of down the toilet, the utensil rinsed and washed in hot water and detergent and dried. Gloves should be worn for handling and cleaning the utensil.
- If en suite toilet facilities are available, they must be flushed after use, cleaned when visibly soiled and at least daily. Disposable toilet seats are not necessary.
- Communal toilets should be avoided where the risk of transmitting the infection is increased, such as when the child has diarrhoea or vomiting. Aerosols may occur and contaminate the environment.
- It is ineffective to soak excreta in a disinfectant. Disinfectants are slow to penetrate organic matter and they may be inactivated.
- In the home setting, faeces from nappies or colostomy bags should be put down the toilet and the nappy or bag wrapped in newspaper or biodegradable polythene and disposed of in the dustbin.

Isolation area

- The area should be uncluttered and thoroughly cleaned at least daily with hot water and detergent (Collins 1988). Domestic staff must be appropriately trained and supervised.
- Disposable gloves and aprons should be used for cleaning and disposed of after use in clinical waste bags.
- Cleaning cloths should be disposable or laundered daily.
- Mop heads should be laundered daily in a washing machine and stored dry. They should not be left soaking in disinfectants as this increases the risk of contamination with organisms such as *Pseudomonas*. The same mop should not be used in other communal areas or kitchens because of the risk of cross-infection.
- Curtains should be laundered frequently and changed if visibly dirty. If shedding of pathogenic organisms such as staphylococci is extensive, as on the skin scales of a child with eczema, then curtains should also be changed on discharge.
- Follow local infection control policies for decontamination of the environment on discharge of the child.
- In the home setting maintain standards of hygiene and cleanliness. Do not use communal washing/bathing equipment such as towels, flannels or toothbrushes as these may be a source of cross-contamination.

Spillages of blood or body fluid

- Any spillages should be cleaned up immediately using a hypochlorite disinfectant (either granules or solution) and disposable towels (see Control of Infection, p. 13). The area should then be washed with hot water and detergent and dried. Care should be taken on carpeted areas as hypochlorites are bleaches and will discolour the area. Steam cleaning is considered appropriate.

Cleaning of equipment

- Examination and other equipment should be thoroughly cleaned according to manufacturers' instructions on discharge of the child. Other clinical equipment should be either disposable or heat treated accordingly. Chemical disinfection should be used for heat-labile equipment only (Oldman 1987, Thomson & Bullock 1992, Wright et al 1995).
- Soft toys used in hospital should be individual use only (or taken home) and laundered where possible or destroyed if contaminated with blood or body fluids. Hard-surface toys can be washed in hot water and detergent and dried thoroughly. Televisions, videos and computer equipment must be kept clean by wiping with a damp cloth.
- Communal play equipment which is easily contaminated with body fluids and is difficult to clean, such as musical wind instruments, should be avoided where the risk of infection to the child is high.
- Bar soap, pots and tubes of creams should be for single patient use only as these may become contaminated and cause cross-infection. They must

be discarded on discharge of the child. Disposable equipment which has not been in contact with infected material generally need not be discarded. This should be discussed with the infection control team according to the likely causative organism and mode of transmission.

Documentation and planning of care

- When preparing the bed area, plan the minimal amount of equipment including disposable items required, to minimise contamination and wastage.
- Plan and document all care around the family and child, taking into consideration their cultural, spiritual, psychosocial and physical needs. Care should be individualised according to the risk of acquiring or spreading infection. Consider age, mobility, understanding, adherence to hygiene, compliance with precautions and the type of infection (Webster & Bowell 1986).
- In consultation with the medical staff and whilst maintaining confidentiality, give the family an honest explanation of hospital-acquired infection or details of outbreaks of infection in the area of the hospital in which their child is receiving care. This helps minimise complaints. Seek advice from the infection control team. Document what has been communicated.
- Explain to the child and parents the need for some infections, such as *Shigella*, to be reported to the environmental health officer with further follow-up at home. Emphasise how nurses and doctors maintain confidentiality. Obtain advice from the infection control nurse or infection control doctor. There are legal obligations for certain infectious diseases to be reported to the environmental health department (see Control of Infection, p. 13).
- Assess daily the need for all the precautions.
- Report to the doctor any changes or deterioration in the child's condition or any signs or symptoms of infection in the family.
- Report to the infection control nurse or infection control doctor any suspicions of secondary cases such as other people with diarrhoea, rashes or chest infections.
- Obtain written information for parents and children about the infection and the need for restricted precautions.
- Medical/nursing notes should be kept safely outside the room where possible to avoid unnecessary entry to the isolation area.
- Inform the infection control team, primary health care team or transferring hospital/unit of any actual or potential infections.

- Consider the need for health education for the child and family. If the child has an infection which could be transmitted through sexual contact, such as human immunodeficiency virus (HIV), then this should be discussed with the parents through the multidisciplinary health care team. Sex education, where necessary, should be given in accordance with government guidelines (DES 1991, DoH 1992, DoE 1994).

Do and do not

- Do remember that handwashing is the single most important point in controlling cross-infection.
- If inoculation or mucosal or non-intact skin contamination with blood or body fluids occurs, do apply first-aid measures immediately and report to your manager and the occupational health department as soon as possible.
- Do keep all cuts and abrasions covered with a waterproof plaster. Wear appropriate protective clothing according to the risk assessment of the task.
- Do discuss with parents and the child all precautions to be taken whilst the child is in hospital. Ensure that there is a means of communication if the child is in a single room, for example a bell, two-way intercommunication apparatus or telephone. Include the need to extend precautions in the home, at school or nursery. Seek help from the infection control team if parents require further explanations.
- Do maintain confidentiality for both children and staff who have an infection or communicable disease.
- Do set a role model for others to follow in basic hygiene principles.
- Do not make the child and family feel responsible, guilty or alienated when involved in issues related to infection.
- Do not avoid your responsibility to adhere to research-based methods which prevent infection occurring or control its spread.
- Do not use laundry or waste bins with swing lids as this may cause aerosols and increases the risk of hand contamination.

References

Ayliffe G A J, Lowbury E J L, Geddes A M, Williams J D 1992 Control of hospital infection, 3rd edn. Chapman and Hall Medical, London

Begg N T 1992 Update – control of meningococcal disease. Communicable Disease Report 2: R65

Benenson A S 1995 Control of communicable diseases manual, 16th edn. American Public Health Association, Washington

Booth B 1995 No time for kid gloves. Nursing Times 91(46): 43–46

Collins B J 1988 The hospital environment: how clean should a hospital be? Journal of Hospital Infection 11(suppl A): 53–56

Department of Education (DoE) 1994 Education Act 1993. Sex education in schools. Circular 5/94. HMSO, London

Department of Education and Science (DES) 1991 HIV and AIDS: a guideline for the education service. HMSO, London

Department of Health (DoH) 1992 Children and HIV. Guidance for local authorities. HMSO, London

Elliot P 1992 Handwashing, a process of judgment and effective decision making. Professional Nurse 7(5): 292, 294–296

Goldmann D A, Huskins W C 1997 Control of nosocomial antimicrobial-resistant bacteria: a strategic priority for hospitals worldwide. Clinical Infectious Diseases 24(suppl 1): S139–145

Gould D 1994 The significance of hand-drying in the prevention of infection. Nursing Times 90(47): 33–35

Health Service Advisory Committee 1991 Safe working and the prevention of infection in the mortuary and post-mortem room. HMSO, London

Helman C 1994 Culture, health and illness. Butterworth-Heinemann, Oxford

Macqueen S 1996 Think globally – act locally: germ invasion and risk analysis. Journal of Neonatal Nursing 2(1): 20–25

Maki D G, Alvarado C, Hassemer C 1986 Double bagging of items from isolation rooms is unnecessary as an infection control measure: a comparative study of surface contamination with single and double bagging. Infection Control 7: 535–537

Niffenegger J P 1997 Proper handwashing promotes wellness in child care. Journal of Pediatric Health Care 11: 26–31

Oldman P 1987 An unkind cut. Journal of Infection Control Nursing, Nursing Times 83(48): 71–74

PHLS Meningococcal Infections Working Party 1989 The epidemiology and control of meningococcal disease. Communicable Disease Report 89/08: 3–5

Professional Development Unit No. 21 1995 Infection control, knowledge in practice. Nursing Times 91(40): part 1/3

Professional Development Unit No. 21 1995 Infection control, the role of the nurse. Nursing Times 91(41): part 2/3

Professional Development Unit No. 21 1995 Infection control, revision notes. Nursing Times 91(42): part 3/3

Rogers T R, Barnes R S 1988 Prevention of airborne fungal infection in immunocompromised patients. Journal of Hospital Infection 11(suppl A): 15–20

Ross S 1993 Creche course in hygiene. Journal of Infection Control Nursing, Nursing Times 89(29): 59–60, 62, 64

Thomson G, Bullock D 1992 To clean or not to clean. Journal of Infection Control Nursing, Nursing Times 88(34): 66–68

Webster O, Bowell E 1986 Thinking prevention. Nursing Times 82(23): 68–74

Wright I M R, Orr H, Porter C 1995 Stethoscope contamination in the neonatal intensive care unit. Journal of Hospital Infection 29: 65–68

Further reading

Edmond M 1997 Isolation. Infection Control and Hospital Epidemiology 18: 58–64

19

Lumbar Puncture

Introduction

Lumbar puncture is an invasive procedure in which a spinal needle is inserted into the subarachnoid space of the lumbar spine for diagnostic or therapeutic purposes.

Learning outcomes

By the end of this section you should be able to:

- state the indications for lumbar puncture
- understand and assess the risks associated with the procedure
- assist the doctor in performing a lumbar puncture
- explain possible side-effects of the procedure.

Rationale for lumbar puncture

Lumbar puncture is used in order to:

- obtain a specimen of cerebrospinal fluid (CSF) for diagnostic purposes, suspected meningitis being the most common indication
- measure the pressure of the lumbar CSF
- instil therapeutic drugs
- instil contrast media during radiological investigations.

The nurse's role is to prepare and comfort the child before, during and after the procedure, assist the doctor with the procedure, and hold and position the child safely during the procedure.

Factors to note

Lumbar puncture is an invasive procedure and therefore should be performed aseptically. It is a procedure which requires the assistance of two nurses in addition to the doctor.

Sick children

- Children with cancer and acute leukaemia in particular, will have to undergo repeated lumbar punctures throughout their treatment and find them painful and distressing (Broome et al 1990, Ellis & Spanos 1994, Klein 1992).

- In some cancer centres, children with cancer will have the procedure performed under general anaesthetic. In America, Schecter et al (1990) recommended conscious sedation or general anaesthesia for the initial lumbar puncture for children suspected of having cancer. Subsequently, the recommendation was that all children under 5 years should have conscious sedation or general anaesthesia, but not necessarily the older children.
- In the child who requires an emergency lumbar puncture as a one-off procedure, the disadvantages (and availability) of general anaesthetic probably outweigh the disadvantages of performing the procedure under local anaesthetic. However, premedication/sedation and analgesia should always be given consideration (Klein 1992).
- If the procedure is planned in advance, a topical, local anaesthetic cream should be utilised in preference to an injected local anaesthetic which will entail further injections in addition to the lumbar puncture.

Guidelines

Parents are not expected to take responsibility for positioning or observing their child. However, lumbar puncture is a painful procedure, so it is appropriate to involve parents to help support the child. Some parents may find the procedure too distressing to watch and their wish not to be present should be respected. The parents and child (if age and cognitive development allow) should be involved in preparation for the procedure. In an emergency situation there will be little time for preparation, but a brief, succinct explanation must be given. Parents must be aware of what the procedure entails. When time allows, therapeutic play and explanations with play equipment should be utilised to help reduce fear of the unknown and promote cooperation with the procedure (see Appendix 1: Play, p. 329).

Equipment

- Dressing trolley (as for performing an aseptic technique)

Note: many hospital sterile services departments provide a lumbar puncture pack which contains most of the equipment listed below (excluding drugs).

- Dressing pack to provide sterile field
- 2 spinal needles (one spare) (see Table 19.1)
- Sterile gloves
- Sterile drape with hole in middle
- Skin cleansing solution, e.g. chlorhexidine 0.5%
- 2 ml syringe and 2 needles (one 21 French gauge (Fg) for drawing up local anaesthetic and one 23 Fg (child) or 25 Fg (infant) for administering it) if local anaesthetic is to be used
- Local anaesthetic if required, e.g. 1% lignocaine
- Manometer tube and three-way tap if CSF pressure is to be monitored
- Specimen collection pots as required (three separate samples for microscopy culture and sensitivity and a sample for CSF glucose content are common; pots should be labelled 1, 2 and 3)
- Waterproof plaster or other suitable waterproof covering, e.g. Opsite spray
- Rubbish bag
- Bravery certificate

Method

One nurse will assist the doctor to draw up the local anaesthetic (if used), and collect and label the specimens.

The second nurse will care directly for the child as described in this methodology.

1. Explain to the child and his parent what is going to happen to reduce fear of the unknown and promote cooperation. This is important even if they have already undergone preparation prior to the procedure and particularly if they have undergone the procedure before (Broome et al 1990).
2. Position the child on his side, at the very edge of the treatment couch, with knees drawn up towards the chest and the head flexed forward, curled into a ball (see Fig. 19.1) and the lumbar area exposed. The

spine should be kept parallel to the edge of the bed. This posture is very uncomfortable, particularly if the child has meningism, so do not position him until you are completely ready (Bacon & Lamb 1988).

This posture widens the intervertebral spaces and facilitates easier access for the spinal needle (Lang 1993). Ensure that the infant has a clean nappy prior to the start of the procedure. The nappy will have to be partly removed to expose the lumbar region. In order to securely hold the child, it may be necessary to wrap his upper torso in a sheet. It is important that he is held securely to prevent sudden movement which could result in the needle moving and damaging nerve roots when in the subarachnoid space (Allan 1989).

3. Talk to and reassure the child throughout the procedure to try to calm him and promote comfort and safety.
4. Explain what is happening (appropriately to the child's age and cognitive ability) to both parent and child, as it is about to occur. The child is unable to see what is happening to him.

Having washed her hands, put on gloves and drawn up local anaesthetic if used, the doctor will place a sterile towel with a gap in it over the child's lumbar region. Through the gap, she will then cleanse the skin and next inject the local anaesthetic if used. She will wait about a minute for the local anaesthetic, if used, to take effect. She then inserts the spinal needle into the lumbar space between either the 3rd and 4th or 4th and 5th lumbar vertebrae (Bacon & Lamb 1988). This point of entry is selected to avoid damage to the spinal cord, which terminates higher up at the level of the first lumbar vertebrae (Hazinski 1992). Once the needle is in place, the stylet which blocks its core is removed and CSF can be observed to drip from the end of the needle; the stylet is replaced to prevent unnecessary loss of CSF. If CSF pressure is to be measured, it is done now before any CSF sample is

Table 19.1 **Sizes of spinal needles commonly used (the doctor will decide the size to use)**

	Age and size of child		
	Infants under 1 year	Children over 1 year	Adult-sized or over 40 kg
Gauge of needle	22 Fg	22 Fg	18–20 Fg
Length of needle	1–1$\frac{1}{2}$ inches	2$\frac{1}{2}$ inches	2$\frac{1}{2}$ – 3 inches
	25–40 mm	60–65 mm	60–90 mm

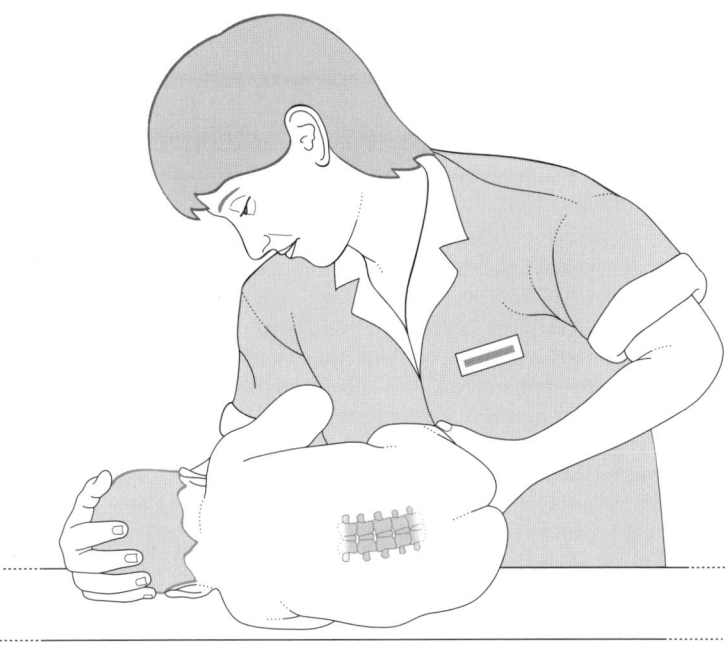

Figure 19.1
*Positioning the child for
a lumbar puncture.*

removed. The manometer, with three-way tap attached, is put onto the end of the needle and a measurement taken. CSF samples are obtained by removing the stylet (or manometer if it has been used) and allowing the CSF to drip into the labelled specimen bottle, held underneath by the first nurse. Between taking samples (usually 5–10 drops of CSF per sample bottle), the stylet should always be replaced to prevent excess CSF being lost. Three samples are commonly taken in case the first sample gets contaminated by blood as the needle is introduced (this is why samples are labelled 1, 2 and 3 in the order that they are obtained). If drugs are to be administered, an equivalent volume of CSF is first removed to prevent increased pressure. To finish the procedure, the doctor removes the needle, immediately applying firm pressure on the lumbar puncture site with a gauze pad for about 30 seconds to prevent CSF leakage (Lang 1993).
A plaster is then placed over the site.

5. Once the procedure is complete, reposition the child more comfortably, re-dress him, return him to his parent and provide praise (bravery certificate), comfort and reassurance.

6. Ensure that the equipment is disposed of correctly, safely and hygienically to prevent injury and cross-infection.

Observations and complications

Observe the child carefully throughout the procedure. Be aware of the possibility of respiratory difficulties. This can be a particular problem for infants because of the position they are required to adopt for the duration of the procedure. An infant has a much softer and more pliable trachea than an older child and this may be liable to collapse when his neck is flexed well forward, resulting in apnoea (Smith 1995). Chest expansion may also be impaired owing to the position of the child. If the child's colour/respiratory rate is seen to deteriorate, inform the doctor immediately. If the child is particularly sick, it would be pertinent to monitor his oxygen saturation level with a pulse oximeter throughout the procedure.

If the child is totally unwilling or unable to cooperate and to continue with the procedure would be to put the child at risk (e.g. he is struggling so much the needle might damage a nerve root whilst in the subarachnoid space), do not proceed. The child may have to be prescribed sedation or undergo a general anaesthetic.

Infection is always a risk of any invasive procedure. Following a lumbar puncture, the child should be observed for any signs of infection either at the site of the lumbar puncture (ideally plasters should not remain in situ for more than 24 hours) or any generalised signs of infection, e.g. pyrexia. If infection has been introduced into the central nervous system as a direct result of the lumbar puncture, the child will exhibit symptoms of meningitis.

If the lumbar puncture was traumatic and a blood vessel accidentally pierced as the needle was introduced, this can result in bloodstained CSF samples and a misleading diagnosis.

By far the most dangerous complication of a lumbar puncture is that of herniation of the brain stem through the foramen magnum (Hazinski 1992) – an event also known as coning. This has very grave consequences and is often fatal. It occurs if there is raised intracranial pressure when the lumbar puncture is being performed. As the stylet is removed from the spinal needle, raised intracranial pressure is suddenly released and the brain stem is sucked downwards into the spinal canal through the foramen magnum and badly damaged as a result. If this occurs and is not immediately fatal, the child will display signs of deterioration in his neurological status (see Neurological Observations, p. 171).

Occasionally, there may be CSF leakage from the lumbar puncture site after the procedure. If this happens, cover the site with a sterile gauze pad, apply pressure and inform the medical staff immediately.

Some children suffer post-lumbar puncture headache which is thought to relate to lost CSF. Allan (1989) explains that it used to be common to advocate bed rest to prevent headache, but since it appeared to make little difference, it is no longer suggested routinely. Analgesia such as paracetamol should be available to offer relief.

Summary of possible complications
- Herniation of the brain stem into the spinal canal
- Infection
- Leakage of CSF
- Respiratory distress
- Damage to nerve roots

Do and do not
- Do ensure that the child is adequately and carefully restrained during the procedure.
- Do observe the child carefully for any signs of respiratory distress and any indication of a deterioration in neurological status.

- Do not allow a lumbar puncture to proceed if the child has any sign of raised intracranial pressure (raised blood pressure, decreased pulse rate, decrease in consciousness). A lumbar puncture undertaken when there is raised intracranial pressure could result in herniation of the brain stem into the spinal canal via the foramen magnum This can be fatal.

References

Allan D 1989 Making sense of lumbar puncture. Nursing Times 85(49): 39–41

Bacon C J, Lamb W H 1988 Diagnosing and treating paediatric emergencies. Heinemann Medical Books, Oxford, pp 268–270

Broome M E, Bates T A, Lillis P P, Wilson-McGahee T 1990 Children's medical fears, coping behaviours and pain perceptions during a lumbar puncture. Oncology Nursing Forum 17(3): 361–367

Ellis J A, Spanos N P 1994 Cognitive-behavioural interventions for children's distress during bone marrow aspirations and lumbar punctures: a critical review. Journal of Pain and Symptom Management 9(2): 96–108

Hazinski M F 1992 Nursing care of the critically ill child, 2nd edn. Mosby Year Book, St Louis, p 619

Klein E R 1992 Premedicating children for painful medical procedures. Journal of Pediatric Oncology Nursing 9(4): 170–179

Lang S 1993 Procedures involving the neurological system. In: Barnardo L M, Bove M (eds) Pediatric emergency nursing procedures, 2nd edn. Jones & Bartlett, Boston, ch 8, pp 152–156

Schecter N L, Altman A, Weisman S 1990 Report of the consensus conference on the management of pain in childhood cancer. Pediatrics 86: 813–834

Smith C 1995 How to do it in paediatrics 2: the lumbar puncture. British Journal of Hospital Medicine 53(6): 273–274

Further reading

Perkins V 1995 Procedures of lumbar puncture in paediatrics. British Journal of Hospital Medicine 54(8): 414

Pinheiro J M, Furdon S, Ochoa L F 1993 Role of local anaesthesia during lumbar puncture in neonates. Pediatrics 91(2): 379–382

Rennick G, Shann F, de Campo J 1993 Cerebral herniation during bacterial meningitis in children. British Medical Journal 306: 953–955

20

Neurological Observations and Coma Scales

Introduction

Neurological observations enable the nurse to assess the neurological status of the child. A coma scale is a tool in which a series of prescribed neurological observations are undertaken and recorded on a scaled chart. Each level of the scale on which results are plotted corresponds to a number. The numbers for different observations can be totalled to give an overall figure known as the coma scale rating, with a maximum score of 15 and a minimum score of 3. The lower the rating, the poorer the child's neurological status.

Learning outcomes

By the end of this section you should:

- understand the importance of an accurate neurological assessment
- be able to list the different elements of a neurological assessment
- be able to explain the significance of any changes in the child's neurological observations
- understand how, when and why coma scales are used and appreciate their limitations.

Rationale

Deterioration in the level of consciousness can occur rapidly with devastating, sometimes fatal consequences which may only be averted with prompt action and treatment. The ability to accurately assess the child's neurological status and interpret the results in order to detect promptly any alteration in conscious level is a vital skill for a children's nurse.

Factors to note

Coma scales

Coma scales were introduced in the early 1970s in a successful attempt to standardise nursing and medical approaches to neurological assessment. Coma scales cover five main areas for assessment, including the patient's ability to:

- open her eyes
- give a verbal response
- effect a motor response

and

- the strength of limb movement
- the size and reaction of pupils to light.

The most commonly used coma scale is the Glasgow Coma Scale (GCS). Devised by Teasdale & Jennett (1974), this is an adult scale but has also been adapted for children in recognition of the fact that verbal and motor responses must be related to the child's age (Campbell & Glasper 1995).

There are various paediatric adaptations of the GCS, for example that of James & Trauner (1985) as demonstrated in Table 20.1.

Another adapted GCS scale is known as the Paediatric Glasgow Coma Scale (PGCS) or Adelaide scale. Physicians at Adelaide Children's Hospital first adapted it for use in paediatrics and their adaptations were to the verbal and motor responses. These were developed to correlate with expected developmental milestones of children of different ages. The adaptations themselves were minor. They expected nurses to be trained to use the tool and those nurses to be able to apply knowledge of normal development when assessing the verbal and motor components of the scale. Table 20.2 demonstrates how a nurse would be expected to interpret a score against normal, verbal developmental milestones.

The Advanced Life Support Group (1997) developed a simplified version of a children's coma scale for use in children under 4 years – see Table 20.3.

Which scale to use is a matter of local choice according to the wishes of the multidisciplinary team. However, the nurse using the tool must be clear that suitable tuition has been given in how to use the tool and interpret results, and be aware of the limitations of each scale.

In addition, it must be remembered that the normal responses of a child who is developmentally delayed may not fall within the specified age range. It has been

Table 20.1   **James & Trauner (1985) paediatric adaptation of Glasgow Coma Scale**

	Children > 5 years	Children < 5 years	Score
Eyes open	▪ Spontaneously – without stimulation	▪ Spontaneously	4
	▪ To speech – when spoken to, not necessarily on command	▪ To speech	3
	▪ To pain – in response to any painful stimulus	▪ To pain	2
	▪ None – no eye opening at all	▪ None	1
Best verbal response	▪ Oriented – able to give name and address in response to verbal question	▪ Usual ability – uses sentences if previously able; recognisable words if not yet able to make sentences; babbles and coos for child not yet able to make words	5
	▪ Confused – able to converse but not oriented in person	▪ Less than usual – confused or no longer able to talk in sentences	4
	▪ Inappropriate – recognisable words but not in an exchange	▪ Cries to pain – cries only in response to painful stimuli	3
	▪ Incomprehensible – grunts, groans, incomprehensible sounds	▪ Only moans – but does not cry in response to painful stimuli	2
	▪ None – no verbal response even to painful stimuli	▪ None – no vocalisation, even to painful stimuli	1
Best motor response	▪ Obeys commands – obeys verbal commands	▪ Normal – normal play or voluntary or spontaneous movements	6
	▪ Localises – hands move above chin in response to supraorbital pressure painful stimulus	▪ Localises – as for > 5 years, or withdraws to painful stimulus	5
	▪ Withdraws – movement of limb away from painful stimulus	▪ Withdraws – as for > 5 years	4
	▪ Flexion abnormal – decorticate flexion at wrist and elbow, and abduction at shoulder to painful stimulus	▪ Flexion abnormal – as for > 5 years years	3
	▪ Extension abnormal – decerebrate extension to painful stimulus	▪ Extension abnormal – as for adults	2
	▪ None	▪ None	1

suggested that it may be more appropriate to identify age-related scales as 'adult/child according to ability' and 'child/infant' rather than 'child over 5 years' and 'child under 5 years', to allow for children who may be developmentally delayed.

Applying a painful stimulus during neurological assessment

In a child who is unconscious, it may be necessary to apply a painful stimulus in an attempt to evoke a motor response. This is done as described by Frawley (1990);

Table 20.2 **Paediatric Glasgow Coma Scale**

	> 1 year	< 1 year	Score
Eye opening	▪ Spontaneously	▪ Spontaneously	4
	▪ To verbal command	▪ To shout	3
	▪ To pain	▪ To pain	2
	▪ No response	▪ No response	1
Best motor response	▪ Obeys commands		5
	▪ Localises pain	▪ Localises pain	4
	▪ Flexion to pain	▪ Flexion to pain	3
	▪ Extension to pain	▪ Extension to pain	2
	▪ No response	▪ No response	1

	> 5 years	2–5 years	0–2 years	
Best verbal response	▪ Orientated and converses	▪ Appropriate words and phrases	▪ Smiles and cries appropriately	5
	▪ Disorientated and converses	▪ Inappropriate words	▪ Cries	4
	▪ Inappropriate words	▪ Cries	▪ Inappropriate crying	3
	▪ Incomprehensible sounds	▪ Grunting	▪ Grunting	2
	▪ No response	▪ No response	▪ No response	1

Reproduced from Lloyd-Thomas 1990 by kind permission of the BMJ Publishing Group.

the child's finger (third and fourth fingers are most sensitive) is placed between the nurse's thumb and a pencil or syringe and gradually increasing pressure is applied to the side of the finger until a response is obtained. Applying pressure to the nailbed with a pencil was frequently used in the past, but Frawley (1990) explains that this often results in bruising or marking.

Supraorbital pressure is another painful stimulus that has been utilised in the past, but it is particularly painful, so very rarely used now. The only exception should be when a child is thought to be in a very deep state of unconsciousness (due for example to a brain stem infarct) or believed to have suffered brain death. In such cases, applying pressure to the finger or nailbed could elicit a reflex response. Therefore in children who are deeply unconscious or undergoing tests for brain stem death, supraorbital pressure is an appropriate painful stimulus to evoke an accurate response. It should only be performed by staff who are competent and confident to do so.

Neonates

Neonates are notoriously difficult to assess neurologically and certainly most existing coma scales, even those that are adapted for infants and children, are not reliably accurate when assessing a child under 6 months of age (Allan 1994). Tatman et al (1997) devised and tested a grimace score for infants and children unable vocalise. It is an assessment of orofacial movement as opposed to a vocal response and has five elements (Table 20.4). Primarily aimed at intubated children in an intensive care unit, it is also used effectively for infants and neonates.

Hazinski (1992) highlights the need to evaluate the baby's alertness and response to his environment and Reeves (1989) the importance of referring to the child's parents who are most cognisant of their child's normal behaviour. Assessment of the fontanelle is also an important part of an assessment in a baby when the nurse feels to see if it is swollen, tense or sunken.

Sick children

Decrease in conscious level can be due to a number of causes, but most commonly will be due to reduced cerebral blood flow causing hypoxia, cerebral oedema, raised intracranial pressure (ICP), encephalopathy or status epilepticus. Common causes of these conditions are listed in Box 20.1.

Table 20.3   **Advanced Life Support Group children's coma scale: < 4 years**

Response	Score
Eyes	
■ Open spontaneously	4
■ React to speech	3
■ React to pain	2
■ No response	1
Best motor response	
■ Spontaneous or obeys verbal command	6
Reaction to painful stimulus	
■ Localises pain	5
■ Withdraws in response to pain	4
■ Abnormal flexion to pain (decorticate posture)	3
■ Abnormal extension to pain (decerebrate posture)	2
■ No response	1
Best verbal response	
■ Smiles, orientates to sounds, follows objects, interacts	5

Crying	*Interacts*	
■ Consolable	Inappropriate	4
■ Inconsistently consolable	Moaning	3
■ Inconsolable	Irritable	2
■ No response	No response	1

Reproduced from Lawton 1995 by kind permission.

It is worth noting that comatose children require and respond to stimulation, both verbal and touch (Hendrickson 1987, Hobdell et al 1989).

In a review of major research studies, Chudley (1994) describes how some nursing interventions can cause an increase in ICP in patients with previously raised ICP. Suctioning an endotracheal tube, repositioning/turning, moving the neck, clusters of care activity and invasive procedures, e.g. passing a nasogastric tube, are all mentioned. This highlights the importance of planning care to ensure minimal handling with periods of rest to allow the ICP to stabilise between care, for any child with a known or suspected raised ICP. However, decisions about timing of care must always be carefully balanced with the need

Table 20.4   **Grimace score (Tatman et al 1997)**

Orofacial response	Score
Spontaneous normal facial/oromotor activity, e.g. sucks tube, coughs	5
Less than usual spontaneous ability or only responds to touch	4
Vigorous grimace to pain	3
Mild grimace or some change in facial expression to pain	2
No response to pain	1

Box 20.1   Possible causes of decreased conscious level in children

- Reduced cerebral blood flow caused by:
  - respiratory insufficiency
  - hypovolaemia
  - gross anaemia
  - poor cardiac output state
- Cerebral oedema caused by:
  - fluid overload
  - multisystem failure
  - seizures
  - hyperpyrexia
  - electrolyte imbalance
- Raised intracranial pressure due to:
  - hydrocephalus
  - space-occupying lesion
  - intracerebral bleeding (traumatic or spontaneous)
  - meningitis
  - trauma/head injury
  - arterial blood gas abnormality, e.g. raised PCO_2
- Encephalopathy due to:
  - infection, e.g. chickenpox, herpes
  - sepsis
  - liver disease
  - renal disease
  - ingestion of toxins
  - hypo/hyperglycaemia
- Blood clots or air emboli caused by intravenous therapy and/or invasive monitoring techniques

---

to monitor closely in order to determine and act swiftly on any detrimental changes in the child's condition.

Guidelines

The important role which parents play in the neurological assessment of a child must be further stressed. A frightened child is unlikely to cooperate initially if strangers ask her to obey commands, whether or not she is physically able to do so. However, she may decide to obey the same command if it is her mother or father who ask, rather than a nurse. Hazinski (1992) describes phrasing questions to the child around people and things which are familiar to her. This information will of course be gained from your initial history taken from the child (if able) and her family (see Assessment, p. 45).

It is also important to remember that head injury in a child or baby could be a child protection issue. In this case, child protection procedures should be instigated and it is important to observe the interaction between the child and her parents. Very occasionally, when it is suspected that a child may have been physically abused, a court order may prevent her parent(s) from being with her.

Equipment
- Thermometer
- Blood pressure monitor
- Pen torch or ophthalmoscope
- Colourful and noisy toys if appropriate
- Neurological observation assessment tool/recording chart

Method
1. Collect equipment together and approach the child.
2. Before undertaking physical observations, assess the child's clinical signs and behaviour generally, taking into account pre-existing conditions and the knowledge gained from the initial history-taking assessment:
   a. Is the child asleep or awake, settled and peaceful or irritable and unhappy?
   b. Is her colour unusual – pallor, redness, mottling or cyanosis?
   c. Does she appear bothered by bright lights (is she photophobic)?
   d. Does she seem reluctant to move her head or cry out if she is made to straighten her legs?
   e. If she is sleeping or quiet, is this appropriate? Is she making any noise at all or is she grunting? Is her breathing regular and easy or shallow, irregular or very slow?
   f. Is there evidence of 'setting sun' eyes – the sclera being visible above the iris?
   g. Does her breath smell of anything unusual, e.g. alcohol, solvents, ketones?
   h. Are there any rashes or skin lesions, e.g. purpuric rash (small red/purple spots, not raised) which does not blanch white if the skin is rubbed/depressed with a finger (suggestive of meningococcal infection), or café au lait spots (coffee-coloured patches on the skin) which could suggest neurofibromatosis?
   i. Is there any evidence of seizures? Any seizure activity must be observed carefully, recorded and reported (see Seizures, p. 249).
   j. If the child is awake and conscious, utilise normal play to assess her conscious level and in particular her eye, motor and verbal responses in accordance with whichever coma scale you are using.
   k. Does she respond to you appropriately for her age and expected development, both verbally and physically?

3. Summarise your initial assessment. Is there any cause for concern such as unusual, unexplained irritability? Severe irritability in any child or baby can be a sign of cerebral irritation and decreasing level of consciousness.

4. If you have any concerns about the above, it is important to inform a senior nurse or doctor and move quickly to take observations to see if there is any further evidence of serious neurological deficit or if there has been any deterioration since observations were last taken.

5. Explain to the child (if able to understand) and parents what you are about to do. Stress that the observations will not hurt.

6. As with any observations, first observe and record those which do not require physical intervention, e.g. respirations (see Assessment, p. 45).

7. Then undertake recordings of temperature, pulse and blood pressure (see Assessment, p. 45).
   a. Temperature. Observe for swings in temperature, e.g. acute pyrexia which could be indicative of raised ICP (causing pressure on the hypothalamus).
   b. Pulse rate. Severe, raised ICP can be indicated by bradycardia caused by excessive pressure on the medulla. Tachycardia could be due to pain, infection or blood loss.
   c. Respiratory rate. Abnormal respiratory rate could be due to pain, infection, pyrexia. Irregular respiratory rate could indicate raised ICP, again because of pressure on the medulla; depressed respiration could be a sign of actual damage to the brain stem.
   d. Blood pressure. Hypertension is a sign of raised ICP (pressure on the medulla), particularly when coupled with bradycardia. Pain could also cause hypertension.
      A very late sign of severe, acute, brain damage is known as Cushing's triad and is indicated by an increased blood pressure and pulse rate with a depressed respiratory rate.

8. If the child has not been able so far to demonstrate eye, motor and verbal responses, e.g. through play or her reactions to your observations, attempt to assess these aspects now.

9. Eye and verbal responses. Confusion and inappropriate words and speech indicate decreasing levels of consciousness as does vigorous or mild grimacing in the non-vocal child.
   a. Are the child's eyes open spontaneously? If her eyes are closed, try to get her to open them by first talking to her. If she does not open her eyes when you talk to her, ask her to open her eyes (if she is old enough). If she still does not open her eyes or is too young to understand the request, try raising your voice a little and give a brief shout (to try to startle her into opening her eyes).
   b. Does a baby fix and follow with her eyes when you dangle a toy in front of her?
   c. Is she able to concentrate on what you are saying to her; is she alert?
   d. Listen to the child. Is she chatting apparently normally, aware of her surroundings and her parents?
   e. Is a baby babbling or cooing?
   f. Is the toddler making words and noises which she would normally make (check with parents)? She may be vocalising, but appear confused. Check that this is not due to her unfamiliarity with her surroundings.
   g. Is any crying appropriate, i.e. because she is scared of what is happening to her and of her surroundings or because she is in pain?
   h. Is she consolable or distressed and irritable?
   i. If a baby is crying, what does it sound like? Is it particularly high pitched? Is she moaning, groaning or irritable for no reason? Grunting noises in any child are a sign that something is seriously wrong. The abnormally high-pitched cry of a baby can be due to raised ICP or cerebral irritation. The child who makes no noise or facial expression could be deeply unconscious.

10. Pupil reactions. Pupils should be of equal size and should both react equally and briskly to light. Any inequality of pupil size or reaction is indicative of a problem on the same side of the brain as the abnormal reaction. Fixed dilated pupils are a very poor sign and can indicate brain death. However, hypothermia and some drugs (e.g. large doses of atropine, some ophthalmic drugs) can cause dilated pupils.
   a. It is important to assess the child's pupils initially, before shining any lights into them. *Before* you start, are her pupils of equal size?
   b. Is there any evidence of a squint which is not normal for her?
   c. If the child is asleep and will not or cannot open her own eyes, the nurse may have to lift her eyelids. It is important that both lids are lifted simultaneously, which may require two people, one to open each eye.
   d. Ideally, pupil reactions are then tested by turning off the main overhead lights and shining a bright, thin beam onto the child's open eye.

e. How do her pupils react to light? Observe the size of the pupil and how it reacts to the light shining on it. Does it contract briskly or is it sluggish or not reacting?

f. A child who has been deeply asleep may also be reluctant to open her eyes and equally her pupils may both be a little sluggish to react at first.

g. If the child cannot or will not cooperate with opening her eyes, you may have to lift the upper lid yourself. If she is unwilling to cooperate, it may help to give her the torch to play with and observe what happens from a little further away or make it into a game with turning lights on and off.

h. Be aware that pupil reactions can be affected (slowed) by severe hypothermia.

11. Motor responses. Assess the child's movements. Observe for decreasing conscious level by assessing any abnormality of motor response.

a. Is the child playing with her toys or feeding from a bottle using both hands?

b. Can she grasp your fingers with equal strength with both her hands?

c. Does she move her legs normally – kicking or reacting if you tickle her feet?

d. If she is not moving, try to get her to move, firstly by asking her to do so, e.g. 'Can you lift your arm for me?' In an infant you would attempt to get her to reach towards you or perhaps move her foot as you tickle it.

e. If there is still no movement, you will have to inflict a painful stimulus to try to evoke a response.

f. If the child is old enough/developmentally capable, ask her to touch her nose with the tip of her finger whilst her eyes are closed (testing her proprioception – awareness of parts of the body without looking).

12. Limb strength and posture. Again, it is inequality of the two sides which can indicate a problem occurring in one side of the brain. Note also if the child is particularly floppy when handled (hypotonia) or stiffer than would be expected (hypertonia) and if this affects one side more than another or both sides equally.

a. Is one of her limbs weaker than the other or stiffer than the other?

b. Again, observe the conscious child at play. Is it obvious that she is not using one limb as much as the others?

c. Is she sitting straight or is she showing a tendency to collapse to one side?

d. In a small baby, put your fingers in her hands and see if she can grasp your fingers equally with both hands.

e. Does she reach for toys?

f. Does she kick her legs?

g. Ask the child who is old enough to understand, to wiggle her fingers and toes, kick with her legs, wave at you with her arms.

h. Is the child assuming an abnormal posture, e.g. opisthotonus (neck retracted fully back and back arched with her head nearing the buttocks), evidence of meningeal irritation?

i. As might be expected from the coma scales, decorticate posturing (abnormal flexion), when a child involuntarily bends her limbs with adduction to the midline, is indicative of a decrease in consciousness. The next sign of deterioration is decerebrate posturing (abnormal extension), when a child involuntarily straightens her limbs which are abducted away from the midline.

j. A child can alternate between decorticate and decerebrate posturing as a result of differing cerebral blood flow to the brain stem and cerebral hemispheres.

13. Record your observations on the coma scale/neurological chart.

14. Interpret your findings. Assess the child's status compared with previous observations and the total of her PGCS on the first occasion. Is she improving or deteriorating? Is there any observation which gives you cause for concern?

15. Report your findings and assess when the next set of observations should be performed.

Complications

There are not really any complications of the procedure of neurological assessment. The dangers lie in:

- an inexperienced practitioner being inaccurate in undertaking the observations
- how the results of the observations are interpreted. If any nurse is unsure of the implications of the results of a set of neurological observations, the advice of a more senior colleague must be sought.

COMMUNITY PERSPECTIVE

This procedure is one that would not often be undertaken in the home. However, there will be occasions when carers and professionals involved in the child's care will need to be aware of altering levels of consciousness. The situation is only likely to occur with the child who is chronically ill where no immediate action is required. It is unlikely that formal recording of observations will be appropriate as it is important that the environment should not become clinical.

The role of the CCN would be to raise the awareness of the carers without causing apprehension, showing them how to undertake any monitoring required. During visits she will routinely assess the child, taking the carer's comments as part of the assessment. Findings will be documented and liaison maintained with medical staff as necessary.

Do and do not

- Do remember that a child's neurological status can deteriorate rapidly. Be alert for signs of raised intracranial pressure.
- Do remember to gain as much information as possible from observing the child and her reaction to her surroundings prior to undertaking observations.
- Do remember that the child's parents are the ones who are most cognisant of what is and is not normal for their child and use this information in your observations.
- Do report any abnormalities or anything of which the implications are unclear.
- Do not miss out on undertaking neurological observations because a child is sleeping, without first checking with a senior nurse. How do you know that the child is asleep and not unconscious?

References

Advanced Life Support Group 1997 Advanced paediatric life support: the practical approach, 2nd edn. British Medical Journal Publications, London, p 119

Allan D 1994 Paediatric coma scale. Surgical Nurse 7(3): 14–16

Campbell S, Glasper E A (eds) 1995 Whaley and Wong's children's nursing, UK edn. Mosby/Times Mirror International, London, ch 31, pp 660–679

Chudley S 1994 The effect of nursing activities on intracranial pressure. British Journal of Nursing 3(9): 454–459

Frawley P 1990 Neurological observations. Nursing Times 86(35): 29–34

Hazinski M F 1992 Nursing care of the critically ill child, 2nd edn. Mosby Year Book, St Louis, ch 8, pp 584–585

Hendrickson S L 1987 Intracranial pressure changes and family presence. Journal of Neuroscience Nursing 19(1): 14–17

Hobdell E F, Adams F, Caruso J, Dihoff R, Neverling E, Roncoli M 1989 The effect of nursing activities on the intracranial pressure of children. Critical Care Nurse 9(6): 75–79

James H E, Trauner D A 1985 The Glasgow Coma Scale. In: James H E, Anas N G, Perkin R M (eds) Brain insults in infants and children. Grune & Stratton, Orlando, pp 179–182

Lawton L 1995 Paediatric trauma – the care of Anthony. Accident and Emergency Nursing 3: 172–176

Lloyd-Thomas A R 1990 Primary survey and resuscitation – II. British Medical Journal 301: 380–382

Reeves K 1989 Assessment of pediatric head injury. Journal of Emergency Nursing 15(4): 329–332

Tatman A, Warren A, Williams A, Powell J E, Whitehouse W 1997 Development of a paediatric coma scale in intensive care clinical practice. Archives of Disease in Childhood 77(6): 519–521

Teasdale G, Jennett W B 1974 Assessment of coma and impaired consciousness. Lancet 2: 81–84

Further reading

Reilly P L, Simpson D, Sprod R, Thomas L 1988 Assessing the conscious level in infants and young children: a paediatric version of the Glasgow Coma Scale. Child's Nervous System 4: 30–33

Simpson D A, Cockington R A, Hanieh A, Raftos J, Reilly P L 1991 Head injuries in infants and young children: the value of the paediatric coma scale. Review of literature and report on a study. Child's Nervous System 7: 183–190

21

Oral Hygiene

Introduction

Maintaining oral hygiene is an essential part of daily living and even in 'healthy' individuals this can be problematic (Thurgood 1994). There is no feeling more uncomfortable than having a sore, dry or dirty mouth or a mouth that tastes unpleasant. There is an important role for the nurse in maintaining good oral hygiene, either directly by providing oral care or indirectly by giving advice and opportunities for self-care (Torrance 1990), thus contributing to the child's overall comfort.

For the nurse to provide a good standard of oral hygiene, knowledge and understanding of the normal anatomy and physiology of the mouth, teeth, gums, tongue and lips is required. In addition to this the nurse must also understand the importance of adequate hydration and nutrition; microbiology and oral infections; the effects of various drugs, treatments and diseases (Thurgood 1994); the implications of physical impairment and altered physical dexterity (Lloyd 1992). Appreciation of these factors will underpin oral assessment and enable the nurse to identify problems amenable to nursing interventions (Krishnasamy 1995).

The nurse has a pivotal role in deciding which form of mouth care to provide, which includes which implement or cleansing agent to use and the frequency with which it is implemented. Oral hygiene is an integral part of the total care; assessment precedes planning, followed by intervention and evaluation, with specific nursing measures instigated to prevent, minimise or reverse changes in the oral cavity (Maurer 1977).

Learning outcomes

By the end of this section the nurse will be able to:

- describe the normal oral physiology of the mouth
- assess the oral cavity, and recognise and describe any deviation from normal
- discuss the factors that may predispose or contribute to oral complications
- describe the various implements and cleansing agents available and how they are used to ensure effective oral hygiene
- recognise the special considerations required by different children, depending on their level of cognitive and physical development
- discuss the nurse's role in oral hygiene as part of a holistic approach.

Rationale for mouth care

'The mouth is important for eating, drinking, speech, communication, taste, breathing and defence' (Thurgood 1994, p. 332). The principal objective of oral hygiene is to maintain the mouth in good condition, that is, comfortable, clean, moist and free of infection (see Box 21.1). To ensure a healthy mouth, all

---

> *Box 21.1* **Aims of oral hygiene (Beck 1992, Clarke 1993, Howarth 1977, MacMillan 1981, Maurer 1977, Richardson 1987)**
>
> - To achieve and maintain a healthy and clean oral cavity
> - To prevent the build-up of plaque on oral surfaces, thus helping prevent dental caries
> - To keep the oral mucosa moist
> - To maintain mucosal integrity and promote healing
> - To prevent infection
> - To prevent broken or chapped lips
> - To promote patient dignity, comfort and well-being
> - To maintain oral function

children, regardless of their age or health status, will require some degree of guidance and assistance, from either their parents or carers, or a member of the nursing team.

Oral physiology

The anatomy and physiology of the mouth are complex. Two of the principal functions of the mouth relate to digestion and defence. The oral cavity is the first part of the gastrointestinal tract. The major structures that are visible on examination are:

The mucosal lining. This is continuous with the gastrointestinal tract and protects the underlying tissues. The mucous membranes, via the salivary glands, secrete mucus and saliva. Saliva is formed mainly of water (99% of total) and normally has a pH of 6.8–7.0. It does, however, become more alkaline as the secretory rate increases during chewing. Saliva contains lysozyme, which has an antiseptic action, immunoglobulin (IgA), which has a defensive function, and a digestive enzyme, salivary amylase (Hinchliff 1988). These properties result in keeping the oral mucosa moist, smooth, clean and shiny with the buffering capacity maintaining the balance of the microbial flora (Campbell et al 1995).

The lips. These form a muscular entrance to the mouth; they are covered by squamous, keratinised epithelial tissue which is vascular and very sensitive. They are necessary for ingestion of food, enunciation of words and convey the mood of a person, e.g. smiling and grimacing (Hinchliff 1988).

The tongue. This is covered with mucous membrane from which project numerous papillae and taste buds on the upper surface. The muscles of the tongue afford it great mobility, which is essential for speech and swallowing; its other main function is interpreting taste sensations.

The teeth. These consist of enamel, dentine, cementum and pulp. The first tooth normally erupts at around 6 months of age with the full complement of 20 deciduous teeth being acquired by the age of $2\frac{1}{2}$ years. Permanent dentition begins between 5 and 6 years; the full number of 28 teeth have normally appeared by 13–15 years (Hall 1995a,b). The four wisdom teeth erupt later, usually by the age of 25, making the full complement of 32 teeth (Hinchliff 1988).

Factors to note

When assessing the oral cavity a thorough and systematic assessment is essential so that any changes are monitored and appropriate treatment implemented.

Disposable gloves and a good source of light should be used when examining the oral cavity. It is also good practice for the child to clean his teeth prior to the examination in order to remove plaque and food debris (Lloyd 1992).

An effective oral assessment should include examination of the components identified in Box 21.2.

Conditions that may compromise oral well-being should also be considered when undertaking an oral assessment. Detailed in Table 21.1 are some specific examples of contributory factors which may affect the ability for oral hygiene to be performed effectively. These factors are considered in the light of subsequent oral complications that may result. Once associated problems have been identified, appropriate advice and support can be given to promote optimal oral health.

Whether 'teething' is a genuine condition resulting from the eruption of a tooth is a controversial issue; hence it is mentioned apart from conditions in Table 21.1. Mothers observe fretfulness, a high temperature or a rash coinciding with tooth eruption in the apparent absence of any other factors (Hall 1995b). Teething would seem to be a physiological rather than a pathological condition, a phenomenon that does not seem to occur with the eruption of second teeth.

Guidelines for implementation of oral care

Dental hygiene should begin as the primary teeth erupt (Bentley 1994, Lloyd 1994). Even babies with no teeth require consideration, as primary teeth can decay like permanent teeth if not looked after (Lloyd 1994). The nurse's role is to facilitate family-centred care; therefore, whenever possible, oral care should be performed by the child or family. However, where there are specific concerns the nurse may be required to assist, support, educate and advise or refer the child or family for more specialised dental assessment or treatment (Casey 1993).

Normal oral care

Teeth should be cleaned effectively twice a day, as soon as possible after meals if eating, and before bedtime, with a soft toothbrush and toothpaste. A cleaning sponge soaked in water may be more appropriate for babies who have no teeth.

The more frequently and the longer teeth are cleaned the greater the probability of effective plaque removal. Even when the child is not eating, such as when he is unconscious, regular and thorough mouth care is vital.

There are occasions when an optimum oral hygiene regime may be sacrificed for patient comfort.

Box 21.2   **Components to be examined during an oral assessment (Eilers et al 1988, Thurgood 1994)**

Voice
- Deep/raspy
- Difficult or painful
- Absent

Palate
- Colour
- Moisture
- Inflammation

Lips
- Cracked
- Lesions
- Bleeding
- Moisture

Tongue
- Texture
- Colour
- Moisture

Swallow
- Difficult or painful
- Inability

Mucous membrane
- Colour
- Moisture
- Ulceration
- Inflammation

Teeth
- Plaque
- Colour
- Cavities
- Loose
- Eruption or exfoliation

Gingiva
- Colour
- Moisture
- Inflammation
- Bleeding
- Ulceration

Saliva
- Thin/watery
- Hypersalivation
- Scanty/absent
- Thick/ropy

Taste
- Impaired
- Altered
- After-taste

Breath
- Halitosis

Positioning

For the younger child (under 7 years), effective positioning should facilitate the carer's access to the child's mouth and stabilise the child's head. One way of doing this is to stand with the child's back towards the adult, using one hand to cup the chin and the other to brush the teeth.

In the case of an ill child, find a position that is most comfortable and reassuring.

Safety

To conform to universal precautions nurses should wear gloves when performing oral hygiene. This is essential as *Candida albicans* can be transmitted between patients on the hands of staff (Burnie et al 1985, cited in Barnett 1991). Oral fungal infections are often asymptomatic; therefore even if the mouth of a patient seems healthy, it is good practice to wear gloves.

Play therapy

Allow the child to handle the mouth care products in a non-threatening environment; perform mouth care on a favourite toy, parent or nurse. This will help reduce anxiety, allow time for questions and ultimately increase compliance.

Play specialists can help provide a supportive role in preparing children for mouth care procedures.

Table 21.1   Assessment of contributory factors which may compromise oral well-being

General conditions that may compromise oral well-being	Specific examples	Oral complications that may be experienced
Impaired/altered physical dexterity	Cerebral palsy Accidents or other illness causing: neurological damage unconsciousness loss of limb maxillofacial injury	Difficulty or inability to perform oral hygiene resulting in: build-up of plaque dental caries halitosis Ataxia or spasticity may increase risk of damage to mucosa and soft tissue structures
Physical complications	Restricted oral access due to: orthodontic or maxillofacial surgery enlarged, protruding tongue respiratory problems epidermolysis bullosa	May cause difficulty in performing oral hygiene (as above) Mouthbreathing causing dry mucosa Increased risk of mucosal deterioration
	Restricted movement of tongue due to: surgery or pain chronic constipation cleft palate (may have prosthesis)	Ineffective removal of debris Foul mouth and odour Lips, gums, palate prone to pressure sores; retention of food debris under prosthesis
Fragile mucosa	Effects of chemo/radiotherapy Epidermolysis bullosa	Mucositis, ulceration, causing: pain infection bleeding
Children with special needs	Down's Syndrome and other disabling conditions Habitual licking or biting of lips	Tendency towards thick, ropy, sticky saliva which adheres to the surface of teeth and forms plaque Deformed teeth may retain plaque Dry, cracked or inflamed lips Discomfort
Immunodeficiencies	HIV Following cytotoxic therapy Combined immune deficiency	Reduced production of protective immunoglobulins in saliva resulting in increased risk of infection Persistent candida infections
Common childhood illnesses and dental habits	Measles Fever Grinding of teeth Thumb sucking	Koplik, white spots Dryness, coated tongue, halitosis Mild/severe loss of tooth surface Alteration to position of teeth (upper, anterior)

Table 21.1 (Contd.) **Assessment of contributory factors which may compromise oral well-being**

General conditions that may compromise oral well-being	Specific examples	Oral complications that may be experienced
Poor nutritional intake	Anorexia	Vitamin deficiency, tissue vulnerability
	Dehydration	Dryness, halitosis
	Metabolic disorders requiring high intake of oral carbohydrates	Increase in dental caries
	Glycoprotein storage disease (some types)	Oral ulceration
Foreign body in nose	Commonly inserted are peas, peanuts and small toys	Sudden foul odour in the mouth
Drugs	Antibiotics	Altered oral flora, increased risk of opportunistic infections
	Antihistamine	Reduced salivary production
	Atropine	Reduced salivary production
	Chlorhexidine-based mouthwash	Temporary brown staining of teeth Stinging/burning sensation Bitter taste, altered after-taste
	Corticosteroids	Delayed healing of tissue
	Cyclosporin	Gum hyperplasia
	Cytotoxic agents	Altered taste perception (often metallic) Saliva absent or ropy
	Diuretics	Altered salivary function
	Insulin	Altered salivary function
	Iron supplements	Temporary green/black staining of teeth
	Long-term, high-sucrose content medication, e.g. lactulose	Increased incidence of dental caries
	Morphine	Dry mucosa
	Nifedipine	Gingival enlargement
	Oxygen therapy	Dry mucosa
	Phenytoin	Gingival hypertrophy

Special consideration for the older child or teenager

These of patients have increased concern regarding body image and sexuality. They may be anxious or embarrassed by changes in their oral cavity, such as gingival enlargement, increased salivation, inability to swallow or speak effectively, halitosis. They may be angry about these changes and direct their anger towards staff or even reject treatment measures. The following issues should always be considered:

- Where possible allow them control; for example, let them choose the timing of mouth care.
- Respect their need for privacy when undertaking any aspect of oral care.
- Involve them in planning their oral care so that they will understand its importance and thus be more receptive to health teaching: 'they should be accepted as a vital member of the health care team' (Brunner & Suddarth 1986, p. 66).
- Ensure that explanations are age appropriate and reinforced with written information.

Children with cancer

Children receiving chemotherapy or radiotherapy may experience specific problems. A number of the chemotherapy agents used are known to cause oral stomatitis: directly, owing to decreased cell renewal, resulting in epithelial thinning, inflammation and ulceration with an added risk of secondary infection; indirectly, because of reduced bone marrow activity, resulting in an increased risk of bleeding (thrombocytopenia) and infection (neutropenia) (Richardson 1987). Radiotherapy exerts a direct effect, decreasing cell renewal with the resulting complications, only when the oral cavity lies within the treatment field (Holmes 1991).

In addition to normal oral care these children may require the use of an antifungal agent and/or an anti bacterial mouthwash (Gibson et al 1997).

Rationale supporting choice of tool and agent

Nurses must be accountable for the care they give, and whenever possible research-based evidence should provide the rationale for that care (see Table 21.2). Effective management will be facilitated by an appreciation of the best agents and implements available, whilst also considering the individual needs of the child.

Not recommended for oral care are:

- glycerin lemon swabs
- hydrogen peroxide

- sodium bicarbonate
- gauze-wrapped fingers or forceps.

The use of glycerine and lemon swabs or solution is actively discouraged. Lemon and glycerine swabs were used routinely for their moisturising and refreshing properties; they also taste pleasant. However, there are no overall benefits in using them as they have little value in either cleaning or moisturising the oral cavity (Beck 1992). Glycerine is hypertonic, drawing moisture from the tissue and causing reflex exhaustion of the salivary process, and lemon contains acid which can irritate the mucosa and decalcify the teeth (Roth & Creason 1986).

The mode of cleansing of hydrogen peroxide is the rapid release of oxygen bubbles when the catalase in saliva reacts with peroxide to produce a froth which exerts a mechanical cleansing action (Beck 1992). Beck also claims that it exerts an antimicrobial effect. These two properties need to be balanced with reports of a burning and stinging sensation, and also a bitter and unpleasant after-taste. In addition, there are potentially more serious implications if solutions are mixed incorrectly, when strong solutions cause superficial burns (Howarth 1977) and alter the oral flora resulting in candidal overgrowth. In children the foaming action is not well tolerated.

Sodium bicarbonate is claimed to be an economical, effective and non-irritating cleansing agent, particularly if crusted sores or a dry coated tongue are present (Campbell et al 1995). It is a mild alkali and therefore has the ability to neutralise the potentially damaging acidic environment produced by bacteria in the mouth, but only when diluted correctly; if the pH becomes too alkaline, it may have adverse effects on the mucosa (Barnett 1991). Poor compliance in children has been attributed to its salty and unpleasant taste (Galbraith et al 1991).

Gauze wrapped around a finger or forceps is ineffective at removing plaque and may even compress debris into crevices and gaps between teeth (Shepherd et al 1987). In addition, if forceps are used it is difficult to assess the amount of pressure being exerted. Where a finger is used, there is an increased risk of transmission of infections between patients, as well as a hazard to the caregiver of a distressed child biting the finger.

Health promotion

Diet

Dietary advice should be given not long after birth, before habits become established. Health visitors are in a prime position to give this advice as well as promoting appropriate oral hygiene and encouraging visits to the dentist at an early age (Bentley 1994).

Table 21.2 **Rationale for use of implement and cleansing agents**

Tool	Action	Advantages	Disadvantages	Comments
Toothbrush	Brushes/cleans teeth and oral tissues. Place tips of bristles at 45 degrees against teeth and gums; move brush backwards and forwards in a gentle but vibratory motion. To clean the inner (lingual) surfaces place toothbrush vertical to the teeth and move it up and down against the gums	Proven ability to clean effectively; provides the most effective method for removing plaque Known to the child	Potential gum haemorrhages Need to keep brush clean	Use a small-headed, soft, multi-tufted, nylon-bristled toothbrush (Gooch 1985, Lloyd 1992, Maurer 1977, Watson 1989) With young children (under 7 years) most effective cleaning is done by parents Important that gums as well as teeth are brushed (Lloyd 1992) Implement of choice even when children are immunocompromised (Tomlinson & Kennedy 1999)
Electric toothbrush	Rotating, oscillating and vibratory action	Useful for physically impaired children	Bristles are hard, not advisable for children with fragile mucosa	
Cleaning sponges	Delivery of fluids to specific places	Soft, malleable, unthreatening, easy to use Can be squeezed into difficult places Useful for removing debris	Ineffective at removing plaque	Local application but no cleaning action (Pearson 1996) Introduced as a temporary measure only, or combined with a toothbrush (Gooch 1985) Preferable in the terminal stages of illness when comfort is the only intended outcome (Holmes 1991)
Dental floss	Pulled gently downwards and upwards between the teeth	Combined with a toothbrush, is the most effective method of removing plaque Reaches parts toothbrush bristles are unable to reach	Need dexterity to manipulate floss, difficult to floss someone else's teeth	Not advised with children under 10 years (Lloyd 1992)

Table 21.2 (Contd.)   **Rationale for use of implement and cleansing agents**

Tool	Action	Advantages	Disadvantages	Comments
Fluoride toothpaste	Use small pea-sized amount on toothbrush	Strengthens tooth enamel and decreases risk of dental caries	Can have a drying effect if left in contact with oral mucosa	Excessive fluoride may result in very tough teeth and produce unsightly spotting – fluorosis (Lloyd 1994) Check fluoride content of water supply prior to introducing supplements Supervise use of toothpaste to prevent swallowing of excessive amounts
Vaseline	Applied to lips providing an occlusive film	Occlusive film retains moisture Easy to apply, will remain in place for many hours if not licked off Soothes dry lips	Highly flammable May trap bacteria on the lips	Not advised for babies under phototherapy Use fresh tube for each child Use sparingly Most acceptable method of preventing dry, cracked lips (Campbell 1987)

Adapted with permission from Campbell et al 1995.

Ensure that the diet contains vitamins B and C to preserve integrity of the mucosa; vitamins A and D and calcium to ensure development of healthy teeth; and protein for repair of cells.

For snacks between meals encourage non-sugary foods such as cheese, fresh vegetables or water. If sugary foods are given, ensure that they are part of main meals and therefore eaten before teeth are brushed.

Do not give prolonged bottled feeds of milk or juice, especially during sleep; this can result in 'bottle caries', a form of very destructive dental disease (Bentley 1994). Encourage the use of a cup or straw, rather than a bottle.

Baby foods given at meal times can be accompanied by a well-diluted natural fruit juice with no added sugar; this will reduce the risk of acid attack on the tooth enamel (Lloyd 1994).

Do not put honey or sweet syrup on a dummy (honey is also a potential source of botulism in babies (Hooton 1995)).

Dental checkups

Encourage children to visit the dentist from an early age. Even very young children can accompany a parent in order to introduce them to the smells and sounds. They can also be encouraged to sit in the dentist's chair in the hope that this preparation will prevent the development of anxiety and fear of the dentist in the future.

Regular dental checks should include prophylactic teeth cleaning.

Promoting sugar-free medicines

Sugar in medicines can contribute to dental caries, especially when given at night (Roberts & Roberts 1979). As saliva flow is greatly reduced at night the sugar remains in contact with the teeth for a longer period (Bentley & Mackie 1995). Paracetamol syrups and cough mixtures are commonly used paediatric medicines and are available sugar-free. Their use should be recommended from an early age.

Injury prevention

Even with the most conscientious supervision, trauma to the teeth is not uncommon in childhood. To decrease the incidence of injury:

- encourage the wearing of mouthguards during contact sports
- use non-slip mats in the bath
- supervise children on play equipment.

Do and do not

- Do involve the child and family in mouth care.
- Do ensure that there is a dentist involved in the care of all children.
- Do individualise the oral care regime; incorporate it into the care plan.
- Do systematically assess the condition of the mouth; include ongoing regular assessment.
- Do minimise mouth problems through introducing systematic care.
- Do consider factors that may compromise oral well-being.
- Do select implements and cleansing agents that are research-based, but also reflect the needs of the child.
- Do remind the child or parent to brush teeth after meals and before bedtime.
- Do use age-appropriate measures to involve children or teenagers in their oral hygiene regime.
- Do promote the use of sugar-free medicines.
- Do, where possible, give non-sugary snacks.
- Do maximise the opportunities presented for health promotion, particularly in relation to dental care and dental checkups for the whole family
- Do not use glycerine and lemon swabs or solution.
- Do not use cleaning sponges in preference to a toothbrush (unless comfort or trauma indicates otherwise).
- Do not use gauze-wrapped fingers or forceps.
- Do not give prolonged breast or bottle feeds (this includes bottles of juice), especially during sleep.
- Do not put honey or sweet syrup on a dummy.

References

Barnett J 1991 A reassessment of oral healthcare. Professional Nurse 6(12): 703–708

Beck S L 1992 Prevention and management of oral complications in the cancer patient. In: Hubbard S M, Greene P E, Knobf M T (eds) Current Issues in Cancer Nursing Practice Updates 1(6): 1–12

Bentley E 1994 Views about preventive dental care for infants. Health Visitor 67(3): 88–89

Bentley E M, Mackie I C 1995 Promoting sugar-free paediatric medicines to parents. Health Visitor 68(8): 327–328

Brunner L S, Suddarth D S 1986 The Lippincott manual of paediatric nursing, 2nd edn. Harper and Row, London

Campbell S J 1987 Mouthcare in cancer patients. Nursing Times 83(29): 59–60

Campbell S T, Evans M A, Mactavish F 1995 Guidelines for mouthcare. The Paediatric Oncology Nursing Forum, Royal College of Nursing, London

Casey A 1993 Development and use of the partnership model of nursing care. In: Glasper E A, Tucker A (eds) Advances in child health nursing. Scutari Press, London

Clarke G 1993 Mouth care and the hospitalized patient. British Journal of Nursing 2(4): 225–227

Eilers J, Berger A M, Peterson M C 1988 Development, testing and application of the oral assessment guide. Oncology Nursing Forum 15(3): 325–330

Galbraith I, Bailey D, Kelly L et al 1991 Treatment for alteration in oral mucosa related to chemotherapy. Pediatric Nursing 17(3): 233–237

Gibson F, Horsford J, Nelson W 1997 Oral care: Ritualistic practice reconsidered within a framework of action research. Journal of Cancer Nursing. 1(4): 183–190

Gooch J 1985 Mouth care. Professional Nurse 1(3): 77–78

Hall A 1995a Children's dental development. 1. Birth to six years old. Professional Care of Mother and Child 5(4): 100–101

Hall A 1995b Children's dental development. 2. Six years old to early teens. Professional Care of Mother and Child 5(5): 129–130

Hinchliff S 1988 The acquisition of nutrients. In: Hinchliff S, Montague S (eds) Physiology for nursing practice. Baillière Tindall, London, ch 5.1

Holmes S 1991 The oral complications of specific anticancer therapy. International Journal of Nursing Studies 28(4): 343–360

Hooton M 1995 Health problems of middle childhood. In: Campbell S, Glasper E A (eds) Whaley and Wong's children's nursing. Mosby, London, ch 17

Howarth H 1977 Mouthcare procedures for the very ill. Nursing Times 73(10): 354–355

Krishnasamy M 1995 The nurse's role in oral care. European Journal of Palliative Care 2(2) (suppl 1): 8–9

Lloyd S 1992 Brushing up on children's mouth care. Professional Care of Mother and Child 2(1): 16–17

Lloyd S 1994 Teaching parents to look after children's teeth. Professional Care of Mother and Child 4(2): 34–36

MacMillan K 1981 New goals for oral hygiene. Canadian Nurse 77: 40–43

Maurer J 1977 Providing optimal oral health. Nursing Clinics of North America 12(4): 671–684

Pearson L S 1996 A comparison of the ability of foam swabs and toothbrushes to remove dental plaque. Implications for nursing practice. Journal of Advanced Nursing 23(1): 62–69

Richardson A 1987 A process standard for oral care. Nursing Times 83(32): 38–40

Roberts I F, Roberts G J 1979 Relation between medicines sweetened with sucrose and dental disease. British Medical Journal 2: 14–16

Roth P T, Creason N S 1986 Nurse administered oral hygiene; is there a scientific basis? Journal of Advanced Nursing 11(3): 323–331

Shepherd G, Page C, Sammon P 1987 The mouth trap. Nursing Times 83(19): 25–27

Thurgood G 1994 Nurse maintenance of oral hygiene. British Journal of Nursing 3(7): 332–353

Tomlinson D, Kennedy H 1999 Introducing the use of toothbrushes for the immunocompromised child. European Journal of Oncology Nursing 3(1): 44–47

Torrance C 1990 Oral hygiene. Surgical Nurse 3(4): 16–20

Watson R 1989 Care of the mouth. Nursing 3(44): 20–24

Further reading

Fayle S A, Duggal M S, William S A 1992 Oral problems and the dentist's role in the management of paediatric oncology patients. Dental Update 19(4): 152–159

Hunter L, Hunter B 1997 Oral health in pregnancy and infancy. Macmillan Press, London

Levine R S 1996 A handbook of dental health for health visitors, midwives and nurses, 2nd edn. Health Education Authority, London

22

Oxygen Therapy

Introduction

Adequate oxygenation is vital to prevent tissue damage. Prolonged hypoxia (a decreased availability of oxygen to the tissues) can result in cell death if allowed to persist (Foss 1990) and could result in damage to the brain and/or heart (Hanna 1995). Administering oxygen to children can be difficult as they do not tolerate oxygen masks well, but nasal cannulae and headboxes are often effective. Oxygen can also be administered via an incubator (see Incubator Care, p. 139).

Learning outcomes

By the end of this section you should be able to:

- assess the most appropriate delivery device for each child according to her age, size, development and condition
- assess whether or not the oxygen delivery system requires humidification
- prepare the equipment necessary to deliver oxygen (humidified where necessary) by both headbox and nasal cannula
- state possible complications of oxygen administration.

Rationale for oxygen administration

Administration of oxygen is a life-saving intervention commonly used in children's nursing and an important skill for a children's nurse to acquire.

Factors to note

Oxygen should be regarded as a drug and planned delivery of oxygen therapy should always be prescribed by a doctor (Bell 1995, Dinesh & Mehta 1996). Administration of an inappropriate concentration of oxygen may have serious or even lethal consequences (Dinesh & Mehta 1996). In any patient, oxygen should be delivered at the lowest concentration possible and for the shortest time possible (Tasker 1995, Wong 1995, Zander & Hazinski 1992). Administration of oxygen to children is usually undertaken using one of three methods: via oxygen mask (which is well covered in other literature: English 1994, Wong 1995, Zander & Hazinski 1992) nasal cannula or headbox. How much oxygen is delivered to the child is expressed as the fractional inspired oxygen concentration (FiO_2): literally, the percentage concentration of oxygen the child is breathing in.

Headbox or body/trunk box

The advantages of these types of device are that they give effective oxygen delivery, it is possible to monitor the FiO_2 and they are totally non-invasive. Disadvantages are that carbon dioxide rebreathing will occur at low oxygen flow rates, < 4–5 litres/minute (Wong 1995), < 7 litres/minute (Zander & Hazinski 1992), removal of the box quickly dilutes the oxygen delivered and a cold gas supply will quickly cool an infant. Therefore, it is important that the gas supply should be warmed. Humidity must always be delivered in addition to oxygen when a headbox or head and body box is used (Tasker 1995, Zander & Hazinski 1992) and for face-mask delivery of over 4 hours' duration. Normally, inspired gas is warmed and humidified in the nasopharynx and reaches the upper trachea with a relative humidity of about 90% and a temperature of 32–36°C, it has reached a temperature of 37°C by the time it reaches the alveoli, (Zander & Hazinski 1992). Mucociliary transport is impaired when relative humidity falls below 75% at 37°C (BCH 1993).

Delivery via a headbox is only really suitable for the smaller baby as it is not well tolerated once the child is over about 8 months of age. However, there are boxes which are integral to a baby chair, e.g. the Manchester and Derbyshire chairs. These enable the child to be seated in the semi-reclined/near upright position and the whole chair is enclosed within a plastic cover into which the humidified oxygen is delivered. The older infant may tolerate this.

Nasal cannula

Advantages of nasal cannulae are that they are reasonably well tolerated by children (particularly in comparison with a face mask) and carbon dioxide rebreathing does not occur. Humidification is not necessary as the gas is entering via the nasal passages where it is warmed and moistened in the normal way. Disadvantages are that nasal cannulae are only suitable for use with a low flow of oxygen, i.e. < 6 litres/minute (Manley 1993) 2L/minute in neonates (Bower et al 1996). Higher flows may be uncomfortable and dry the nasal mucosa. In addition, a child who mouth breathes will dilute the FiO_2 with air.

Healthy children

Healthy children should have an arterial oxygen saturation level of 95–98% (Sims 1996). Some children who have underlying heart conditions may have an oxygen saturation level well below this, even when otherwise healthy.

Neonates

Administration of continuous oxygen therapy to neonates must be monitored very carefully. High oxygen concentrations could raise the infant's partial pressure of oxygen (PO_2) abnormally high. A PO_2 of greater than 15 kilopascals (kPa) can cause the formation of fibrous tissue which damages the retina resulting in permanent sight impairment or blindness (retinopathy of prematurity, previously known as retrolental fibroplasia (Foss 1990)). Prolonged exposure to high oxygen tensions can cause pulmonary oxygen toxicity and permanent lung damage, e.g. bronchopulmonary dysplasia (Foss 1990, George & Gordon 1995).

Sick children

Children with respiratory problems may benefit from being nursed upright, well supported with pillows. An infant may benefit from being placed in a baby chair for periods of up to 4 hours or longer if absolutely necessary. Any child should have a change of position 4-hourly if possible, to relieve pressure areas. If the child is too ill to sit up, consider tilting up the head of the bed or cot.

Occasionally, in children with chronic lung disease, too high a concentration of oxygen can lead to respiratory failure. Normally, the respiratory centres stimulate breathing in response to a rising concentration of carbon dioxide. In chronic lung disease, the respiratory centres become so used to the higher levels of carbon dioxide that they adapt. The increased concentration of carbon dioxide is no longer sufficient to stimulate breathing. Instead, the centres respond to low oxygen concentration in the blood itself. To give high concentrations of oxygen to these individuals is dangerous as it

will remove the stimulus (hypoxaemia) to which their respiratory centres respond to initiate breathing (Tasker 1995, Bower et al 1996, Wong 1995). These children must only receive low-concentration oxygen therapy.

Guidelines

Careful explanation to parents and child (if age and cognitive development allow) about the need for oxygen therapy will help to maximise cooperation. Careful explanation of all the equipment involved is important to minimise anxiety by reducing fear of the unknown.

Parents can be taught how to perform oral care to help maintain a moist, clean mouth if oxygen therapy is causing drying of the mucosa (see Oral Hygiene, p. 179).

Equipment for headbox and body/trunk box delivery

- Oxygen supply (even if supply is piped, consider the need for a spare portable cylinder in case of emergencies, loss or failure of supply)
- Humidifier: preferably a warmed, water bath humidifier such as Aquapak; some humidifiers have temperature controls to enable the water to be heated to varying temperatures
- Nipple to connect humidifier to oxygen supply
- Apparatus to connect humidifier, water and oxygen together (usually supplied as a complete, sterile unit for once-only use, e.g. Aquapak)
- Sterile water for humidification (tap water must not be used as it increases the risk of contamination with *Legionella pneumophila* (Stevenson 1992))
- Elephant tubing
- Oxygen analyser
- Headbox of a size sufficient to enclose the baby's head whilst sitting over the baby's neck (see Fig. 22.1) or Manchester/Derbyshire chair
- Oxygen saturation monitor and probe

Equipment for nasal cannula delivery

- Oxygen supply
- Nasal cannula
- Oxygen saturation monitor and probe
- Tape for fastening the cannula in place
- Low-flow oxygen meter if required

Method for headbox delivery

1. Explain the procedure to the parents to reduce fear of the unknown and aid compliance with the therapy.
2. If using a portable oxygen supply, ensure that the cylinder is full or nearly full. Determine how many hours' supply will be provided by the cylinder.

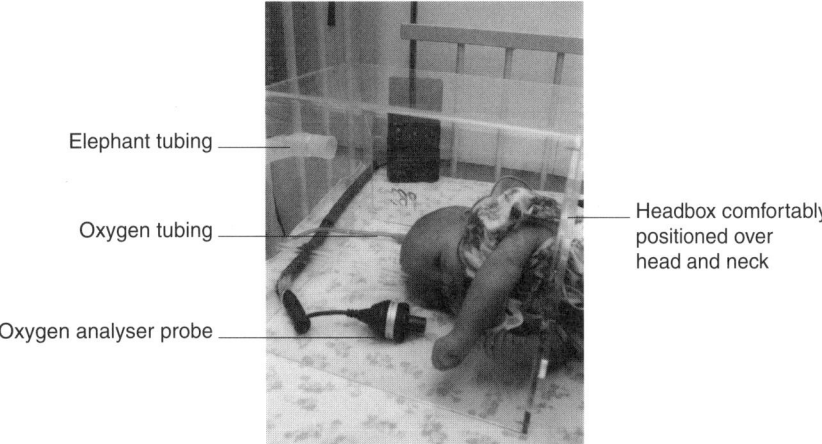

Elephant tubing

Oxygen tubing

Oxygen analyser probe

Headbox comfortably
positioned over
head and neck

Figure 22.1
*Delivery of humidified
oxygen via a headbox
(viewed from above).*

3. Set up the humidification system according to the manufacturer's instructions.
4. Test the alarm and set upper and lower alarm limits on the oxygen analyser. Put the probe of the oxygen analyser into the headbox via the purpose-built (smaller) hole.
5. Position the baby on her back or side in the cot and attach the oxygen saturation monitor probe. Turn on the saturation monitor. Set the upper and lower limit alarms for oxygen saturation and pulse rate (according to medical staff instructions) and record the child's oxygen saturation and pulse rate.
6. Place the headbox, carefully on top of the baby's head, preferably with her shoulders outside. Sometimes the shoulders have to go inside the box as well, particularly in a smaller infant. Ensure that the box does not exert undue pressure anywhere on the baby's body.
7. Position the elephant tubing so that it delivers the oxygen through the purpose-built, larger hole and is behind the head or to one side of the baby's face.
8. Position the oxygen analyser probe so that it is at the opposite side of the box to the point at which the oxygen is being delivered, near to the baby's face.
9. From the prescription sheet, determine the percentage oxygen to be delivered and turn on the oxygen to flow at 4.5 litres/minute minimum.
10. Read the oxygen analyser and regulate the flow of oxygen until the prescribed percentage of oxygen is attained.

11. Monitor the effect on the baby's saturation level and record frequently (every 1–4 hours depending on the child's condition). Report to medical staff if the prescribed percentage of oxygen does not maintain the baby's saturations at a level predetermined by the doctor. Report to medical staff if the saturations are decreasing despite prescribed oxygen flow.
12. Monitor the baby's respiratory rate and effort.
13. Monitor the amount of oxygen remaining in a portable oxygen cylinder at least hourly. Ensure that a replacement cylinder is available before the one in use empties.
14. Monitor the level of water in the humidifier bottle.

Method for nasal cannula delivery

1–2. Follow steps 1 and 2 of headbox delivery.
3. Ensure that the child's nose is cleaned of any dried mucus. Take the nasal cannula and place it over the child's head. Position it so that the prongs slant towards the child's face and each of the two prongs sits in a nostril (see Fig. 22.2).
4. Tighten the cannula to fit closely, by sliding up the movable sheath at the back of the tubing.
5. If necessary, fasten the cannula in place by taping the tubes onto the child's cheeks. Ensure that the child is not allergic to the tape. If the skin is particularly delicate or sore, consider using a protective barrier such as a piece of extra-thin hydrocolloid sheet (e.g. Granuflex).

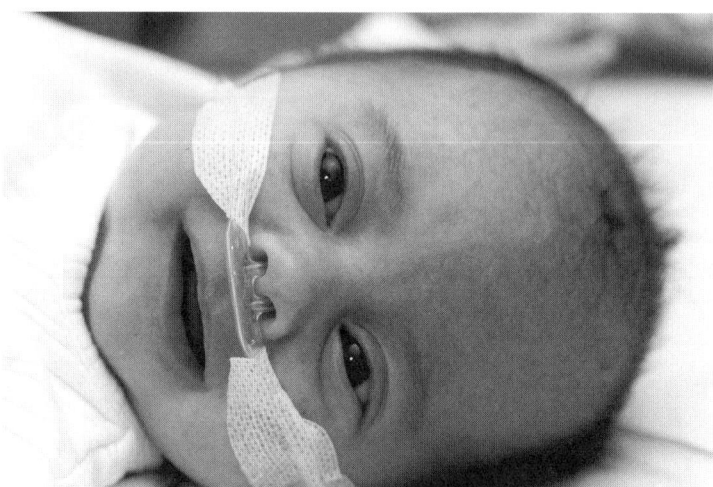

Figure 22.2
Delivery of oxygen via nasal cannula: nasal prongs in situ.

6.   Attach the oxygen saturation monitor probe. Turn on the saturation monitor. Set the upper and lower limit alarms for oxygen saturation and pulse rate (according to medical staff instructions) and record the child's oxygen saturation and pulse rate.

7.   Attach the end of the nasal cannula tubing to the oxygen supply.

8.   From the prescription sheet, determine the oxygen flow rate to be delivered and turn on the oxygen accordingly.

9–10.   Follow steps 11 and 12 of headbox delivery.

Observations and complications

A child requiring oxygen therapy should always be monitored carefully. Oxygen saturations should be monitored continuously while oxygen is being delivered, using a pulse oximeter. Pulse oximetry will detect hypoxia long before clinical signs become apparent (Hanna 1995). The child's oxygen saturation level, respiratory rate and effort and percentage/flow rate of oxygen delivered should be monitored and recorded regularly, between 1- and 4-hourly depending on the stability of her condition. Report any decrease in saturations, increase in respiratory rate and/or effort. If using a portable supply, check the cylinder regularly to ensure that sufficient oxygen remains in it. Even if piped oxygen is supplied, it may still be prudent to have a spare, portable cylinder close by in case of emergencies/loss of supply. Remember to change the humidifier water bottle at least once every 24 hours to prevent infection (Mehtar 1992). Humidifiers are a common source of Gram-negative bacilli and viruses associated with the respiratory system (Mehtar 1992). The highest incidence of hospital-acquired pneumonia occurs amongst patients who have had respiratory therapy, and bacterial contamination is a particular problem when gases are mixed with water as in humidifiers (Wilson 1995). Check the humidifier regularly (4-hourly) to ensure that it has not emptied. Ensure that the nostrils remain free from dried mucus; they may need gentle cleansing with warm water. Remember that some infants will not tolerate being removed from the headbox for washing, feeding, etc. They may require a source of oxygen close to their face during the time that they are removed from the headbox.

Risks of oxygen therapy

- There is a risk of eye damage associated with PO_2 above 15 kPa (see Factors to note, p. 190).
- There is a risk of lung damage associated with prolonged, continuous administration of high-pressure oxygen therapy (see Factors to note, p. 190).
- There is a risk of respiratory depression in children who have chronic obstructive respiratory disease (see Factors to note, p. 190).
- Whenever oxygen therapy is administered, remember that there is an increased risk of fire as oxygen is highly flammable.

COMMUNITY PERSPECTIVE

Prior to discharge

- Ensure that the parents are aware of all the constraints and problems that caring for a baby/child on long-term oxygen therapy can pose and consent to take on this role.
- Initiate a teaching programme for parents. This will need to cover:
  - recognising normal and abnormal respiratory patterns in their child, including signs of desaturation
  - knowing what action to take in the event of problems occurring
  - training in resuscitation
  - familiarisation with the use of an oxygen concentrator (electrical machine that can extract oxygen from surrounding air) and oxygen cylinders
  - knowing what action to take should there be problems with the apparatus; they will need the telephone number of an oxygen supplier and an engineer in case of emergencies
  - competence in caring for their baby/child with nasal prongs in situ and being able to change the prongs when necessary
  - familiarisation with the use of an apnoea monitor if one is in use
  - information on the need to inform their insurance companies and the local fire station that they will be storing oxygen at home, and may carry cylinders in their car
  - ensuring that they recognise the need for no smoking and are prepared to enforce this
  - having the contact numbers of the children's community nurse and the children's ward readily available.
- A home visit by the CCN or SCBU liaison nurse will need to be arranged to check the suitability of the home and discuss the positioning and storage of the oxygen concentrator and the large spare oxygen cylinder (this is required in the event of a power failure).
- The parents will need to have a telephone and arrangements should be made to install one if necessary.
- Liaison with the primary health care team is necessary, and the GP will need to prescribe the oxygen concentrator, the back-up cylinder and low-flow metre. The GP will also need to prescribe the number of hours of oxygen required and the flow rate.
- The CCN should liaise with the company supplying the concentrator and inform them of the name, address and likely discharge date of the child.

Equipment required

- Apnoea monitor and possibly baby alarm
- Nebuliser/nebuhaler if necessary
- Portable oxygen cylinder
- Low-flow head compatible with the cylinder and a carrying bag
- Spare nasal prongs and tape
- Humidifying device if necessary
- Prescribed drugs including saline nasal drops as required
- Equipment to measure oxygen saturation and heart rate if the child needs monitoring overnight

The family will need to be in touch with the social worker to claim any benefits to which they are entitled, e.g. payment of telephone, electricity payment for the concentrator. They will be entitled to a disability living allowance, but may require help to complete the appropriate forms.

They may find it helpful to be given the name of a family in a similar situation (Golder 1993).

Initially the family will need frequent home visits as they often feel very isolated at home and may experience a delayed reaction to their baby's admission to a SCBU (Golder 1993).

Ongoing support is essential to enable the parents to cope with the oxygen-dependent baby or child. As they become more proficient and the child more stable, the nurse can advise the parents on future management to enable them to be more mobile.

Community perspective
Do and do not

- Do ensure that the oxygen is prescribed.
- Do remember to check whether or not humidity is required.
- Do check whether the child has any chronic lung disease which could affect the normal functioning of her respiratory centre and therefore her response to oxygen therapy.
- Do monitor the duration and concentration of oxygen therapy at all times.

- Do not administer high concentrations of oxygen over prolonged periods without discussion with senior medical staff (particularly to the neonate or premature infant).
- Do not administer more than 6 litres/minute of oxygen via a nasal cannula 2L/minute in neonates and infants <6 months (Bower et al 1996).

References

BCH 1993 Oxygen administration within children's services unit. Birmingham children's Hospital Procedure Manual. Steelhouse Lane, Birmingham p132–137

Bell C 1995 Is this what the doctor ordered? Professional Nurse (Feb): 297–300

Bower L, Barnhant S L, Betit P 1996 Selection of an oxygen delivery device for neonatal and pediatric patients. American Association of Respiratory Care, Clinical Practice Guideline. Respiratory Care 41(7): 637–646

Dinesh A B, Mehta D K (executive eds) 1996 Oxygen. British National Formulary 32(Sept): 145

English I 1994 Oxygen mask or nasal catheter? An analysis. Nursing Standard 8(26): 27–31

Foss M A 1990 Oxygen therapy. Professional Nurse (Jan): 188-190

George C D, Gordon I 1995 Imaging the paediatric chest. In: Prasad S A, Hussey J (eds) Paediatric respiratory care.

Chapman and Hall, London, ch 3, pp 34–35

Golder S 1993 Parents support group. Paediatric Nursing 5(3): 14

Hanna D 1995 Guidelines for pulse oximetry use in pediatrics. Journal of Pediatric Nursing 10(2): 124–126

Manley L K 1993 Procedures involving the respiratory system. In: Barnardo L M, Bove M (eds) Pediatric emergency nursing procedures, 2nd edn. Jones & Bartlett, Boston, ch 5, pp 64–67

Mehtar S 1992 Hospital infection control. Oxford University Press, Oxford, ch 5, pp 121–123

Sims J 1996 Making sense of pulse oximetry and oxygen dissociation curve. Nursing Times 92(1): 34–35

Stevenson G 1992 Infection risks in respiratory therapy. Nursing Standard 6(18): 32–33

Tasker R 1995 Management of the acutely ill child in respiratory failure. In: Prasad S A, Hussey J (eds) Paediatric respiratory care. Chapman and Hall, London, ch 4, pp 43–45

Wilson J 1995 Infection control in clinical practice. Baillière Tindall, London, ch 5, pp 235–238

Wong D L (ed) 1995 Whaley and Wong's nursing care of infants and children, 5th edn. Mosby Year Book, St Louis, ch 31, pp 1346–1348

Zander J, Hazinski M F 1992 Pulmonary disorders. In: Hazinski M F Nursing care of the critically ill child, 2nd edn, Mosby Year Book, St Louis, ch 6, pp 395–420

23

Pain Management

Introduction

Pain is a subjective experience which is inherently difficult to assess, particularly in children, who often lack the verbal or cognitive ability to express their feelings of pain. However, pain assessment is essential, not only to detect pain but to evaluate the effectiveness of our pain management interventions if we are to provide optimal pain control.

Learning outcomes

By the end of this section you should:

- be aware of the myths surrounding pain in children
- recognise how your own feelings and beliefs may affect your assessment of pain in children
- have developed an awareness of the different types of assessment tools and the factors affecting their application
- understand the importance of routine pain assessment and documentation, involving the parent and, more importantly, the child where possible
- be aware of the commonly used analgesic drugs and the different routes of administration
- understand the importance of administering balanced analgesia.

Rationale

The treatment and alleviation of pain is a basic human right that exists regardless of age (Schechter et al 1993). The consequences of untreated pain include a delay in mobilisation, psychological trauma, an increase in the risk of infections, slower recovery and a delay in discharge from hospital. The undertreatment of pain in children is evident in the literature (Beyer et al 1993, Schechter et al 1986); however, over recent years, the problems of managing pain in children are beginning to be addressed. In 1993 in a publication entitled *Children first: a study of hospital services* the Audit Commission identified pain relief as an indicator for measuring quality of care for children in hospital. Assessment of a child's pain is problematic but it is essential if we are to provide effective management and therefore it must be an integral part of our nursing care.

Assessment of pain

Guidelines

Parents have a part to play in the assessment of their child's pain (Dearmun 1994). Where the situation permits, this involves determining a child's past pain experiences and whether these were good or bad. Children have been found to use a variety of words to describe pain (Jerrett & Evans 1986) and these should be identified prior to potentially painful experiences. A description of the child's behaviour which would normally indicate the presence of pain should be sought from the parents. The family may already employ certain coping strategies; these, along with analgesics used at home, should be discussed. Parents can also be helpful in identifying the pain assessment scale that may be appropriate for their child.

Pain is difficult to measure accurately and reliably in children. There are several pain scales available for paediatric use; however, development of verbal skills and cognitive ability show wide variation in children and this must be taken into account. Sociocultural and environmental factors must also be noted. In addition, to selecting the appropriate scale for an individual child, the nurse must consider several issues:

- the period of time that is available to teach the child how to use the assessment scale
- whether the child is able to grasp the function of the scale, enabling the nurse to achieve an accurate assessment
- whether the child is comfortable with using the scale; it is important that the nurse obtains the child's commitment to working with it
- if the child has a choice of pain scales, the nurse must abide by the choice and preference of the child.

It is vital that the nurse is completely familiar with the use of the pain assessment scale. A problem identified by Harrison (1991) is the need to differentiate between inaccuracy and bias when assessing pain. Harrison suggests that to overcome this problem nurses and observers should be trained to use assessment techniques more skilfully, thus helping to increase their sensitivity to pain cues. This is particularly important with children who are too sick to use self-reporting scales, neonates/infants and children with special needs. Pain assessment should be part of a holistic approach to the child. The nurse should be able to take the information the child gives her and interpret it with skill. For example, a report of pain described in a particular manner may indicate a full bladder and urinary retention rather than wound pain. This should be treated in a different way and it is important therefore that the information given is channelled correctly.

It is also vital that children who can comprehend the pain scale and self-report are made aware that if they are in pain the treatment of that pain is patient friendly. Mather & Mackie (1983) found that some children may lower their pain intensity report because of fear of treatment, for example an intramuscular injection being administered. Harrison also concluded that children are capable of providing an accurate pain assessment but that the consequences of doing so may prevent them.

It is widely recognised that self-reporting pain scales are the most accurate, when children can describe their pain in an appropriate manner and relevant language for their age and development. However, for certain patients this will not be possible.

Factors to note

Sick children

A very sick child may be too ill to comprehend instructions regarding the use of a pain scale. A child in an intensive care setting, who is perhaps ventilated, sedated or paralysed, will be unable to use a self-reporting scale that would normally be used for his age and development. With these patients, physiological and behavioural factors should be considered jointly to enable the nurse to judge whether the child is distressed by pain. The child may also become distressed by the requirement for suction, position change or oral hygiene and this should be taken into consideration. As the nurse develops a relationship with the patient she will be able to differentiate between distress and pain and the pain scale will be an aid to this nursing skill.

Neonates

Neonates can not communicate by verbal report so they are dependent on caregivers to recognise that they are in pain. Physiological and behavioural factors must be observed and interpreted as an indication of pain being present. Again the requirement for other nursing/clinical interventions should be considered, e.g. suction etc. A variety of scales have been made available for neonates, taking into consideration features such as facial expression, body position, mobility, colour, oxygen saturation (SaO_2), respiratory rate, blood pressure, heart rate and crying. However, it should be noted that these observations can be affected by a variety of factors as well as pain. The scales that take this into consideration may be more accurate.

Infants/toddlers

Similar problems occur with infants and toddlers regarding the use of pain scales. Again the nurse should be able to pick up pain cues from the infant and toddler by observing physiological and behavioural signs and then act appropriately. Toddlers may clutch at the site of the surgery. They may also display the characteristic signs of frustration and unhappiness that they cannot communicate verbally.

Children (preschool to 7 years)

Studies have shown that many 3-year-olds can identify the presence and absence of pain and can report a pain intensity. It is recommended that the choice of pain intensity scores for this age group should be limited to around four choices. They can usually verbalise in appropriate language, to the nurse or their parents, a description of 'their hurting'. It is important to remember that younger children may choose extremes of measurement and some may even confuse the scales with measurements of happiness. Some children in this age group may experience behavioural disturbances due to the trauma of hospital admission. Regression to earlier stages in development, such as loss of speech, clinging to parents or a return to bed wetting, may be noticed. Aggression may be a form of identifying pain. Children may be in pain but unable or reluctant to indicate that it is present. Their behaviour becomes aggressive as a response to this pain. It is important that nursing staff can recognise this and educate parents to avoid a child being labelled as naughty.

Older children (7 years to adolescence)

Older children of a normal developmental level can usually self-report their pain and understand the use of visual analogue scales.

Adolescents, however, are developing quickly physically but emotional development can be at a different rate. It should be remembered that they will be anxious and often frightened about hospitalisation. They may be aware of peer group pressure and may not admit pain because of fear of ridicule or comparison to another child. Fear of treatment may also be a problem. The nurse should ensure that adolescent patients have complete privacy and quiet to report any pain and that they are aware of the 'patient-friendly' treatments.

Conducting a pain assessment

History taking

It is vital that the nurse, on admitting a child to the ward or unit, takes a pain history from the parents or guardian. The nurse should record the child's reaction to pain, the usual method for reporting pain (if developmentally able) and what happens in response to pain at home. This information should be incorporated into the nursing care plan. The appropriate scale should be selected at this time, if possible taking into account:

- age
- mechanical interventions that may be necessary
- special needs
- clinical condition
- type of pain, i.e. acute, chronic or recurrent.

Documentation of pain assessments should occur and guidelines recommend that they be recorded on the routine observation chart (Royal College of Surgeons and the College of Anaesthetists 1990). This is important because there is evidence to suggest that accurate documentation increases the assessment of pain and the administration of analgesia (Goddard & Pickup 1996, Savedra et al 1993, Stevens 1990). For postoperative pain, for example, a pain scale should be used to assess a child's pain with the routine postoperative observations, decreasing in frequency as the observations decrease but more regularly if a child is complaining of pain or analgesia has been administered.

Pain assessment scales usually incorporate one or more of the following:

- behavioural assessment
- physiological assessment
- self-report techniques.

Behavioural assessment

This involves looking at how a child behaves in response to pain.

Facial expression, together with cry, has been reported as the most widely accepted sign of pain in infants (Porter 1993). A unique pain cry has been suggested but there is consensus that cry does not appear to be a simple discrete signal with a single meaning (Porter 1993).

Coding systems have been developed; however, intense crying with high motor activity could indicate pain, whilst equally an infant that is withdrawn and quiet could also be in pain, highlighting the difficulties.

Body movements have also been examined, but no specific response has been shown to indicate pain.

It must be remembered that behaviour can be affected by many things including drugs, splints, ventilation and prematurity.

Behavioural pain assessment has some advantages in that it is non-invasive, does not put any demands on the child nor does it depend on his cognitive ability or language skills.

Assessment of behavioural signs could indicate the presence of pain and help determine the effect the pain is having on the child or infant.

Physiological assessment

Physiological signs vary greatly, particularly in premature infants.

Different parameters have been examined, includ:

- pulse rate
- respiratory rate
- blood pressure
- neurochemical and neurohormonal activity
- palmar sweating
- SaO_2.

There is a debate surrounding the reliability of using physiological signs to determine the presence of pain (Carter 1994). There is in fact insufficient evidence to suggest that physiological signs are directly related to the pain experienced. Like behavioural responses, physiological responses can be affected by many things, resulting in problems of interpretation.

Self-report techniques

As pain is a subjective experience, self-reporting techniques are acknowledged as the most accurate indicators of pain; however, they rely on children having the relevant language for their age and development and the ability to describe their pain in an appropriate manner. It must be remembered, that a child's self-report of pain may be affected by contextual factors or concerns regarding the pain-relieving interventions that may be offered.

There is agreement that multidimensional assessment is essential.

Ross & Ross (1988) suggest that the three pain assessment components, behavioural assessments, physiological assessments and self-report techniques, taking into account contextual factors, 'enable us to draw some conclusions about the child's pain'.

An approach that takes these factors into account is QUESTT (Baker & Wong 1987):

Question the child
Use pain-assessment scales
Evaluate behaviour and physiological signs
Secure the parents' involvement
Take the cause of pain into account

Take action and evaluate results.

Some of the pain scales that are available for children are listed in Table 23.1. Other scales are:

- Poker Chip Tool (Beyer & Wells 1989)
- Oucher (Beyer & Wells 1989)
- Colour Scales (Beyer & Wells 1989)
- Coloured Vertical Analogue (McGrath et al 1996)
- Horizontal Linear Analogue (Beyer & Wells 1989)
- Adjectival Self Report (Morton 1993)
- Sheffield Children's Hospital Pain Assessment Tool (Goddard & Pickup 1996) (see Fig. 23.1).

Table 23.1 **Children's pain scales**

Scale	Age range	Comments
OPS (Broadman et al 1988)	Neonate to 7 years	Easy to use Follows pain over a period of time Accurate between assessors Cannot be used with intubated or paralysed patients
CRIES (Krechel & Bildner 1995)	Neonate	Easy to use Reliable down to 32 weeks gestational age Uses SaO_2 as a measure, which can be affected by many other factors
COMFORT (Ambuel et al 1992)	Neonate to 7 years	Complicated scale to use Cannot be used with intubated or paralysed patients
TIPPS (Tarbell et al 1992)	Infant/toddler	Correlates with nurse and parent assessment Pain scores follow the effects of the analgesia, i.e. decrease if analgesia satisfactory, increase when more is required
FACES (Beyer & Wells 1989)	Child 3–7 years	Younger children may choose extremes Some children may confuse with happiness measurements
CHEOPS (McGrath et al 1985)	Child 3–7 years	Complicated behavioural scale May not track postoperative pain adequately in children of this age who are experiencing behavioural disturbances due to trauma of hospital admission
NPS (Lawrence et al 1993)	Neonate	Cannot be used in intubated or paralysed patients Six categories but two of these very similar

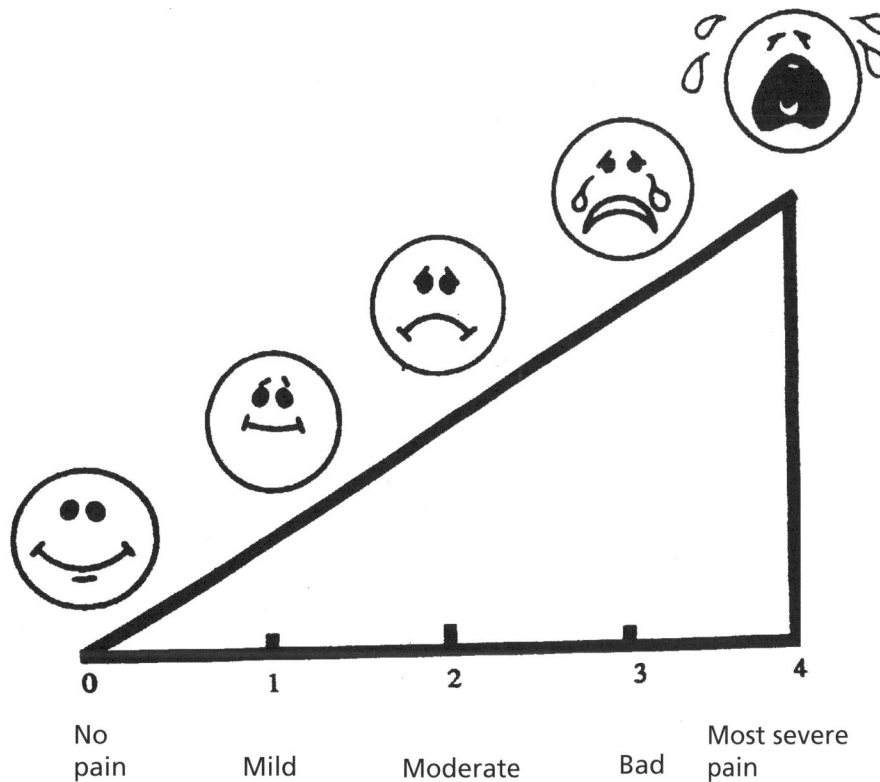

Figure 23.1
Sheffield Children's Hospital pain assessment tool (adapted from Brown & Fisk 1992).

0	1	2	3	4
No pain	Mild	Moderate	Bad	Most severe pain

Management of pain

Pain has both physical and psychological components and as a result both physical and psychological methods of pain management can be employed.

Non-drug methods of pain management

Psychological techniques include distraction, using interactive toys and games, e.g. pop-up books, music books, blowing bubbles and guided imagery, where the child is encouraged to imagine something pleasant, e.g. a favourite holiday destination. These techniques can help distract and relax a child. Transcutaneous electrical nerve stimulation (TENS) machines can relieve pain and be useful in reducing conventional analgesic requirements.

Massage, aromatherapy and reflexology have a role to play in pain management. For further information on these methods, please refer to Appendix 2: Complementary Therapies, page 335.

Drug methods of pain control

Broadly speaking there are two types of analgesics, centrally acting and peripherally acting; these terms describe their specific sites of action in the nervous system. Centrally acting drugs act on the opioid receptors in the brain and spinal cord and peripherally acting drugs inhibit the production of prostaglandins, which sensitise the nerve endings to pain.

Analgesics are generally described as either opiates or non-opiates.

Methods of analgesia administration

Oral
This tends to be the preferred route of analgesia administration in children because of their dislike of needles.

Rectal

This route is useful when children are experiencing nausea and vomiting or are permitted nil by mouth.

Intravenous

Analgesia can be administered via this route as a bolus dose, a continuous infusion or as patient-controlled analgesia (PCA).

Intramuscular

This is the least preferred route of analgesia administration, often causing pain and anxiety.

Subcutaneous

The subcutaneous route, through a subcutaneous cannula, can be used as an alternative to intramuscular injections. Analgesia can be administered continuously or as a bolus dose when required.

Topical

The use of a topical local anaesthetic cream, e.g. EMLA or Ametop, can reduce the pain and discomfort a child may experience during intravenous cannulation or blood sampling.

Local/regional

For postoperative analgesia, blocks, including femoral nerve blocks, lumbar plexus blocks, penile blocks and ilioinguinal blocks, are performed by the anaesthetist whilst a child is anaesthetised. Wound infiltration with local anaesthetics is also used for postoperative pain and for procedures in the accident and emergency department.

Inhalation

Entonox is a self-administered inhaled gas that will provide analgesia for procedural pain of short duration.

Intrathecal

This is the instillation of drugs into the subarachnoid space to produce an analgesic effect.

Epidural

This is the instillation of drugs into the epidural space (extradural space). A caudal block is an epidural block using a sacral approach.

Transdermal

This is where an analgesic drug is absorbed through the skin creating a systemic effect. Fentanyl patches are an example of transdermal analgesia.

Transmucosal

Drugs are rapidly absorbed from the oral and nasal mucosa. The analgesic buprenorphine utilises this route.

Analgesia

EMLA and Ametop

These are topical local anaesthetics that are used to reduce the pain experienced during blood tests and venous cannulation. When using either EMLA or Ametop, they need to be applied to the skin and then covered with an occlusive dressing. EMLA needs to be applied at least 60 minutes before the procedure and can be used for children over 1 year of age. Ametop works more quickly, needing to be applied 30 minutes before blood taking and 45 minutes before venous cannulation. Ametop can be used with children and infants from 1 month of age upwards.

Paracetamol

Although paracetamol is highly toxic in overdose, it is a safe and effective analgesic when administered in therapeutic doses. It has antipyretic properties but no recognised anti-inflammatory effects.

Ibuprofen and diclofenac

These are non-steroidal anti-inflammatory drugs (NSAIDs). They produce an analgesic, antipyretic and anti-inflammatory effect. NSAIDs should be administered with caution to children who are asthmatics. There is a theoretical risk of an allergic reaction to these types of drugs. Extreme caution should be taken if a child has renal disease or any renal impairment.

Opiates

There are several methods of administering opiate analgesia, with the subcutaneous and intravenous routes currently increasing in popularity. Morphine remains the most widely used opiate in children.

Some children, although not requiring opiates continually to control pain, may still require one or two doses of opiate during the postoperative period. To avoid the use of intramuscular injections, a subcutaneous cannula can be sited in theatre or on the ward, after applying EMLA or Ametop. Nursing staff can then administer bolus doses of morphine as required. Morphine can also be administered continuously via this route. This method of analgesia administration should be used with caution in a child who has impaired peripheral circulation.

Patient-controlled analgesia (PCA) is a method of intravenous analgesia administration. The child (usually aged 5 and over) controls his own analgesia by means of a hand-held button attached to a computerised pump. The pump is set up with a suitable dose of opiate calculated on the child's body weight and age. The pump permits the child to self-administer a small pre-set amount of analgesia by pressing the button. A maximum dose per hour and a lockout interval is programmed into the pump so that the child cannot overdose, thus ensuring safety. The child is then able to titrate his own requirements of analgesia in an efficient and safe manner.

For children in whom PCA is not appropriate, an intravenous infusion of opiate can be connected to run continuously. Nurse- or parent-controlled analgesia may also be an option, following specifically produced guidelines.

The aim of morphine administration is to achieve the optimum level of analgesia with minimal side-effects. Side-effects include excessive sedation, respiratory depression, nausea, vomiting, pruritus and urinary retention. A child's vital signs should be monitored for complications and the child observed for side-effects. Regular pain assessments are necessary to determine if the morphine is having the desired effect.

Codeine phosphate and dihydrocodeine are opiates most commonly administered orally.

Entonox

Entonox (50% nitrous oxide and 50% oxygen) is an effective inhalation method of managing procedural pain of short duration. The gas is self-administered through a demand apparatus which safeguards the child from overdose. The onset of analgesia is rapid, usually within 2–3 minutes and the effects wear off quickly.

Balanced analgesia

Pain control can be enhanced by using a combination of analgesic approaches. A child using a morphine PCA pump, for example, will have his pain more effectively managed if an NSAID and/or paracetamol is administered. This will reduce the child's opiate requirements and therefore the potential for side-effects, whilst attacking the pain both centrally and peripherally. Also, the use of local and regional analgesia techniques can significantly reduce the amount of analgesia required postoperatively.

Evaluation

It is necessary to evaluate and document the efficacy of any pain-relieving interventions regularly. It is also important to observe that the child is not experiencing side-effects as a result of analgesia administration. It must be remembered that other factors can increase the pain experienced by a child, for example anxiety and muscle tension, and this must be taken into account as we plan our pain-relieving interventions.

Summary of complications

- There may not be consistent behavioural and physiological changes in all infants and children experiencing pain.
- Many factors, including distress, can affect both behaviour and the physiological signs used to assess pain.
- It is difficult to distinguish between stress and pain, particularly in the infant or neonate.
- The ability to self-report depends on the cognitive ability and language skills of a child and may be affected by clinical condition, drugs or mechanical interventions.
- Children may report lower pain intensity than they are experiencing for fear of the consequences.
- A child's pain can be affected by previous pain experiences, cultural and social expectations and levels of anxiety.
- As nurses, our own experiences of pain and our preconceived ideas about how much an injury or certain type of surgery should hurt may affect our interpretation of a situation.

COMMUNITY PERSPECTIVE

Parents are likely to be more 'tuned in' to their child in pain than professionals. However, there will be times when parents lose their objectivity about this, especially during terminal care. Denying the level of pain may be a coping strategy for a parent but this takes away the rights of the child.

The role of the CCN is to be aware of the dynamics within the family and sensitively to lead the parents to a more objective assessment. For this to be possible, the family must have developed trust in the CCN and, when appropriate, other members of the team. Once their cooperation has been gained in titrating analgesia and they are able to recognise that the child is more settled and possibly able to participate in family life, a hurdle will have been surmounted, the child's pain will be better managed and the relationship between family and nurses strengthened.

Each individual case will need consideration as to whether the use of pain scales will be helpful. Whereas it may be appropriate to use them in an acute pain situation, for example the child with a fractured femur, it may be less so for the terminally ill child. Ongoing assessment of pain, however, is essential, whether this is undertaken using pain scales or as an ongoing assessment as part and parcel of family life. The preference of the child must be valued.

For the child with communication difficulties, the parents are almost without exception those who recognise when their child is in pain. The role of the CCN here is to listen and learn from the parents and take action accordingly.

Do and do not

- Do involve the parents and, more importantly, the child himself.
- Do take into account the child's age, clinical condition, type of pain, and any special needs or mechanical interventions.
- Do use a multidimensional scale where possible.
- Do evaluate any pain relief given.
- Do not let your own beliefs and values cloud your judgement when assessing pain.
- Do not let the common myths and misconceptions surrounding pain in children affect your assessment strategies. They include:
  – babies and infants do not feel pain
  – children do not remember pain
  – children who are playing or sleeping cannot be in pain
  – children always tell the truth about their pain.

Remember that pain is a subjective experience which is not solely dependent on the amount of tissue damage involved. It can be affected by many things which should be reflected in our assessment strategies and choice of assessment scales.

References

Ambuel B, Hamlett K W, Marx C M, Plummer J L 1992 Assessing distress in pediatric intensive care environments. The COMFORT scale. Journal of Pediatric Psychology 17: 95–109

Audit Commission 1993 Children first: a study of hospital services. HMSO, London

Baker C, Wong D 1987 Q.U.E.S.T.T.: a process of pain assessment in children. Orthopaedic Nursing 6(1): 11–21

Beyer J E, Wells N 1989 The assessment of pain in children. Pediatric Clinics of North America 36: 837–853

Beyer J E, DeGood D E, Ashley L C, Russell G A 1993 Patterns of post operative analgesic use with adults and children following cardiac surgery. Pain 17: 71–81

Broadman L M, Rice L H, Hannallah R S 1988 Testing the validity of an objective pain scale for infants and children. Anesthesiology 69: A770

Brown T C K, Fisk G C 1992 Anaesthesia for children, 2nd edn. Blackwell Scientific Publications, Oxford, p 129

Carter B 1994 Child and infant pain. Chapman and Hall, London

Dearmun A K 1994 Why involve the parents? Child Health 2(4): 166–170

Goddard J M, Pickup S E 1996 Post operative pain in children: combining audit and a nurse specialist to improve management. Anaesthesia 51: 588–590

Harrison A 1991 Assessing patients' pain: identifying reasons for error. Journal of Advanced Nursing 16: 1018–1025

Jerrett M, Evans K 1986 Children's pain vocabulary. Journal of Advanced Nursing 11: 403–408

Krechel S W, Bildner J 1995 CRIES: a new neonatal postoperative pain measurement score. Initial testing of validity and reliability. Paediatric Anaesthesia 5: 53–61

Lawrence J, Alcock D, McGrath P, Kay J, MacMurray S B, Dulberg C 1993 The development of a tool to assess neonatal pain. Neonatal Network 12: 59–65

McGrath P J, Johnson G, Goodman J T, Schillinger J, Dunn J, Chapman J A 1985 CHEOPS: a behavioural scale for rating postoperative pain in children. Advances in Pain Research and Therapy 9: 395–402

McGrath P A, Seifert C E, Speechley K N, Booth J C, Stitt L, Gibson M C 1996 A new analogue scale for assessing children's pain – an initial validation study. Pain 64: 435–443

Mather L, Mackie J 1983 The incidence of post operative pain in children. Pain 15: 271–282

Morton N S 1993 Development of a monitoring protocol for the safe use of opioids in children. Paediatric Anaesthesia 3: 179–184

Porter F 1993 Pain assessment in children: infants. In: Schechter N L, Berde C B, Yaster M (eds) Pain in infants, children and adolescents. Williams & Wilkins, Baltimore

Ross D M, Ross S A 1988 Assessment of pediatric pain. Issues in Comprehensive Pediatric Nursing 11: 73–91

Royal College of Surgeons and the College of Anaesthetists 1990 Commission on the provision of surgical services. Report on the Working Party on Pain After Surgery. Royal College of Surgeons, London

Savedra M C, Holzemer W L, Tesler M D, Wilkie D J 1993 Assessment of post operation pain in children and adolescents using the Adolescent Pediatric Pain Tool. Nursing Research 42: 1, 5–9

Schechter N L, Allen D A, Hanson K 1986 Status of pediatric pain control: a comparison of hospital analgesic use in children and adults. Pediatrics 77: 11–15

Schechter N L, Berde C B, Yaster M 1993 Pain in infants, children and adolescents. Williams & Wilkins, Baltimore

Stevens B 1990 Development and testing of a pediatric pain management sheet. Pediatric Nursing 16(6): 543–548

Tarbell S E, Cohen I T, Marsh J L 1992 The Toddler-Pre-school Postoperative Pain Scale: an observational scale for measuring postoperative pain in children aged 1–5. Preliminary report. Pain 50: 273–280

Further reading

Broadman L M, Rice L H, Hannallah R S 1988 Testing the validity of an objective pain scale for infants and children. Anesthesiology 69: A770

Lawson R A, Smart N G, Gudgeon A C, Morton N S 1995 Evaluation of an amethocaine gel preparation for percutaneous analgesia before venous cannulation in children. British Journal of Anaesthesia 75: 282–285

McNicol L R 1994 Local anaesthesia. In: Morton N S, Raine P A M Paediatric day case surgery. Oxford University Press, Oxford, ch 4, pp 24–50

Morton N S 1996 Pain assessment in children. Paediatric Anaesthesia 7: 267–272

Wolf A R, Lawson R A, Fisher S 1995 Ventilatory arrest after a fluid challenge in a neonate receiving s.c. morphine. British Journal of Anaesthesia 75: 787–789

24

Phototherapy

Introduction

Phototherapy consists of the application of fluorescent light to reduce the serum bilirubin level of an infant. This light is normally a mixture of blue and white radiant light and is not in the ultraviolet range.

Learning outcomes

By the end of this section the nurse will be able to:

- identify the infant with a raised serum bilirubin level
- initiate phototherapy, as directed by medical staff, safely and appropriately
- understand the needs of the infant undergoing phototherapy
- recognise any adverse reactions
- explain the need for phototherapy to the parents/primary caregivers.

Rationale

The primary aim of phototherapy is to prevent kernicterus, that is mental retardation caused by persistent raised serum unconjugated bilirubin.

Factors to note

Normal red blood cell life in the adult human is approximately 120 days. In the neonate this is reduced to 80 days; in the premature neonate it is even shorter, reducing to 30–40 days (Bennett & Brown 1993, Edwards 1995).

Red blood cells are broken down in the spleen (by the reticuloendothelial system) and to a lesser extent in the liver. Bilirubin is one of the end-products of red blood cell breakdown, being derived from the haem part of haemoglobin (see Fig. 24.1). Bilirubin, unconjugated, is not water-soluble and is toxic to the body at high levels. If not converted to the water-soluble (conjugated) bilirubin, the unconjugated bilirubin will be deposited in the brain cells, which will lead to a condition called kernicterus.

Unconjugated bilirubin is transported in the bloodstream bound to albumin, a plasma protein, to the liver where, following a complex process of enzyme actions, it is converted to conjugated bilirubin.

Conjugated bilirubin is water-soluble and is excreted by the liver via the biliary system into the intestine.

In the intestine the bilirubin is converted to urobilinogen, some of which is absorbed by the enterohepatic circulation and is eventually excreted in the urine. The majority of the urobilinogen is oxidised in the colon to a brown pigment, urobilin, which is excreted in the stool (Marshall 1995).

An increase in serum bilirubin causes jaundice, a yellow/amber discoloration of the skin, also seen in the sclera of the eyes and mucous membranes. This is seen when the serum bilirubin rises above 80 micromoles per litre (Bennett & Brown 1993). It is often the nurse who notices the infant's jaundice and this initiates the checking of the serum bilirubin level.

Jaundice is relatively common in both term and preterm infants because of the increased haemolysis of fetal haemoglobin (Kedzierski 1991). In the majority of cases this is relatively benign; however, close monitoring of the serum bilirubin level is important because of the risk of kernicterus.

An early high level of serum bilirubin, normally within the first 24 hours of life, may indicate ABO or rhesus incompatibility.

Persistent jaundice after the first week of life must be fully investigated to determine the cause. Biliary atresia is one condition where the prognosis is improved with an early diagnosis (Hussein et al 1991).

Breast milk jaundice is a benign condition, which may persist up to 3 months after birth and is thought to be caused by a factor within the breast milk which inhibits bilirubin conjugation (Bennett & Brown 1993, Wong 1997).

Estimations can be made using a transcutaneous bilirubin monitor; however, the serum level should always be obtained before phototherapy is commenced (Ruchala et al 1996).

Phototherapy is ineffective before the infant is jaundiced; hence it cannot be used prophylactically. However, early use in infants with known haemolytic disease is indicated as a means of control of the serum

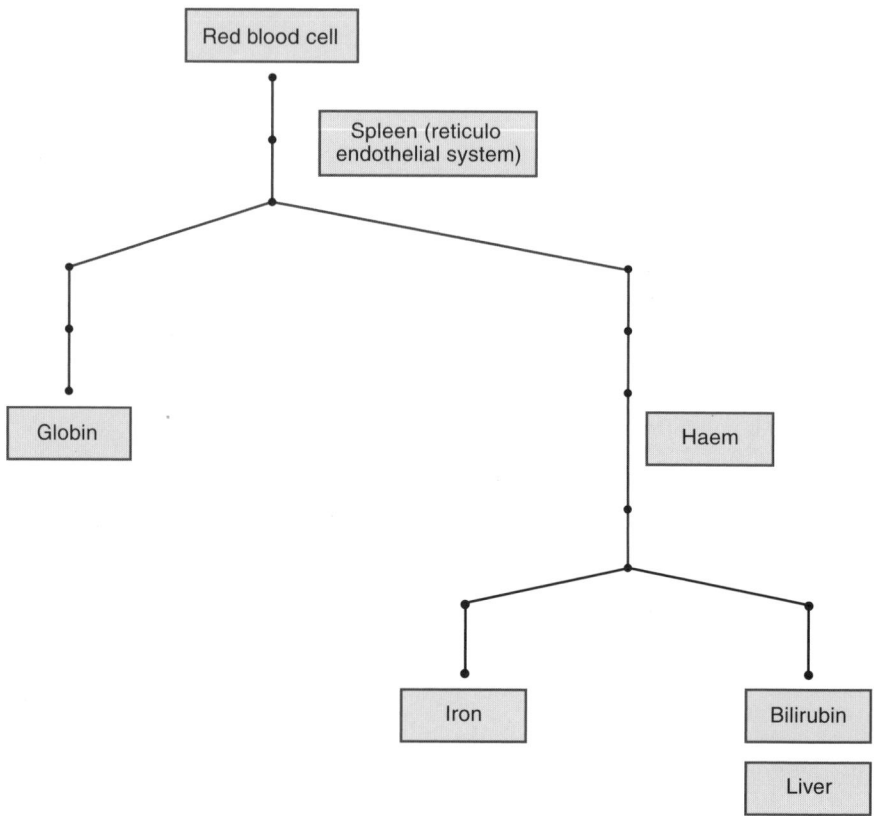

Figure 24.1
Breakdown of red blood cells.

bilirubin level. Initiation of therapy is dependent not only on the serum bilirubin, but also the gestational age at birth of the infant (Bennett & Brown 1993).

Preterm and sick infants are more prone to the complications of jaundice; hence phototherapy is initiated at lower serum bilirubin levels.

Equipment
- Open cot, Baby Therm or incubator
- Phototherapy unit(s)
- Eye shield/cover

Method
Commencement of phototherapy is determined by the serum unconjugated bilirubin level (Dodd 1993).

The following guidelines refer to the use of a phototherapy unit (Fig. 24.2). Some neonatal units, however, use fibreoptic blankets, known as 'bile blankets', which are wrapped around the infant (Hart, Day & Hainsworth 1997, Hamlin & Seshia 1998).

- The infant is placed naked, with gonads protected, into an open cot, Baby Therm or incubator.
- The phototherapy unit is placed over the infant, approximately 45 cm above the body. (*Note:* The units are normally fixed onto stands at this height.) More than one unit may be used.
- The infant's eyes are covered to prevent retinal damage.
- The phototherapy unit is switched on. The treatment can be given continuously or intermittently.
- The infant should be turned on a regular basis, every 2 hours, to ensure that all of the skin is exposed.
- The phototherapy unit should be switched off when the infant is being fed or the eye shields are removed.
- The duration of treatment will be determined by the level of serum unconjugated bilirubin.
- In some areas the nursing staff may be responsible for checking the serum bilirubin level by capillary heel stab.

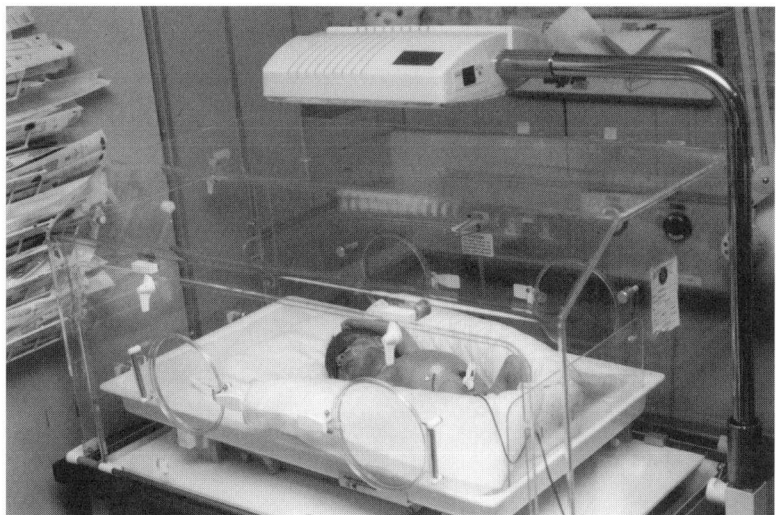

Figure 24.2
Infant under the phototherapy unit.

- Where the infant is being constantly observed, protective glasses should be available for staff use.
- Care should be coordinated (clustered care) to ensure minimal disruption to the infant.

Observations and complications
- Check the infant's temperature regularly as infants are prone both to hypothermia (due to being naked) and to hyperthermia because of heat radiated from the phototherapy unit.
- Increase fluid intake by 25–30% (or as determined by local policy) to maintain hydration, as the infant's insensible losses are known to rise (Edwards 1995, Kedzierski 1991, Mathew 1995).
- Cover the gonads of the very and extremely low birthweight infants; this has to be balanced with maximum skin exposure. DNA mutations and breaks have been reported with the use of phototherapy (Edwards 1995). Theatre masks worn by the infant as bikini bottoms may be used.
- Check skin colour using daylight, as assessment of jaundice is often difficult under artificial light (Hart, Day & Hainsworth 1997).
- Loose green stools are common during treatment. Stools should be monitored, as fluid loss may increase as a result of frequent loose stools.
- Ensure that the infant's eyes remain closed when shields are in place, as corneal abrasions may occur. The shields should be removed and the eyes checked on a regular basis.
- The effect of phototherapy on the eyes is uncertain. However, animal studies indicate that retinal

degeneration can occur if there is continuous exposure (Sisson 1970).
- The infant may become lethargic, irritable and develop poor feeding.
- Tanning and rashes are common. This is referred to as 'bronze baby syndrome'.

Dos and do nots
- Do encourage parents to be involved in care.
- Do ensure that care is clustered.
- Do encourage mothers to continue with breastfeeding.
- Do ensure that the position of the infant is changed to ensure maximum exposure.
- Do not use creams, lotions or oils on the infant's skin, as they may cause burning.
- Do not remove the eye shields while the phototherapy unit is in operation.

References
Bennett V R, Brown L K 1993 Myles textbook for midwives, 12th edn. Churchill Livingstone, Edinburgh
Dodd K L 1993 Neonatal jaundice – a lighter touch. Archives of Disease in Childhood 68: 529–533
Edwards S 1995 Phototherapy and the neonate: providing safe and effective nursing care for jaundiced infants. Journal of Neonatal Nursing (Oct): 9–12
Hart G, Day C, Hainsworth A 1997 Phototherapy for neonates: Drager phototherapy 4000. Journal of Neonatal Nursing 3(4)
Hamelin K, Seshia M 1998 Home phototherapy for uncomplicated neonatal jaundice. The Canadian Nurse 94(1): 39–40
Hussein M, Howard E R, Mieli-Vergani G et al 1991 Jaundice

at 14 days of age: exclude biliary atresia. Archives of Disease in Childhood 66(10): 1177–1179

Kedzierski M 1991 Liver disease in babies and children. Nursing Standard 5(43): 30–33

Marshall W 1995 Illustrated textbook of clinical chemistry, 3rd edn. Lippincott/Gower, London

Mathew R 1995 Nursing care of infants on phototherapy. Nursing Journal of India LXXXVI(9): 197–198

Ruchala P L, Seibold L, Stremsterfer K 1996 Validating assessment of neonatal jaundice with transcutaneous bilirubin measurement. Neonatal Network 15(4): 33–37

Sisson T 1970 Retinal changes produced by phototherapy. Journal of Paediatrics 77: 251

Wong D 1997 Whaley and Wong's essentials of pediatric nursing, 5th edn. Mosby, St Louis

Further reading

Blackburn S T 1996 Research utilisation: modifying the NICU light environment. Neonatal Network 15(4): 63–66

Campbell S, Glasper E A (eds) 1995 Whaley and Wong's children's nursing. Mosby, London, ch 13

Rose B S 1990 Phototherapy: all wrapped up? Pediatric Nursing 16(1): 57, 58, 72

Schooebel A, Sakraidas S 1997 Hyper bilirubinaemia: new approaches to an old problem. Journal of Perinatal and Neonatal Nursing 11(3): 78–97

25

Plaster Care

Introduction

Plaster casts are used to obtain complete immobilisation, protection and correction of bony or tissue damage or deformity.

Correct care is essential to prevent complications arising.

Learning outcomes

By the end of this section you should:

- understand the principles of plaster care
- develop an understanding of the factors which predispose to common complications
- be able to recognise common complications
- be able to explain nursing interventions required when complications arise
- be able to advise carers and their children on future plaster care.

Rationale

It is essential that children and carers are adequately prepared and understand the necessity for the application of the cast, its subsequent care, and the recognition of possible complications. It is therefore necessary that the nurse has the required skills of cast application and knowledge of the principles involved, including possible complications which may arise.

Factors to note

Plaster materials

Plaster of Paris and fibreglass cast tape are the most commonly used materials today. Each has its own advantages and disadvantages for use.

Plaster of Paris. This is a gypsum salt mixture which is impregnated into gauze rolls (Lane & Lee 1982). It has been the most common choice for immobilisation for many years. It is relatively inexpensive, pliable and easy to mould, smoothing to conform almost exactly to the extremity.

However, despite starting to set in 15–20 minutes, it may take up to 2 days for the plaster cast to dry completely. This means no weight bearing or use of the casted limb can take place before the cast is completely dry, without causing damage to the surface or denting (Kelly 1983).

Fibreglass. A fibreglass cast is usually a knitted fibreglass fabric impregnated with a polyurethane resin which hardens on exposure to water in a matter of minutes. It usually takes 10–15 seconds in water to initiate the chemical reaction (Kelly 1983).

It comes in a variety of colours, is radiolucent, lightweight and, as noted by Leach (1974) and Lane & Lee (1982), is three times stronger than plaster of Paris, making it more resistant to damage from repetitive use.

It takes approximately 30 minutes to dry completely, making weight bearing and use of the casted limb possible much sooner. Unlike plaster of Paris, once hardened, the cast can be re-exposed to water without damage. However, the underlying padding can pose a problem if exposed to water, and may result in excoriation of the skin or formation of a pressure sore.

The resilience of the material makes it more difficult to conform well to the extremity and, unlike plaster of Paris, it does not mould specifically. The extremity must be in the correct position before application; if not, wrinkles may develop which cannot be smoothed out and can result in pressure sores.

The resin becomes tacky when in contact with water and may make the material resist coming off the roll. If pulled too hard on application, it may result in compromising the circulation. The tacky resin is also difficult to remove from equipment, skin and clothing, so gloves and aprons should be worn when applying the fibreglass tape (Kelly 1983).

It is more expensive than plaster of Paris, and for this reason is often not the initial cast of choice following trauma or surgery, when removal may be necessary because of swelling or wound inspection. The surface is rougher and, as noted by Lane & Lee (1982), may cause abrasions to the patient when in contact with other areas of the body. It may also cause snags to some clothing.

Non-fibreglass tape is used in some areas; it is radio-lucent, lightweight and is more environmentally friendly.

Both materials generate heat initially; therefore it is advisable to use cool or tepid water for dipping the tape, otherwise the patient may sustain a plaster burn.

Contact dermatitis or an allergic skin reaction has been reported in the past by Leach (1974) and Roof & Hodgkinson (1975, cited in Lane & Lee 1982), but occurred in such a small percentage of patients (approximately 0.5%) that it is not considered to be a marked disadvantage for use.

Effects of application on the patient and family

The cast is most often applied following trauma. However, it can also be applied to correct bony or tissue deformities which may be present at birth, e.g. developmental dysplasia of the hip and congenital talipes equinovarus.

No matter what the reason is for a cast being applied, nurses must be aware that although the procedure may be routine for them, it can be very stressful for both the child and his carers. This is why clear explanation of the reasons behind the application and its subsequent care are essential.

Very often carers are not prepared for the frustrations, fears and difficulties associated with the child's cast confinement (Cuddy 1986). As noted by Benz (1986), preparation of the family for the reality of home care could help to make what may be a difficult recovery period more acceptable to all concerned. Problems cannot be eliminated, but prior warning enables the carers and child to deal with them in whatever way is convenient to their circumstances. What makes these problems overwhelming is learning about them after discharge when lack of knowledge, equipment and support becomes apparent.

A simple explanation of what is normal and what is not can be very helpful, for example the psychological aspects of cast confinement: a once independent child may now be totally dependent, causing insecurity, frustration, tantrums and demanding behaviour. Educating the family will help to eliminate this (Benz 1986).

Casting can be used over a prolonged period. This is often age and disease related and may be for a number of years rather than weeks or months. This can cause major disruption to family life at home.

Written as well as verbal reinforcement of cast care is essential.

Types of cast

There are many different types of cast which can be altered as dictated by the orthopaedic medical staff to meet the individual's needs.

The most common casts used in paediatrics are:

- below elbow – distal radius and ulna fractures (Fig. 25.1)
- above elbow – proximal radius and ulna fractures supracondylar fractures (Fig. 25.2)
- scaphoid – scaphoid bone injuries (Fig. 25.3)
- below knee – fibula and tibial fractures metacarpal fractures, ligament and tendon injuries, talipes equinovarus (Fig. 25.4)
- above knee – fibula and tibial fractures, patella fractures, tendon and ligament injuries (Fig. 25.5)

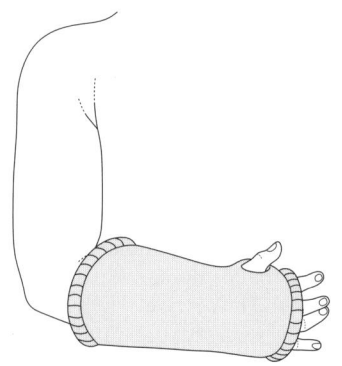

Figure 25.1
Below-elbow cast.

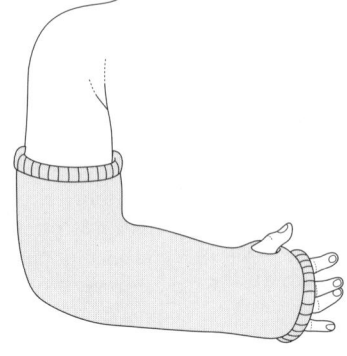

Figure 25.2
Above-elbow cast.

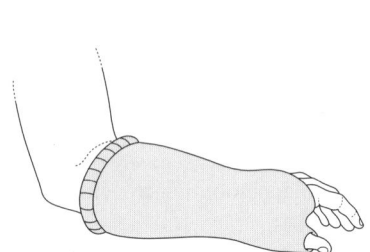

Figure 25.3
Scaphoid cast.

- cylinder – patella fractures, ligament and tendon injuries (Fig. 25.6)
- hip spica – femoral fractures, developmental dysplasia of the hip (Fig. 25.7)
- broomstick – developmental dysplasia of the hip (Fig. 25.8).

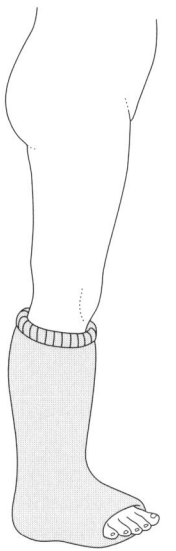

Figure 25.4
Below-knee cast.

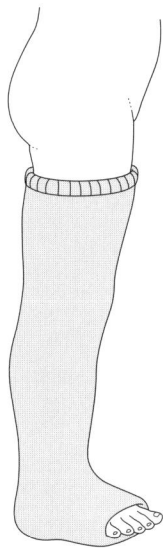

Figure 25.5
Above-knee cast.

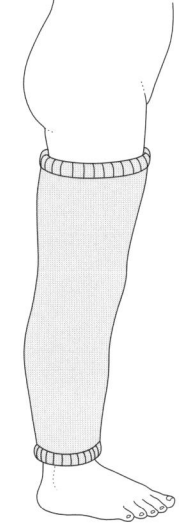

Figure 25.6
Cylinder cast.

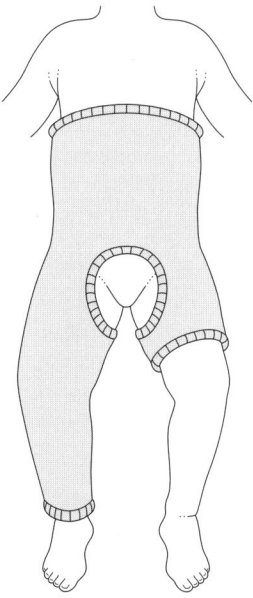

Figure 25.7
Broomstick cast.

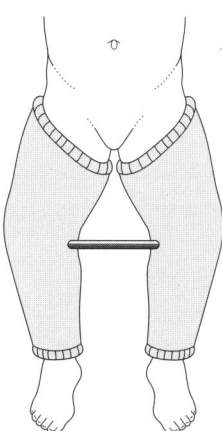

Figure 25.8
Hip splica cast.

The multidisciplinary team

The child in a cast may require input from various members of the multidisciplinary team whilst in the hospital and in the community.

Physiotherapists.   Advice can be given to the carers on lifting techniques, sitting, turning and carrying of the child, especially those whose needs prevent them doing it themselves. Many carers experience low back pain as a result of not being taught how to lift correctly (Cuddy 1986, Newman & Fawcett 1995).

Physiotherapists may also provide wheelchairs, reclining or ordinary, leg extensions and extra-wide pushchairs.

Teaching the correct method and use of crutches may also be carried out by them.

Occupational therapists.   They may be required to assess the home circumstances and provide various aids to caring for the child at home, e.g. a wheelchair ramp, plastic bedpans, etc.

Application of the cast

Equipment

Whatever the type of cast or reason for application, there is usually little variation in the equipment used.

- Stockinette
- Velband/Softband
- Plaster of Paris or fibreglass (Scotchcast)
- Disposable apron
- Disposable gloves
- Protective sheet
- Plaster bucket and stand
- Plaster sink
- Limb support
- Tepid/cool water

Method

The nurse applying the cast needs to assess the necessity for appropriate prescribed analgesia prior to application, e.g. oral or inhalational (Entonox).

1. Prepare the child and carer for the procedure, explaining why the cast is being applied and what the equipment is for. This is to minimise anxiety and gain cooperation.
2. Ensure that any administered analgesia has taken effect. This is also to reduce anxiety and gain cooperation.
3. Ensure privacy and protect the child's and carer's clothes using a protective sheet.

4. Position the child comfortably using a limb support if necessary. This is to facilitate progress of the procedure.
5. Apply the stockinette first and then the Velband, paying particular attention to bony prominences. This is to protect the skin from plaster burn on application, pressure sores caused by the rigid cast during the period of immobilisation, and from the plaster saw when the cast is being removed.
6. The nurse should protect her own clothes with a plastic apron and use disposable gloves, especially if a fibreglass cast is to be used as it may be an irritant to the skin.
7. Position the affected limb correctly or as directed by the orthopaedic medical staff. Persuade children to achieve the position themselves if possible; if not, seek the assistance of someone to hold the position so that smooth application of the cast is achieved.
8. Unwind the cast bandage for approximately 10 cm before immersing it in the water. This prevents the end of the bandage becoming lost in the roll. If fibreglass is used, immerse totally in the water for 10–15 seconds to initiate the chemical reaction of the resin, allowing the material to be shaped and eventually become rigid (Barrett & Bryant 1990).
9. Withdraw the bandage from the water, gently compressing it to remove excess water. Do not wring out the bandage, especially if plaster of Paris is being used, as this will result in a loss of the plaster cream.
10. Apply the wet cast bandage with even pressure around the correctly positioned limb, taking care not to pull too tightly, as this may compromise circulation. Warn the child that the bandage may feel warm and explain that it is the chemical reaction which will eventually harden the cast.
11. Turn back the ends of the stockinette and apply the casting material, allowing enough padding to remain visible at each edge. This will ensure patient comfort and reduce the risk of the cast rubbing against the skin and causing a sore. If necessary, trim rough edges and pad with tape or moleskin.
12. When handling a wet cast, use the palms of the hands and not just the fingers. Supporting the cast thus will minimise the risk of indentations which may cause pressure sores, and the developing of cracks in the cast which will weaken the support it provides.
13. The limb should be elevated for the first 24–48 hours, and circulation checks maintained. This

will minimise swelling of the limb and aid early detection of any possible circulatory problems.

14. On discharge, all carers must be given written as well as verbal instructions about their cast to ensure continuity of care.

Observations and complications

Frequency of observations varies from centre to centre depending on the reason for the application of the cast and the severity of the injury.

Circulatory, motor and sensory checks are essential, as trauma to a limb can affect the circulation, muscles and nerves. These checks may be performed every 30 minutes to 1 hour initially for up to 24–48 hours, depending on the severity of the injury.

Circulation. Indication of a problem in the circulation to the limb is noted by a change in colour to a blue or pale appearance, a change in the temperature of the peripheries from warm to cool, and by the absence of a distal pulse. (It may not be possible to feel the distal pulse as it may be covered by the cast.)

Muscle. Damage to muscle following injury, if neglected, may be irreparable especially if a condition known as Compartment Syndrome develops. Observations to detect this are referred to as the five Ps.

1. Pain – increasing in nature
2. Pallor – of the extremities with swelling
3. Pulse – diminished or absent
4. Paraesthesia – altered sensation, often tingling
5. Power loss – inability to move the associated extremities.

Nerves. Damage to nerves is indicated by altered sensation, pins and needles or numbness.

Any of the above changes must be reported immediately.

Swelling. Swelling usually peaks in 24–48 hours, which is why elevation is important during this period. This helps to prevent venous pooling and oedema (McConnell 1993).

Wound infection and pressure sore. Assess for the following signs and symptoms:

- drainage/seepage at the ends of the cast or over the wound site
- foul odour
- tingling or burning sensation under the cast
- pain under the cast, particularly over bony prominences or pins.

If wound infection or a pressure sore is suspected, a window may be cut out of the cast. If a sore or infection has developed, this enables dressings to be changed and the window can be replaced and held in position with tape or a bandage.

Too tight/loose. Too tight a cast will lead to circulatory problems. If it is too loose, it will not support the limb and may cause friction.

Skin. Inspect the skin regularly for signs of irritation or rubbing around the edges of the cast. To avoid this occurring, ensure that adequate padding is used on application of the cast.

Advice to carers

Hygiene and skin care

Information about keeping a cast clean, particularly around the perineal area for those in a hip spica, is very important. Excreta can seep inside the cast and cause skin and odour problems (Newman & Fawcett, 1995).

Shesser & King (1986) suggested using a smaller-sized nappy than usual, tucking it between the skin and the cast and ensuring that the plastic backing is next to the cast's inside surface. Observation of the area immediately under the cast is needed to ensure that the nappy is not causing any pressure sores. However, this very much depends on whether adequate space has been left around the perineal area to allow for this. Where possible, do not place the nappy over the cast as excreta will be absorbed into the cast causing odour and softening.

Also suggested by Shesser & King (1986), was the use of a sanitary towel inserted into the nappy to absorb more urine, particularly at night. Carers are also advised to check and change the nappy more frequently and as necessary.

For the older child in a hip spica, the use of a bedpan and urinal is recommended. As highlighted by Benz (1986), carers need to be made aware that they will need these items before discharge home. Waterproof tape (sleek) can be placed around the edges of the cast and replaced as necessary.

A thorough wash from head to toe may replace normal bathing. Hairwashing may be a problem and require two people – one to hold the child's head over the sink/bath, and the other to wash. An alternative is to use dry shampoo.

Positioning and safety

The affected limb should be positioned on cushions or pillows initially when at rest.

A hip spica cast often extends up to the diaphragm, so enabling the child to sit up requires special consideration. The use of pillows and cushions or a bean bag may assist in achieving this.

Turn the child from front to back several times a day to prevent pressure sores. The change in position also encourages different play activities.

Safety straps on pushchairs and highchairs, and side rails on cots/beds, will be required as children soon learn how to manoeuvre themselves. A car seat may require alterations to ensure safe transportation.

Eating and drinking

The extension of a spica cast may cause eating and drinking to be awkward, and the child may experience discomfort after meal times because of the restriction caused by the rigid cast. As Benz (1986) noted, it is better to ask carers to give smaller, more frequent meals to avoid discomfort, than let them discover this through experience.

If the cast reduces mobility, it may be necessary to increase the fibre content in the diet and give more fluids to prevent constipation.

A closed cup or the use of a flexible straw may be the best method for drinking to prevent too many accidents and spillages on to the cast.

Sleeping

Sleeping may be affected as a result of the effects of trauma and/or hospitalisation. Cramp and itching may occur, causing the child to become restless and only able to sleep for short periods.

The inability to turn over easily may also interrupt sleep.

Mobility

Balance may be affected by lower limb casts. If a weight-bearing cast has been applied, crutches may be advised initially, but the child must not be discharged home until shown the correct use of crutches by an appropriately trained person, e.g. a physiotherapist.

The ability to get out of the house is important for both the carers and the child to prevent social isolation. Input from the physiotherapist and occupational therapist is necessary for the provision of ramps, wheelchairs and wide pushchairs, etc.

Transportation may be a problem, especially with hip spica casts. A hospital taxi or ambulance may be required for discharge and follow-up appointments. If the child cannot safely be strapped into a car seat, a seat belt extension may need to be obtained.

Clothing

Shirts, shorts, dresses and skirts can usually be worn normally. However, a larger size may be necessary for those in a spica cast. Underwear, trousers, etc. for lower limb casts, spica and broomstick casts can be split at a side seam and Velcro strips, poppers or zips inserted for ease of access.

Removal of a cast

Equipment
Tools for removal of cast:
- plaster saw
- plaster shears
- plaster spreaders
- bandage scissors.

Method
1. Ensure that the equipment you require is available.
2. Explain to the child and carer what you will be doing, and give reassurance regarding the use of the saw and the noise it makes. The blade oscillates, so an explanation is needed to tell the child that the blade will not cut through the protective padding. Children should also be told that they may experience a vibrating or tickling sensation and slight warmth, especially during the removal of a large cast. This will help minimise anxiety and gain cooperation for the procedure to continue.
3. If necessary, mark the cast with a pen for exact lines to be cut, avoiding bony prominences and wound sites. This will minimise the possibility of trauma.
4. Position the child comfortably, enabling easy access to the cast on a secure and steady surface. Remove any clothing covering the cast, and if necessary protect other clothing with an apron or protective sheet.
5. When applying the saw to the cast, support the neck of the saw with one hand to avoid too much pressure being exerted downwards. Each time the blade cuts through the cast it should be lifted out, and the procedure repeated so a series of small cuts are made. The blade should not be run up and down the length of the cast, as this causes a great deal of heat to be generated by the blade because of friction.
6. Avoid using the saw on the extreme edges of the cast. These areas should be cut with the plaster shears.
7. When cutting is complete, open the cast with care using the plaster spreaders, avoiding too much disturbance to the limb.

8. Use the bandage scissors to cut the padding.
9. Note any signs of pressure from the cast on the skin or damage from the saw. If any, notify the doctor.
10. *Note:*
    – lower limb plasters – the child should not weight bear until seen by a doctor
    – upper limb plasters – arms should be supported until seen by a doctor.
11. Carers and child should be advised that once the cast is removed it may take some time for life to return to normal. A rehabilitation period may be necessary, as muscles and joints have been inactive for some time.

Adapting to mobilising in a cast, and losing the security of this immobilisation, can cause anxiety and discomfort for the child, as well as frustration at not being able to use the limb normally immediately (Cuddy 1986).

COMMUNITY PERSPECTIVE
The CCN will liaise with the family on the ward to ensure that they feel confident to take the child home.

Home visits may be arranged to advise on adaptations in the home, e.g. moving the child's bed downstairs.

Discharge planning should ensure that there is sufficient equipment at home, e.g. pillows, a pram sufficiently large to take the child in the plaster, a tummy trolley where necessary, vacuum cushions, bedpans/urinals.

The family should be given information concerning the charity STEPS (National Association for Children with Lower Limb Abnormalities) which may be able to provide additional equipment such as pushchairs or a low table with attached seat for a child with a hip spica.

The CCN will need to visit to ensure that the parents are coping with the physical care as well as the frustrations of restricted mobility and changed pattern of family life. She may be required to trim casts and apply sleek plaster to the edges.

Where there is a community play specialist, visits may be helpful in showing parents ways in which to occupy the child and the use of play techniques to relieve frustration and encourage normal development.

School-age children will need the involvement of the education department to supply a home tutor.

Results of findings by STEPS showed that 'High levels of emotional distress associated with diagnosis and treatment were often exacerbated by lack of information and equipment at the point of discharge.' (Hinde 1996). The provision of equipment for children with hip spicas and splints was found to be both uncoordinated and patchy. Often the first problem for parents is that of safety in the car, which is likely to occur immediately on discharge. They require access to appropriate harness devices or car seats. The problems for children with hip spicas are ongoing, as there appears to be a national lack of suitable equipment. Even where families are able to acquire a suitable pushchair, there may be a problem of access to the home as adaptations such as ramps are not usually available because this is not a long-term need.

Do and do not

- Do carry out observations for complications.
- Do exercise extremities as well as joints proximal to the cast. This will encourage venous return and thus help to reduce swelling. It will also help to prevent muscle wasting and joint stiffness.
- Do use the palms of the hands when moving a newly casted limb for the first 24 hours if plaster of Paris is used, and for 30 minutes if fibreglass material is used.
- Do elevate the limb whenever possible, especially during the first 24–48 hours after application.
- Do instruct the patient and carers to return to the hospital if:
  – pain is experienced that is disproportionate to the injury
  – there is marked swelling or discoloration of the peripheries
  – there is altered sensation or inability to move fingers or toes
  – the cast cracks, becomes soft, loose or uncomfortable.
- Do inspect the skin around the edges of the cast.
- Do advise the patient to use the crutches as instructed.
- Do give written cast care instructions.
- Do not allow the patient to weight bear until the cast is completely dry, or as instructed by orthopaedic medical staff.
- Do not permit any writing on the cast until it is completely dry, and advise the use of felt tip pens

only as ball point pens may cause cracks to develop in the cast.

- Do not allow the cast to get wet.
- Do not encourage anything to be poked down inside the cast such as pencils, knitting needles, etc., as sores may develop as a result.
- Do not allow the cast to become too hot, e.g. sitting too close to a fire or radiator. Once hot, the cast will take some time to cool down and may cause a burn beneath the cast.

References

Barrett J B, Bryant B H 1990 Fractures – types, treatment, perioperative implications. AORN Journal 52(4): 755–771

Benz J 1986 The adolescent in a spica cast. Orthopaedic Nursing 5(3): 22–23

Cuddy C M 1986 Caring for the child in a spica cast, a parent's perspective. Orthopaedic Nursing 5(3): 17–21

Hinde S 1996 Provision and availability of equipment for children in hip spicas and splints. STEPS, Lymm Court, Lymm, Cheshire WA13 0LP

Kelly D J 1983 The use of fibreglass as reinforcement with plaster casts. Orthopaedic Nursing 2(6): 17–21

Lane P L, Lee M M 1982 New synthetic casts: what nurses need to know. Orthopaedic Nursing 1(6): 13–20

Leach R E 1974 New fibreglass casting system. Clinical Orthopaedics and Related Research 103: 109–113

McConnell E A 1993 Providing cast care. Nursing 23(1): 19

Newman D, Fawcett J 1995 Caring for a young child in a body cast: impact on the care giver. Orthopaedic Nursing 14(1): 41–46

Shesser L K, King T F 1986 Practical considerations in caring for a child in a hip spica cast. An evaluation using parental input. Orthopaedic Nursing 5(3): 11–15

Further reading

Blaney A R 1985 Practical problems of managing a child at home in splints and plasters. Physiotherapy 71(9): 395–397

Jolleys J V Caring for a child in a cast. Presented by Orthopaedic Products, 3M Healthcare

Kelly A, Miljesic S, Mant P, Ashton N 1996 Plaster checks by nurses: safe and efficient? Accident & Emergency Nursing 4(2): 76–77

Monk H L 1993 Fractures are never simple. Registered Nurse 56(4): 30–36

Williamson M J 1994 Paediatric forearm fracture. Orthopaedic Nursing 13(3): 65–68

26

Positioning, Handling and Exercises

Introduction

Correct positioning is an integral part of the care of sick children or those with a physical disability, and can be used to enhance their speed of recovery, promote normal development and prevent deterioration in their condition. Competent handling is a crucial part of holistic care, as is the provision of appropriate opportunities for exercise, both active and passive.

Learning outcomes

By the end of this section you should:

- understand the benefits of correct positioning
- be able to assess the most appropriate positions and specific handling needs for children according to age, size, developmental level and condition
- recognise the dangers of incorrect positioning
- be able to determine whether specialised advice and equipment is necessary
- be aware of the need to assess the risk of lifting and handling
- be aware of the child's exercise requirements according to age, developmental level and condition.

Rationale

Any child with limited ability to move herself, whether because of age or condition, requires assistance to ensure appropriate and comfortable positions are achieved. This will maximise recovery and minimise deterioration. Some children have specific handling requirements, for example premature infants or those with certain conditions such as cerebral palsy. Others may require intervention by means of active or passive exercise.

Factors to note

Positioning

In order to practice good positioning it is necessary to understand how it is used and the benefits it affords. Variations in position will allow the child to be comfortable and ease the pressure exerted on any one area. This will help prevent the skin becoming sore or breaking down and the subsequent pain and limitation of movement which might result. Certain positions can be used to help facilitate play. Allowing the child to experience movement in a range of different positions encourages normal development (Bly 1994).

Specific positioning may be an important part of training a child to feed by ensuring correct head-on-body alignment. Positioning can assist the child with respiratory difficulties to drain secretions or reduce the work of breathing (Hough 1984). Positioning can have an influence on an infant's ability to lose heat and on the speed of gastric emptying (Hallsworth 1995). Children who have limited ability in movement need regular alterations to their positions in order to prevent the formation of muscle contractures and deformities (Dubowitz 1969). It has also been shown that children with abnormal movement patterns and involuntary movements can have their problems reduced by correct positioning (Finnie 1974).

Normal infants. Extensive research by the Foundation for the Study of Infant Deaths (Epstein 1993) and the Department of Health (1993) has shown that the risk of sudden infant death syndrome is significantly reduced by ensuring that young babies are not positioned to sleep on their fronts. The risk is further reduced by ensuring that they are positioned on their backs. Recent guidelines also suggest that babies should be positioned with their feet close to the foot of the bed so that they can not slide down under the covers.

Remember 'Back to sleep', 'Feet to foot'.

The judicious and considered handling of children can bring many benefits to certain situations, helping to build trust and promote psychological well-being as well as, at times, being an integral part of their treatment.

Manual handling

The risks of musculoskeletal problems to which all who work with children are exposed should be recognised, whether they come from continual lifting, stooping or working at an awkward level (Alexander 1997). With the advent of the Manual Handling Operations Regulations (1992), employees' responsibilities for their own safety are clearly set out. In summary these are:

- to avoid manual handling where there is risk of injury so far as is reasonably practicable
- to assess the risks in those operations that can not be avoided
- to take action to reduce risks to the lowest level reasonably practicable.

In order to undertake risk assessment, there are many factors that must be taken into account. These can generally be classified into four categories as follows:

- the load (the child) – weight, age, muscle tone, compliance/comprehension, drips/drains, plasters/splints, wound site, pain level, required oxygen, mobility
- the task – frequency, duration, distance, posture, fatigue, individual capability
- the environment – space, floor surface, nurse's uniform/footwear, patient's clothing, furniture (height and stability)
- the equipment available – hoists, transfer sliding boards/sheets (Chartered Society of Physiotherapy 1994).

It is important to note that this is only a brief guide to risk assessment and that each employer will have its own local code of practice with which its employees have a duty to cooperate (Royal College of Nursing 1993) (see Concepts p. 8).

Exercise

Exercise is the practice or training of a movement, and is a natural and essential part of development. It provides children with an outlet for energy and enables them to learn about themselves, their environment and others (Eckersley 1993).

Guidelines

Whenever possible all carers should be aware of the specific positioning, handling and exercise needs of their child, and careful explanation should be given at all times to the family to maximise their support.

Preterm babies

A full-term infant spends the last 4–6 weeks in utero in an increasingly compressed position. A preterm infant does not experience this time in flexion and so when born exhibits a floppy, extended posture. Babies who are born early, typically, have low muscle tone (Downs et al 1991) and often require special life-supporting care. This, together with immature development at birth, is likely to limit their ability to move against gravity and hence encourage them to lie in a flattened, frog-shaped posture (Fig. 26.1). Meanwhile, hypotonic neck muscles cause the head to rest flat on the side, resulting in narrow elongated head shape moulding. The aim of positioning must therefore be to:

- stimulate active flexion of the trunk and limbs
- encourage midline orientation
- minimise facial moulding and ensure full range of active head rotation
- encourage a balance between extension and flexion
- allow more symmetrical postures and enable postural stability
- facilitate smooth antigravity limb movements (Updike et al 1986).

Preterm babies should be cared for in a variety of positions mimicking normal development. However, some babies may be given specific positions by a physiotherapist because of 'particular concerns following a birth history indicating abnormal factors that are likely to cause handicap' (Murphey 1984).

When a baby is first admitted to a neonatal intensive care unit, the primary goal of care is to achieve physiological stability. Commonly, the prone position is best able to facilitate this, leading to improved oxygen saturation, heart rate and pulmonary resistance, and also helping to prevent gastric reflux and aspiration. Energy expenditure and heat loss are less in the prone position and babies are found to sleep better and startle and cry less.

When positioning a baby prone, Turrill (1992) suggests that the arms should be placed close to the body with the hands symmetrically brought up close to the mouth; the head unfortunately has to be turned to one side. The legs should be encouraged to flex, with the knees brought up towards the chest raising the hips slightly. This position is best maintained by using a soft rolled blanket to make a boundary (Fig. 26.2).

There are times when sick, preterm babies will be nursed in a supine position, for example to enable necessary equipment to be placed on the baby, for medical procedures or to make observation easier. This position does nothing to assist with the acquisition of a flexed posture, and so should be avoided whenever possible. To minimise the detrimental effects of this position the baby should be 'nested', i.e. given adequate support using small fabric rolls (Fig. 26.3). This will help to achieve the following desired position:

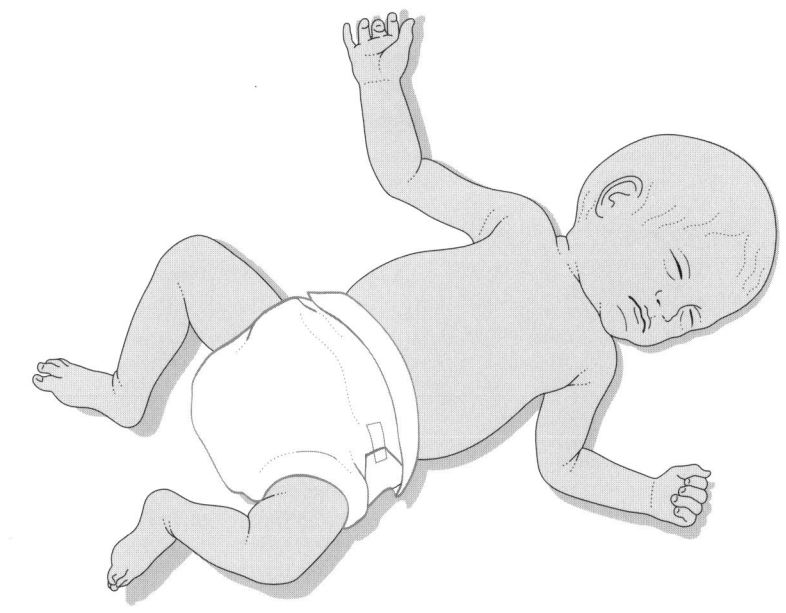

Figure 26.1
A typical frog-shaped posture adopted by a preterm infant.

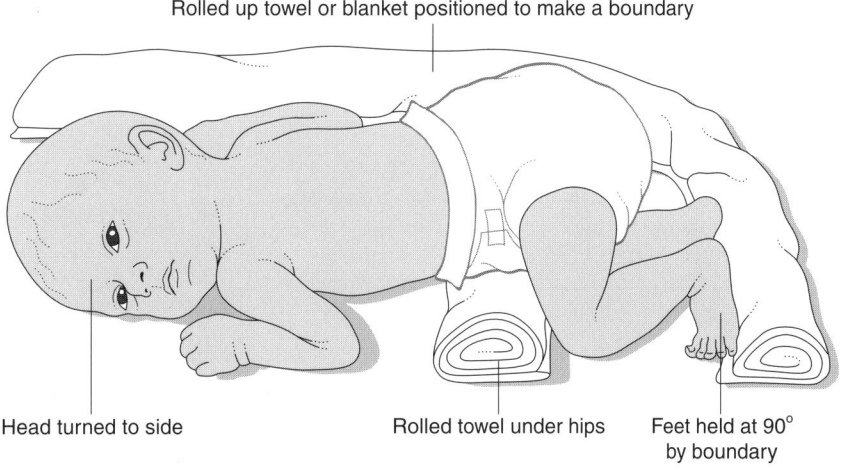

Rolled up towel or blanket positioned to make a boundary

Figure 26.2
A preterm baby positioned in prone.

Head turned to side   Rolled towel under hips   Feet held at 90° by boundary

- head in midline
- shoulders protracted
- hands to midline
- hips abducted and flexed (supported in neutral)
- knees flexed
- feet 'neutral' (Hallsworth 1995).

From this position the baby will be able to begin to develop head control, maintain a symmetrical posture, achieve normal flexor tone and establish visual skills. It will also encourage her to bring her hands together in the midline and to kick against gravity (Merenstein & Gardiner 1993).

Side-lying is a valuable position that can be used to encourage flexion and symmetry in the preterm infant. It is important to ensure that the trunk is held perpendicular to the cot surface by the use of a roll along the baby's back (not touching the back of the head as the baby may be stimulated to push back into it). The legs

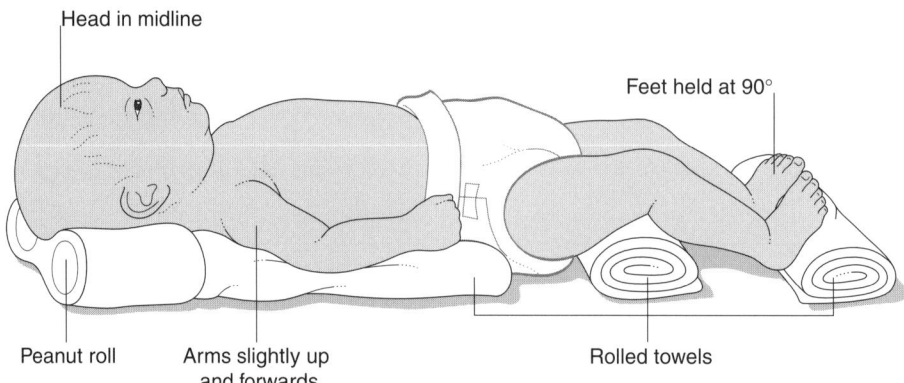

Figure 26.3
A preterm baby positioned in supine.

Head in midline

Feet held at 90°

Peanut roll

Arms slightly up and forwards

Rolled towels

should be flexed, and the upper leg supported in a neutral position, by the use of a folded nappy or roll between the legs (Fig. 26.4). In this position, the head is already in the midline and the arms can be placed forwards and up towards the mouth. It is also suggested that a thin soft towel can be placed for the baby to hold between the arms to give a stimulus to flex towards (Turrill 1992).

Note that 'the baby's position can affect the parents' perceptions. A comfortable curled baby with hands touching face looks far more appealing than a flat, extended baby' (Warren 1993).

When handling preterm babies, it is important to consider certain principles:

- Handling of sick, preterm babies should be kept to a minimum, as handling in any way will usually cause their condition to deteriorate, typically by making them hypoxic (Parker 1993).
- It is valuable to maintain positions of flexion during handling, either by lifting babies in a side-lying or prone position, with appropriate head support, or by swaddling them before they are lifted (Turrill 1992).
- Massage therapy has been found to be beneficial in terms of increased weight gain in certain medically stable preterm infants (Scafidi et al 1993) (see Complementary Therapies p. 335).

Acutely sick children

The positioning of an acutely sick child will often be a compromise in order to allow two or more body systems to be cared for simultaneously. However, it is important to understand the rationale for positioning for each of the different problems encountered.

Respiratory system

Drainage of secretions.   The child is positioned to assist the drainage of secretions from specific areas of the lungs by means of gravity. The positions relate to the anatomy of the bronchial tree. A physiotherapist may choose to leave a child in a certain position, the relevance of which is indicated in Table 26.1.

Improving gaseous exchange:

- Lung volume can be increased by helping a child to sit upright rather than slumped, or by positioning in side-lying when the abdominal contents will fall forwards away from the diaphragm (Hough 1984).
- Adequate gaseous exchange is dependent on adequate ventilation and adequate perfusion. Inadequate ventilation can be caused by pneumonia, paralysed hemidiaphragm or pneumothorax. Inadequate perfusion can be caused by pulmonary vasoconstriction or pulmonary embolus. In unilateral disease (only one lung affected), gas exchange is optimum when the child is side-lying with the good lung uppermost and the child should therefore be positioned thus.

Reducing the work of breathing.   When in respiratory distress there are six relaxed positions a child could adopt: high side-lying; forward lean sitting; forward lean kneeling; relaxed sitting; forward lean standing; and relaxed standing (Davis 1983).

Central nervous system

Control of raised intracranial pressure.   These children may be nursed in a head-up position in order to reduce cerebral blood flow and with the head in midline in order to prevent any compression of the cerebral vessels.

Skin

- The avoidance of breakdown of pressure areas demands frequent changes in position. Children who are at particular risk are those with reduced

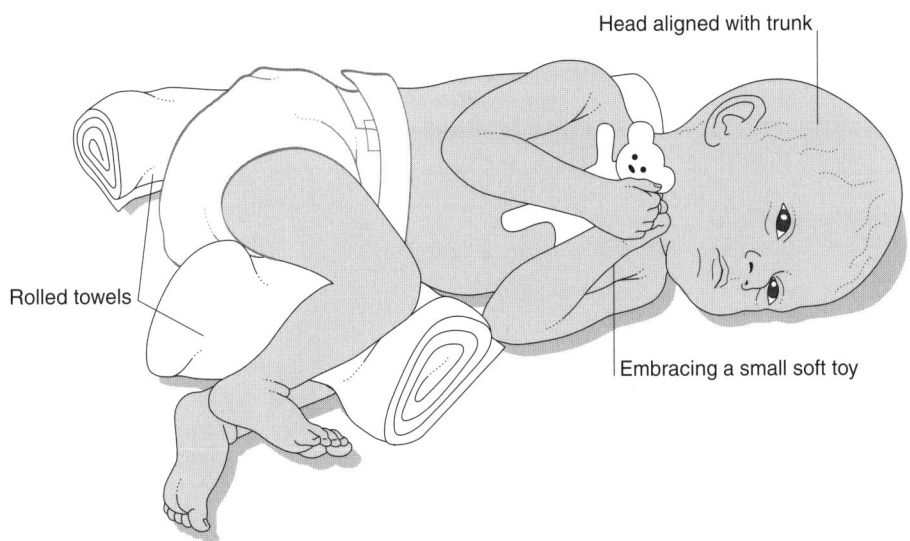

Head aligned with trunk

Rolled towels

Embracing a small soft toy

Figure 26.4
*A preterm baby
positioned in side-lying.*

Table 26.1 **Positions to aid postural lung drainage**

Area of lung to be drained	Possible positions
Right or left upper lobes	Sitting
	Supine lying – flat
	Three-quarters prone lying – flat
Right middle lobe	One-quarter left side-lying – head down 15 degrees
Lingula	One-quarter right side-lying – head down 15 degrees
Right or left lower lobes	Prone – head down 20 degrees
	Supine – head down 20 degrees
	Left or right side-lying – head down 20 degrees

active movement, diminished sensation or poor circulation. Often a regular 30 degree turn is all that is necessary (see Pressure Area Care p. 235).

■ Following a burn, skin or joint contractures may develop. Collagen formation and contraction begin before the wound is healed and continue until the scars are fully mature. A child in pain will assume a position of comfort, generally a position of flexion (Sadowski 1992). Therapeutic positioning and exercises must therefore be performed as soon as possible and continued with regular monitoring throughout rehabilitation, to prevent the onset of contractures and subsequent disability. The use of splints and/or pressure garments may be necessary.

Chronically/long-term sick babies

Chronically sick babies often suffer from delayed development due to inadequate nutrition, recurrent illnesses and lack of stimulation. It is important to try to provide them with a position and environment from which they can get satisfaction in play with minimal effort. This should then increase their motivation to further explore their environment. Side-lying with a roll behind the back, to stop them falling back, helps to bring their hands together and position their head in midline, which is crucial in the development of coordination between the two sides of the body (Bly 1994). Sitting in a car seat, bouncy chair or tumble form chair enables them to be able to see their surroundings and toys more easily, and will encourage them to try to reach out for them.

In addition, prolonged hospitalisation may interfere with parental bonding. The parents may be reluctant to be involved with the normal care of the child (cuddling, feeding, changing, playing, etc.). When medically stable, these babies should be exposed to as much handling and interaction during such activities as possible.

The floppy child

A child may be floppy for many reasons, for example:

- acute illness (infection, dehydration)
- paralysis
- neuromuscular diseases (muscular dystrophy, spinal muscular atrophy, neuropathies)
- other disorders of the central nervous system (some types of cerebral palsy, Down's syndrome)
- metabolic disease.

When positioning these children, special consideration should be given to the prevention of deformities, which could eventually prove to be a greater disability than their weakness (Dubowitz 1969). They must therefore have regular changes of position throughout each day (sitting, prone, supine and side-lying) with an emphasis on providing enough support through the use of pillows, cushions or rolled towels to maintain a symmetrical posture. Floppy children, because of their inability to move against gravity, will find side-lying and sitting helpful positions to enable them to develop their skills.

In order to help prevent the development of contractures, active movement, coupled with passive movement of the joints through their full range should be encouraged. Spinal braces or foot splints where provided must be worn.

When lifting a floppy child, remember that such children are likely to be unstable (owing to their lack of trunk control) and difficult to grasp (characteristically 'falling through' when lifted from under the arms). Therefore special care should be taken by the lifter to ensure that there is no accidental damage to the child's lax joints.

The neurologically impaired child

Disorders of the central nervous system are the result of either abnormal development of the central nervous system itself or an insult to the brain or spinal cord, commonly affecting the sensorimotor activities of the child (Bedford & McKinlay 1993). The largest group with these problems will be children who have or are developing cerebral palsy. The principles of positioning and handling for these children can be extended to other children with neurological impairment such as head injury, cerebrovascular accident, cerebral tumour or

other acute insults including meningitis and encephalitis.

The main feature of this type of disorder is abnormal movement which may be:

- limited, stiff and in stereotyped patterns due to spasticity
- floppy, feeling loose and with greater range than one would normally expect
- athetoid – almost continuous and unwanted movement which the child can not control
- ataxic, jerky and uncoordinated.

Children with neurological impairment may have various combinations and distributions of any of these abnormal movements, and the first step towards effective handling and treatment calls for a full assessment of the child by a physiotherapist (Finnie 1974). Good positioning and handling are vital to help to:

- reduce abnormal movements
- break up and control stiffness
- maintain the normalised tone achieved through active treatment.

Poor positioning will worsen these children's problems.

A general guideline is to place and carry children in a different position from that which they assume naturally, but abnormally.

The extending child should not be left supine. In this position, the force of gravity pulls the body into an increasingly extended posture, making it more difficult for the child to move. Side-lying, with the inclusion of semi-flexion at the neck, hips and knees, the legs separated by a towel or pillow and the arms placed forwards, is helpful. In addition, sitting in a chair may be useful. It can provide support to ensure a position with 90 degree hip and knee flexion, trunk and head alignment in the midline, and the shoulders prevented from being retracted. When carried, the child should first be moved into a more flexed and symmetrical position (e.g. sitting) and then held facing the lifter, with the legs apart and flexed at the hips and with the arms up and forwards on the lifter's shoulders.

In contrast, predominantly flexed children should be carried on their side or front in an extended position, with arms reaching up and legs held apart. It may also be appropriate for them to be positioned to sleep on their tummy, but it is important that they are fully assessed by a physiotherapist before this is attempted.

A child who is strongly asymmetrical and usually holds her head turned to one side is helped most if her bed or seating is positioned so that all stimulation is from the opposite side.

Both athetoid and ataxic children need stability when they are being lifted or carried, and so handling should be steady and firm and the child usually responds well to generally flexed positions.

Observations and complications

Having positioned any child, always stand back and observe the child in the new position:

- Have you achieved what you were aiming for?
- Is the child comfortable?
- If you are having difficulty making the child comfortable, contact a physiotherapist for advice at the earliest opportunity.

COMMUNITY PERSPECTIVE

Prior to the discharge of a child who has a specific problem of mobility, it must be ensured that the parents are aware of any special procedures and that they have been taught how to carry them out. Lifting techniques should be explained, demonstrated and assessed.

Consideration should be given to the fact that one parent is likely to be on his or her own for the majority of the time and that the average home is not designed to cater for carrying older children from one room to another, or up and down stairs. These factors may pose a considerable risk to both carer and child.

An assessment should therefore be made of the home, involving other members of the multidisciplinary team as necessary, for example the occupational therapist to advise on bath aids, hoists and possible adaptation/extension of the home.

Many of the children who require long-term care at home will need to wear nappies. The nappy service may only call once every 8 weeks, leaving a bulky delivery, causing storage problems. Equipment needed for the child's care may also be difficult to manoeuvre and therefore pose a risk to the carer's back.

Part of the role of the CCN is to monitor the impact that constant moving and handling is having on the carers and to act accordingly. The families may have no-one else who can help and the CCN may need to organise respite care or press for a speedy implementation of adaptations and provision of equipment.

Do and do not

- Do think before you start: 'What am I trying to achieve for the child?'
- Do keep the handling of acutely sick children to a minimum.
- Do remember to involve a physiotherapist.
- Do remember to assess any manual handling/lifting situation for risk.
- Do not ever put a baby to sleep on her front, unless medically advised to do so.
- Do not ever put a stiff extended child onto her back.

References

Alexander P 1997 Handling babies and young children. In: The guide to the handling of patients, 4th edn. National Back Pain Association/Royal College of Nursing, London

Bedford S, McKinlay I 1993 Disorders of the central nervous system. In: Eckersley P M (ed) Elements of paediatric physiotherapy. Longman, London, pp 115–155

Bly L 1994 Motor skills acquisition in the first year. Therapy Skill Builders, Tucson, Arizona

Chartered Society of Physiotherapy 1994 Manual handling training. Factsheet 9. CSP, London

Davis A J 1983 Medical chest physiotherapy. In: Downie PA (ed) Cash's textbook of chest, heart and vascular disorders for physiotherapists. Faber & Faber, London, pp 298–329

Department of Health (DoH) 1993 Cot death. HMSO, London

Downs J A, Edwards A D, McCormick D C, Roth S C, Stewart A L 1991 Effect of intervention on development of hip posture in very preterm babies. Archives of Disease in Childhood 66: 797–810

Dubowitz V 1969 The floppy infant. Heinemann, London

Eckersley P M 1993 Elements of paediatric physiotherapy. Longman, London, pp 343–375

Epstein J 1993 The Foundation for the Study of Infant Deaths campaign to reduce the risk of cot death. What is the research evidence? Maternal and Child Health 18(1): 6–8

Finnie N R 1974 Handling the young cerebral palsied child at home. Butterworth-Heinemann, Oxford

Hallsworth M 1995 Positioning the preterm infant. Paediatric Nursing 7(1): 18–20

HMSO 1992 Manual handling Operations regulations and guidance on regulations L23. HMSO, London

Hough A 1984 The effect of posture on lung function. Physiotherapy 70(3): 101–104

Merenstein G, Gardiner S L 1993 A handbook of neonatal intensive care. Mosby, St Louis

Murphey F 1984 The physiotherapist in the neonatal unit. In: Levitt S (ed) Paediatric development therapy. Blackwells, Oxford, 63–75

Parker A 1993 Neonatal problems and the neonatal unit. In: Eckersley P M (ed) Elements of paediatric physiotherapy. Longman, London, pp 79–96

Royal College of Nursing (RCN) 1993 Code of practice for the handling of patients. RCN, London

Sadowski D A 1992 Care of the child with burns. In: Hazinski M F (ed) Nursing care of the critically ill child. Mosby, St Louis, ch 13, pp 875–927

Scafidi F A, Field T, Schanberg S M 1993 Factors that predict which preterm infants benefit most from massage. Journal of Developmental and Behavioural Pediatrics 14(3): 176–180

Turrill S 1992 Supported positioning in intensive care. Paediatric Nursing 4(4): 24–27

Updike C, Schmidt R E, Macke C, Cahoon J, Miller M 1986 Positional support for premature infants. American Journal of Occupational Therapy 40(10): 712–715

Warren I 1993 How to place a baby. MIDIRS Midwifery Digest 3(4): 452–453

27

Postoperative Care

Introduction

Postoperative care commences as the patient leaves the operating theatre and ends when he is discharged from the ward.

Learning outcomes

By the end of this section you should:

- understand the three stages of postoperative care
- be able to understand fundamental postoperative care
- recognise the role of the patient/carer and family in the child's recovery
- recognise the involvement of the multidisciplinary team.

Rationale

Care of the child in the postoperative phase is aimed at preventing complications and ensuring as quick a recovery from the operation and anaesthetic as possible. Postoperative care covers many different surgical specialities; however, the fundamental principles of care can be applied to any surgical procedure.

Factors to note

There are three stages of postoperative care:

- the immediate recovery period
- the intermediate stage of dependency
- returning to normality (Lyon & Best 1994).

These three stages are not perhaps thought of consciously but are planned for from the moment the child is admitted. Surgery can be planned, emergency or day case (see Preoperative Care, p. 231).

A good preoperative preparation can make a difference to the child and his family postoperatively.

If children are treated honestly with realistic values and expectations, they can begin to accept the surgery and the consequences of it.

The immediate recovery period

Immediate recovery from anaesthesia should be in a fully equipped recovery area with one-to-one ratio of personnel trained in children's nursing (McConchie et al 1989). Recovery units may be known by a different name in some areas, such as reception or post-anaesthetic care units (PACU). Recovery is usually situated near to the operating theatres. This enables easy access to the patients by the surgical and anaesthetic staff should an emergency arise.

Whilst the child has been in theatre and recovery the bed/cot area should have been prepared for his return to the ward. In some areas the bed may have been transferred to the recovery unit perioperatively to minimise pain and distress for the child postoperatively. All beds must have a tilt facility and must be able to be raised up and down. (The tilt facility is important if children are experiencing postoperative shock or vomiting as it allows the child's head to be lowered or raised according to need.) It is imperative that the bed space has access to working oxygen and suction. It may also be necessary for the child to be moved closer to the nursing station for closer observation. Neonates may need to be transferred in an incubator or Baby Therm and the same principles must apply to them. Equipment that may be required postoperatively such as infusion pumps and monitoring equipment should be tested and ready when the child is transferred back to the ward. During the perioperative phase of nursing, the theatre nurse is responsible for the child whilst he is under anaesthetic and serves as the patient's advocate.

Once the theatre nurse has handed the child over to the recovery unit, his immediate postoperative management is the responsibility of the anaesthetist involved in the surgery and the unit staff. Handover should incorporate the condition of the child whilst under anaesthetic, any problems which may have occurred, and any analgesia which may have been administered.

Serious complications can occur during the initial stage after surgery; hence the child receives short-term intensive care nursing whilst in the recovery area. The duration of a child's stay in the recovery area depends on the type of surgery undertaken and the child's reaction to anaesthesia. If the child's condition indicates further intensive nursing intervention, the child will be transferred to the high-dependency unit (HDU) or the intensive care unit (ICU).

In the recovery unit the child is attached to a multifunctional monitor which monitors the following: heart rate, ECG, respiratory rate, oxygen saturation, non-invasive blood pressure, rectal temperature and skin temperature. This kind of monitoring reduces disturbance to the child yet provides more detailed information for the nurse. Not all children will need all these facilities, as this depends on their condition and the type of surgery undertaken (See Reference on p. 45).

All vital signs, e.g. temperature, pulse, blood pressure, respirations and conscious level, are affected by the surgery and anaesthetic. On recovery from anaesthesia initially, the child will be supine with the head tilted; this ensures that the jaw is kept forward, positioning the tongue so that it does not obstruct the airway.

Airway management is one of the most important areas of recovering a child from anaesthesia and should only be undertaken by appropriately trained staff. The airway requires support and this usually entails the administration of oxygen via a face mask and continuous monitoring of oxygen saturation.

If the child has an airway in situ, the nurse waits for signs of returning consciousness.

Anaesthesia-induced unconsciousness will mean normal reflexes are absent and respiration must be supported. During semi-consciousness the reflexes, e.g. breathing, coughing, swallowing and blinking, begin to return and finally the patient should be awake and orientated with the return of all normal reflexes.

The airway is usually removed when the patient coughs it out or tries to remove it. It should be stressed that monitoring is only an aid to continuous nursing observation. One of the most common surgical complications is haemorrhage, which can lead to shock. Any deterioration in condition is usually rapid and demands urgent attention. When shocked, the child will be pale, tachycardic and not responding as normal. In children, and especially neonates, it only takes a small amount of blood loss to make transfusion or rapid fluid replacement essential.

It is imperative that each bed/trolley space has working oxygen and suction, an emergency buzzer and easy access to the resuscitation trolley. The nurse should observe the colour of the child, and whether it is good for that particular patient. This type of information is often gained during the preoperative visit or from the ward's nursing documentation. Many children with special needs or those with cardiac/pulmonary problems can be pale or even cyanosed. Their oxygen saturations may also be lower than is normal. The promotion of safety and comfort is paramount and the use of cot sides is universal.

Although the child may feel alert and capable of moving, the remaining effects of the anaesthesia and sedation may mean that his movements are uncoordinated. Special consideration should be given to children who have had spinal and epidural anaesthesia. Frequent assessment of the lower extremities should be made to determine the return of function. Temperature, colour and range of sensation and movement should be observed. In recovery, the relief of pain and encouragement to rest are also of high priority. The inclusion of parents in the recovery area is a relatively new idea. The child has to be sufficiently recovered, e.g. fully conscious and maintaining his own airway, for the inclusion of the parent.

The presence of the parent affords reassurance and comfort and is effective in reducing postoperative distress and anxiety. However, the presence of parents who are themselves visibly distressed or anxious can have an adverse effect on the child's emotional condition. It must also be stressed that not all recovery units may allow a parent into the recovery area, although this is becoming more common.

Before the child is transferred back to the ward certain criteria must be fulfilled:

- the child is conscious (but may be asleep)
- the protective reflexes have returned
- the child is maintaining his own airway and respirations are satisfactory
- the child's colour is good for that particular patient
- postoperative observations have been stable
- the child is comfortable and pain is adequately controlled
- the child's temperature is above 36°C
- the child is clean and tidy.

The intermediate stage of dependency: return to the ward

Postoperative observations may include some of the following: temperature, pulse, respirations, blood pressure, colour and conscious level of the child; monitoring of the wound site; maintenance of intravenous infusion; and monitoring of drains and urinary catheters. The frequency of routine postoperative observations may vary and is dependent on the child's condition. Observation of pulse and respirations is more frequent when intravenous opiate analgesia is in progress. One of the side-effects of opiates is respiratory depression, so the rate, depth and quality of respiration is monitored. Reduction in frequency of postoperative observation is based on the nurse's assessment of the child's condition.

Research has shown that the nurse often carries out more frequent observations than the patient's condition dictates, mistakenly believing that the regime had been prescribed by the hospital or by nursing policy (Botti & Hunt 1994).

Hydration

Normally, the reintroduction of oral fluids is left to the discretion of the nurse and is determined by the type of surgery undertaken. However, if the child has had surgery which requires him to have no fluid or dietary intake for a long period of time, e.g. following bowel surgery, his hydration needs will have to be met by intravenous means until he can tolerate fluids orally.

In this instance a fluid balance chart is crucial to monitor all input and output. Output includes urine, vomit, wound leakage, gastric aspirate and stool.

The nurse should also observe for signs of dehydration, e.g. decreased urine output, dark sunken eyes and dry mucous membranes.

Oral fluids should be reintroduced once the child is sufficiently awake. However, in more complex surgery it is common to wait until bowel sounds have returned, and fluids should be commenced as advised by the surgeons. Should it be anticipated that the child is going to be nil orally for some time, e.g. after bowel surgery, the child will have a nasogastric tube for the purpose of draining the stomach of bile and secretions. These losses are replaced millilitre for millilitre with intravenous fluid to prevent the child from becoming dehydrated. Enteral feeding is usually commenced within 24 hours of surgery unless contraindicated. For example, a child having undergone a fundoplication and/or gastrostomy may have to wait 48 hours prior to commencing enteral feeds to allow primary healing. Parenteral nutrition may be administered to children who have been poorly for some time and have no expectation of being able to tolerate diet and fluids normally within a few days. Again, bowel surgery is a good example of this.

Pain (see also Pain Management, p. 195)

Many hospitals have a pain management policy for children which focuses on pain prevention and, where possible, children should be involved in assessing their own pain level. Pain assessment tools rely on the child's understanding of numbers, colours and drawings, so a selection of pain assessment tools is helpful in finding the right one to suit the child's level of understanding (Twycross 1995).

Parents play an important role in communication with the child and for those who cannot communicate verbally, pain control is something that should be discussed preoperatively.

As well as pharmacological pain relief, alternative methods include distraction, massage and snoozelen therapy. The latter works with all the senses, using aids such as soft music, optic fibre lights and tactile toys.

Pain is not just a consideration in the immediate postoperative period. The nurse has to prepare the child and family for potentially painful procedures such as removing drains and mobilisation. On these occasions, the play specialist can provide valuable input. It is important where possible to carry out such procedures away from the bedside as the bed should be seen as a safe haven and a place of comfort. Privacy and dignity should be maintained at all times.

Method

1. Establish baseline information. Record temperature, pulse, respirations and blood pressure. Vital signs should be monitored and recorded regularly to detect any complications such as haemorrhage or compromise of the airway. They may also indicate that the child is experiencing pain. Assess consciousness level. Report any changes or concerns.
2. Observe the pallor of the skin. If oxygen is to be administered, ensure that the mask is correctly positioned and that the oxygen is delivered at the prescribed rate. Mouth care is essential to ensure patient comfort (see Oral Hygiene, p. 179).
3. Check wound sites and drains. Monitor wound sites at regular intervals for signs of leakage and mark as necessary; change dressings or add additional padding as required. Report any excessive leakage. If drains are in situ, record output regularly and note the characteristics of the fluid. e.g. haemoserous fluid. (*Note:* Aim to observe the wound site at the same time as these observations to reduce disturbance to the child.)
4. Commence fluid balance chart. If an intravenous infusion is in situ, maintain it at the prescribed rate and record the amount infused hourly. Check the access point for signs of extravasation or phlebitis and report immediately. Reintroduce oral fluids as advised and increase intake as tolerated. All intake and output should be recorded. In the absence of

oral fluid intake, ensure that adequate mouth care is provided.

5. Observe for signs of dehydration. Look for decreased urine output, poor skin turgor, dark sunken eyes, sunken fontanelle (in babies), dry mucous membranes and prolonged episodes of vomiting. Inform the medical staff of concerns. If an intravenous infusion is not in progress, it may be necessary to site one. Anti-emetics may help to reduce nausea and vomiting and need to be prescribed and monitored as to their effectiveness.

6. Assess pain. Use a pain tool relevant to the child's age and development to assess the need for analgesia. All analgesia should be given as prescribed and monitored for any adverse reactions and effectiveness. If intravenous analgesia is in progress, such as a patient-controlled analgesia (PCA), maintain it at the prescribed rate and record pulse and respirations hourly, as some opiates may cause respiratory depression. Report any significant changes immediately. Liaise with the pain management team, if available, to regularly manage the child's pain safely and effectively.

7. Remember reduced mobility. Observe and relieve pressure areas at regular intervals. Encourage the child to move himself where possible, but nursing staff should be there to assist. Changing position can also help to relieve any pain or discomfort the child may be experiencing. If appropriate, and if parents feel confident, babies and young children can be nursed on a knee or in a pushchair.

   Encourage older children to cough and deep breathe. It may be necessary to involve the physiotherapist to relieve any chest problems and help with mobilisation. This type of involvement is usually for those who have had more major surgery, e.g. appendicectomy, nephrectomy. It is usual to mobilise as soon as the child's condition allows.

   Reduced mobility can also affect bowel movement. Monitor signs of constipation and give aperients as prescribed if necessary. When diet and fluids have been re-established, encourage a good fluid intake and a diet which contains roughage. Depending on the type of surgery undertaken, for example following fundoplication, it may be advisable for the child to have smaller meals more frequently until normal dietary intake is re-established.

The family

Following the acute stage of surgical nursing care the priority is to encourage a safe return to normality.

It should be stressed to the parents and the family that the child still needs periods of rest. Sometimes this can be hard, especially when many paediatric wards and hospitals encourage an open visiting policy. Again it must be stressed that not all wards will have this policy.

The paediatric nurse should always take account of the different ages of the children she is caring for. Adolescents have specific needs too and provision should be made to keep children of similar age together where possible. Privacy and dignity should be maintained at all times.

Discharge planning

The nurse should begin planning for discharge from the time of admission whenever possible. Usually, the initial assessment will identify potential problems, such as transport home and referrals to community nurses. Effective discharge planning can reduce any delay once the decision has been made to allow the patient home. Many areas have pre-printed discharge plans which form part of the nursing documentation, and these often extend to printed discharge advice leaflets. The discharge plan should include any supplies that may be required, e.g. dressings, catheter bags, etc. Drugs required on discharge and specific instructions are important. Examples of such information are when the child should resume school and physical exercise. Information should also be given regarding pain relief, observation of the wound site and who to contact in an emergency.

Personal experience has shown that parents find it useful to have written instructions for reference, and contact numbers should be included for advice if they are having any problems.

If a child is a day case, it may be appropriate to arrange a district nurse, probably a paediatric community nurse, to visit the child the following day to perform a post-operative check and ensure that the parents are happy with their child's recovery. Again it should be noted that this is not always the case; local policy may dictate this practice.

COMMUNITY PERSPECTIVE

The role of the CCN in postoperative care can vary, particularly in reference to day surgery, from maintaining telephone contact with the family to check that all is well, to regular visiting to help with nursing care and monitor progress, ensuring that

---

recovery is at the expected rate. This can be reassuring for parents, should any unforeseen problems occur. In some areas this routine postoperative care may be undertaken by district nurses, who can refer cases to the CCNs if they feel this to be appropriate.

It may be necessary to visit to change dressings or remove sutures.

Do and do not

- Do encourage the parents to participate in their child's care.
- Do explain the planned care to the child and his family.
- Do explain the use of any equipment, e.g. infusion pumps, and also the purpose of any drains in situ.
- Do encourage the child to rest.
- Do explain discharge arrangements to the parents prior to discharge.
- Do outline the limitations, if any, when the child returns home, i.e. return to school and exercise.
- Do not allow the child to be discharged without arranging follow-up or community nurse input, if required.
- Do not forget that surgery is never routine for the child or his family.
- Do not assume that the parent or carer will want to participate in postoperative care. This should always be negotiated.
- Do not forget to give parents a contact number for advice should they have any problems.

References

Botti M A, Hunt J O 1994 The routine of post anaesthetic observations. Contemporary Nurse 3(2): 52–57
Lyon M H, Best B J 1994 Immediate postoperative recovery: management and care. British Journal of Nursing 3(17): 866, 868–870
McConchie I W, Day A, Morris P 1989 Recovery from anaesthesia in children. Anaesthesia 44: 986–990
Twycross A 1995 Children's nursing in Canada. Paediatric Nursing 7(4): 8–10

Further reading

Campbell I R, Scaife J M, Johnson J M 1988 Psychological effects of daycase surgery compared with inpatient surgery. Archives of Disease in Childhood 63: 415–417
Chitwood L B, Crister Swan D 1992 Perioperative nursing. Springhouse, USA
Drain C B 1994 The post anaesthetic care unit (PACU). W B Saunders, Pennsylvania
Fairchild S S 1996 Peri-operative nursing: principles and practise, 2nd edn. Little Brown, Boston
Hatfield A, Tronson M 1992 The common recovery room book. Oxford Medical Publications, Oxford
Hawthorne J 1995 Understanding and management of nausea and vomiting. Blackwell Science, Oxford
Hogg C 1994 Standard setting for children undergoing surgery. Action for Sick Children, London
Jacobson W K (ed) 1992 Manual of post-anaesthetic care. W B Saunders, Pennsylvania
Morton N S, Raine P A M 1994 Paediatric day case surgery. Oxford Medical Publications, Oxford
Smith F 1995 Children's nursing in practice – the Nottingham model. Blackwell Science, Oxford
Whaley L F, Wong D L 1994 The essentials of paediatric nursing, 4th edn. Mosby, St Louis

28

Preoperative Care

Introduction

Effective preparation of children who are to undergo anaesthesia and surgical intervention is an important factor in reducing the anxiety experienced by the child and her family during hospital admission (Taylor 1991).

Learning outcomes

By the end of this section you should:

- recognise the need for safe preparation for theatre
- understand the role of the parent in the preoperative phase
- be able to identify the needs of different age groups and their level of understanding
- recognise stressors affecting both parent and child
- be able to identify multidisciplinary involvement in preoperative care
- be able to assist in the safe preparation of a child for theatre

Rationale

Children, regardless of age, need to be appropriately prepared for theatre. This involves both physical and psychological aspects of care. Children who are familiar with their surroundings and are informed of events associated with surgical procedures, are more likely to cope with the overall experience (Newman & Scott 1990).

Factors to note

Planned surgery

- Planned, or elective, surgery lends itself very well to good preparation. There is time to involve other disciplines who can make a contribution to the overall readiness of both the child and her family for forthcoming surgery.
- Psychological preparation can begin at home well before the planned date of admission. There is a wide range of books and other visual aids available from libraries and book shops which offer the opportunity to talk through the need for

hospitalisation and what to expect. Schools and nurseries will often facilitate role play which involves dressing up and acting out the nurse/doctor roles. These are all recognised as ways of allaying fears and anxieties of children and can help those parents who have little experience of hospitals themselves (Eiser & Hauson 1989).

- The development of pre-admission programmes, such as Saturday morning clubs, allows interaction between hospital staff and parents and allows the opportunity to discuss pain control and the admission procedure. Efforts made at this stage of contact promote a feeling of well-being and aid in the speedy recovery of the child (Cooper & Harpin 1991).
- On admission, there is the opportunity to involve play specialists and theatre staff. Action for Sick Children (1991) highlighted the value of play in hospital and this role has been developed well in paediatric areas. The benefit of the involvement of play specialists in overcoming operation anxiety, the use of photograph albums and visits made by recovery staff, all give a broader view of what the child will experience, and what the parents' role is in the process (See Play p. 329).

Emergency surgery

- Unplanned surgery often means that there is little time for the psychological preparation of the parent or child. Some children go to theatre directly from the accident and emergency department, and so there may be limited time for explanations or time for premedications. Sudden loss of contact with parents and siblings can cause additional stress to the child. The nurse should be aware of these factors and deal with them sensitively.
- When the child has been transferred to theatre it is usual that the parents will be taken to the admitting ward to wait for the surgery to be completed. It is during this time that additional information and emotional/psychological support is given.

- When a child is transferred to the ward only a short time prior to surgery, emphasis is mainly on physical preparation, with medical staff completing tasks such as obtaining consent and examination of the child. There may be an opportunity for the parents to speak with the anaesthetist or surgeon, but this is not always possible. Fuller explanations of procedures and planned care usually take place whilst the child is in theatre and upon return to the ward.

Day care surgery

- Day surgery has many advantages for both the child and her family. The report, *Caring for Children in the Health Service* (Action for Sick Children 1991) explored the benefits of paediatric day care from an economic viewpoint, and from the child's needs with regard to avoiding the need for overnight admission. This was reinforced by the Audit Commission report, *Children First* (1993), which encouraged the development of such facilities.
- Morton & Raine (1994) defined some of the benefits as: absence of parental separation; less disruption to the family; and an increase in the amount of parental involvement. All of these should be supported by care being available for children in the community following attendance at a day care facility.
- The National Association for the Welfare of Children in Hospital (NAWCH, now known as Action for Sick Children) produced advice and 12 quality standards for children admitted as day cases in a report entitled *Just for the Day* (Thornes 1991). This covered the need for pre-admission programmes, literature available outlining the parental responsibilities, and a friendly environment. Some hospitals may have a designated area for children within an adult setting. In these instances great care must be taken to provide adequate facilities suitable for both children and their families.
- To shorten the admission time it is preferable that routine preoperative investigations are completed during outpatient visits so that all necessary results are available on the day of admission.
- Written instructions for preoperative fasting should be given to the parents along with information about giving routine medications, e.g. inhalers. The parents should be encouraged to bring any medications with them on the day of admission.
- At some centres, children can travel to theatre on bicycles and in motorised cars which makes the journey much more acceptable and exciting. The wearing of their own clothes is becoming more widespread, but parents should be advised to bring a change of clothes as a precaution.
- Most areas now use topical anaesthetic creams such as EMLA, and this can sometimes negate the need for oral premedications. The use of local anaesthesia (e.g. nerve blocks) during surgery was shown to reduce the complications of pain, nausea and vomiting, and the children were awake more rapidly following anaesthesia, allowing diet and fluids to be accepted (Cohen et al 1990). This enables discharge to occur earlier, therefore minimising the children's stay in hospital.
- It should be stressed to the parents that there may be the possibility of an overnight stay if events change. This enables the family to make further arrangements if necessary.
- Arrangements should be made in advance for transport home (according to local policy), a discharge letter to be sent to the GP and, in some instances, a postoperative home visit.

Children with disabilities

- The preparation of children with disabilities may place more emphasis on the parents' or carers' involvement depending on the degree of disablement. However, the basic principles of preoperative care still apply and the methods by which the children are prepared for theatre may need only slight adjustment. For example, the preparation of a child with visual impairment will be verbal rather than visual, but although photograph albums are of little use to the child, they may be helpful to the parent or carer who in turn may help you to explain procedures in a language that the child can understand.
- Distraction therapy may be useful to reduce the anxiety of the child and involvement of play specialists is helpful in this instance (Honeyman 1994) (See Play p. 333).
- For those children who cannot communicate verbally, one of the most important discussions which should take place prior to surgery is that of pain control. The non-verbal signs used by the child to convey pain or discomfort are more readily known by the parent; similarly they usually know what comforts the child, such as rocking, stroking or talking. Richardson (1992) highlighted the fact that professionals sometimes underestimate the amount of pain experienced by children; it is therefore desirable to secure parental involvement when possible in pain control.

General points

Policies for allowing parents into the anaesthetic room vary from hospital to hospital. However, adequate preparation of the parents as to their role in the anaesthetic room should remove one of the main reasons for their exclusion (Pethen 1990). Parents who do accompany their child to theatre are the responsibility of the ward nurse. She will ensure that the parent is not becoming distressed and will take the parent back to the ward with her once the child is asleep. Any toys or comforters with the child will either be given to the parent or taken to the recovery room in readiness for the child being received from theatre. Where parents are excluded, the role of the named nurse or primary nurse has great importance in reducing separation anxiety (Gahan & Rogers 1993).

Whenever possible, the child should have every opportunity to be prepared for theatre by both professionals and parents. Their involvement may affect the level of cooperation the child is willing to give, and will lessen the amount of anxiety and stress felt by the child and family alike.

Age-appropriate preparation

- Age-appropriate preparation is vital. Children have different attention spans and their ability to take in information and make sense of it may be limited. In these instances it is more appropriate to direct most of the educational efforts towards the parents.
- Older age groups are looking for answers; knowledge gives them a sense of control and the ability to cooperate. They are more able to contribute to their own care by becoming involved in the planning and negotiating of preoperative care. Explanations of the planned surgery and the sensations they will experience are appropriate.
- In the physical preparation, involve the parents as much as possible whilst giving them the opportunity to opt out of any part of the process that they do not feel comfortable with. Callery & Smith (1991) emphasised the importance of negotiating care delivery with parents to benefit the child and to help them adapt to their parental role during their hospital stay.

Method

1. Introduce yourself to the child and family as the nurse designated for the child's care.
2. Familiarise the child and family with the ward environment and the child's allocated bed.
3. Complete the admission procedure including baseline observations and current weight. Assist the medical staff with any preoperative investigations, e.g. haemoglobin levels if necessary.
4. Encourage the child to bathe if not already done and remove any nail varnish. The fingertip colour is a good indication of the level of oxygenation in the bloodstream and is observed during the operative stage.
5. Remove any jewellery, or tape it if it cannot be removed, and either give it to the parents for safekeeping or lock it in the hospital safe. (Jewellery can act as a conductor of electricity and may result in contact burns if not managed appropriately.)
6. Encourage the child to empty the bladder or put on a clean nappy prior to giving any premedication.
7. Make a note of any loose teeth and inform the anaesthetist. If a tooth is very loose, the anaesthetist may suggest that they remove it when the child is asleep to safeguard accidental ingestion or inhalation during the operation. Remove any dentures or plates.
8. If the child has long hair, tie it up using a non-metallic device.
9. Remove any prosthesis, hearing aids or spectacles. The latter two may be removed in the anaesthetic room at the last moment.
10. Some hospitals may allow children to wear their own clothes. If this is the case, ensure that they do not restrict access to the operation site; otherwise make sure that a suitable theatre gown is available for the child to wear. Small babies and neonates may also need to wear a hat as they lose most of their body heat through the scalp.
11. Check that the child has been fasted for a specified time. There are many views as to the safe recommendations for fasting, ranging from nil orally from midnight before surgery, to no clear fluids from 4–8 hours before the procedure. Schreiner et al (1990) showed that clear fluids up to 2 hours before surgery for children of any age posed no additional risk of pulmonary aspiration during elective surgery. Miller (1990) highlighted the dangers of hypoglycaemia induced by excessive fasting, particularly in children under 4 years of age or below 15 kg. Be aware of your hospital policy or protocol on fasting, and if unsure check with the appropriate anaesthetist.
12. Check that the child's name and hospital number are correct and legible on the wrist band as sometimes these can become unclear after bathing.

13. Ensure that the premedication has been given by the prescribed route and at the prescribed time. If there are any queries relating to the premedication, check with the anaesthetist.
14. Check that the case notes, X-rays (if applicable) and nursing documentation are available, and that the consent form has been completed correctly.
15. Ensure that the operation site, if previously marked by the medical staff, is still clearly visible.
16. Complete the theatre checklist, as per local policy, and await confirmation that theatre is ready to receive the child. (The checklist should be complete immediately prior to the child going to theatre.)
17. Accompany the child to theatre having first checked the patient details with the theatre slip brought by the theatre porter. Some hospitals may check the details in theatre reception to confirm the identity of the child.

Do and do not
- Do involve the parents in the preparation if they wish.

TCOMMUNITY PERSPECTIVE
Owing to time constraints, input from the community children's nurse is only likely in exceptional or complex cases unless the team is already involved with the child's care. There are some cases where parents can be helped to organise specific equipment prior to admission, for example when a child is to have a hip spica plaster applied. It is always important to ensure that parents are well informed because any anxiety of the parent will be transmitted to the child.

Preoperative therapeutic play can be undertaken in the home environment by community play specialists, where these are available (Shipton 1997). In this way potentially traumatic situations can be defused by familiarising the child with medical equipment. Children with needle or hospital phobia may be referred prior to admission and, in the safe environment of the home, be helped to overcome their fears by various play techniques. In some centres the play specialist can meet the children in the hospital on admission and continue to work with them.

Children who are on the waiting list for a renal transplant can be prepared in advance in the home (Wilson 1992). This can be done by storytelling, playing with dolls and introducing medical equipment. In this way, children are helped to cope with some of their anxieties.

- Do be honest in answering the child's questions.
- Do remember that this is not routine to the family and be aware of their fears and anxieties.
- Do give clear and concise information.
- Do not assume that children who have had previous operations are not in need of support.
- Do not devolve total responsibility to parents to enforce fasting. Sometimes this can be misunderstood as meaning food only.

References
Action for Sick Children 1991 Caring for children in the health service. Action for Sick Children (formerly NAWCH), London
Audit Commission 1993 Children first: a study of hospital services. HMSO, London
Callery P, Smith L 1991 A study of role negotiation between nurses and parents of hospitalized children. Journal of Advanced Nursing 16(7): 772–781
Cohen M et al 1990 Paediatric anaesthesia morbidity and mortality in the perioperative period. Anaesthesia and Analgesia 70: 160–167
Cooper A, Harpin V 1991 This is our child. Oxford University Press, Oxford
Eiser C, Hauson L 1989 Preparing children for hospital: a school-based intervention. Professional Nurse 4(6): 297–300
Gahan B, Rogers M 1993 Recent advances in child health nursing. In: Glasper A, Tucker A (eds) Advances in child health nursing. Scutari, London, pp 91–105
Honeyman L 1994 Play for children with special needs. Paediatric Nursing 6(3): 18–19
Miller D C 1990 Why are children starved? British Journal of Anaesthetics 64: 409–410
Morton N S, Raine P A M 1994 Paediatric day case surgery. Oxford Medical Publications, Oxford
Newman J, Scott G 1990 Preoperative care. In: Paediatric nursing. Springhouse Clinical Rotation Guides. Springhouse, Pennsylvania, pp 219–224
Pethen C 1990 Involving the parents. Nurse 4(19): 12(5): 22–25
Richardson J 1992 Acute pain in childhood. Surgical Nurse 22
Schreiner M S, Treibwasser A, Keon T P et al 1990 Ingestion of liquids compared with pre-operative fasting in paediatric outpatients. Anaesthesiology 72(4): 593–597
Shipton H 1997 Play at home. Cascade. Action for Sick Children (formerly NAWCH), London, pp 8–9
Taylor D 1991 Prepare for the best. Nursing Times 87(1): 64
Thornes R 1991 Just for the day. Action for Sick Children (formerly NAWCH), London
Wilson L 1992 The home visiting programme. Paediatric Nursing (July): 10–11

Further reading
Department of Health 1991 The patient's charter. HMSO, London
Department of Health 1996 Services for children and young people. DoH, London

29

Pressure Area Care

Introduction

Many nurses do not believe children get pressure sores, but clearly they do. In 1997, Waterlow studied 302 children from 0–16 years in multicentre trials, and found 17 patients who developed 33 sores. In 1993 the Department of Health produced a report highlighting key issues in pressure sore management. Whilst collection of data on the prevalence of pressure sores is often a purchaser requirement as part of quality assessment, in many trusts paediatric data are not included. Many of the principles of pressure area management are taken from adult practice and may not in fact be appropriate to paediatric care (Waterlow 1997).

Learning outcomes

After reading this section, you should be able to explain:

- the causes of pressure sores
- the principles of risk assessment
- prevention.

Risk assessment

Guidelines

When asked which children are at risk of pressure sores, most nurses will immediately think of children in intensive care, those who are terminally ill, are severely disabled, or have orthopaedic problems. In adult practice, a scoring system is used, which assesses known risk factors. The most well-known system is probably the Waterlow score (Waterlow 1985), but Waterlow herself, in a recent study, found this score inappropriate for children and recommended instead drawing attention to risk factors and appropriate preventive measures (Waterlow 1997).

Risk factors to note

Waterlow (1997) identified that extrinsic rather than intrinsic factors predispose the child to increased pressure sore risk. She argues that it is the fact that adult scores measure intrinsic as well as extrinsic factors that makes them less suitable for children.

Extrinsic factors include:

- pressure: compression on a local point (e.g. due to immobility)
- shearing: whereby skin is distorted beyond its ability to adapt (e.g. poor positioning) (Wienke 1987)
- friction: where skin is moved along the supporting surface (e.g. poor manual handling techniques)
- moisture.

Waterlow (1997) recommends that each child should be assessed using a questionnaire. She recommends the use of infant and child body maps and full documentation. It is helpful to assess the following:

Body weight. Overweight children may have difficulties mobilising, or the excess weight may be due to fluid overload; underweight children, for example neonates, may have less subcutaneous fat and therefore be at risk of high local pressure, especially over bony prominences.

Incontinence. Contamination of the skin with urine or faeces may result in moist and dirty skin, which predisposes to infection and ulceration.

Skin condition. Dry skin tends to be brittle and cracks easily. Equally, very sweaty skin can become sore and chafe. If the tissues are oedematous, the skin surface becomes fragile and can tear easily. Neonates have particularly fragile, almost translucent skin.

Mobility. The natural response to prolonged pressure in any body part is to shift position spontaneously. This may not be possible if the child has an altered level of consciousness, is disabled, in pain, in a plaster cast (see Plaster Care, p. 209), or is very young. A child who has been in theatre for a long operation may be at risk, as may the child in intensive care who has an ECG lead or intravenous line inadvertently pressing on any body area.

Nutrition. Malnutrition increases the skin's vulnerability to pressure sore formation. Ascorbic acid (vitamin C) is essential for collagen synthesis; protein deficiency delays wound healing and predisposes to oedema (see above). Zinc deficiencies also delay wound healing. Malnutrition is common in the chronically ill child.

Dehydration.   This can lead to dry skin (see above) and inadequate tissue perfusion.

Tissue hypoxia.   Anaemia, shock and hypoxia may all cause poor peripheral circulation, causing greater risk of skin breakdown.

Medication.   Long-term steroid use will cause papery, dry skin. Steroids and other anti-inflammatory drugs suppress the inflammatory response, the essential first stage in healing. Steroids and other cytotoxic drugs inhibit the body's immune system, increasing susceptibility to infection. Some inotropes cause peripheral vasoconstriction. Sedation can lead to altered consciousness, where the child is less likely to alter his position to relieve pressure. Paralysis will totally inhibit the child from moving.

Pressure sores

Pressure sores can occur anywhere, depending on the cause, but typical sites for pressure sores in children will include any of the bony prominences, including the sacrum, buttocks, ear, back of the head, heels. Waterlow (1997) particularly noted the risks inherent in plaster casts, splints (e.g. intravenous splints), tubing or long lines.

Several scales are used in adult practice for grading the severity of the ulcer; an example is given in Box 29.1.

Prevention

Risk assessment for each child should form part of the normal admission and ongoing assessment (see Assessment, p. 45). The purpose of assessment is to identify interventions that may be made to reduce any risk. These interventions may be the subject of local policy, which rationalises use of scarce or expensive pressure-relieving equipment. Waterlow (1997) recognises that pressure sores can occur even when preventive aids are in use.

Positioning of the baby or child is crucial, especially if mobility is limited. If a child at risk is lying on something hard, such as a monitor lead or toy, even for a short time, a pressure sore can develop. In a child the back of the head is particularly at risk, and often forgotten. Regular turning, if possible given the child's clinical condition, is important; if turning is not possible, pressure-relieving aids may be of even more importance.

Identifying, and if possible correcting or avoiding risk factors, is the most important aspect of prevention and care. For example, malnutrition may be slowly or quickly corrected by use of appropriate supplements, as advised by the dietitian. For a child who is incontinent, regular changing and good hygiene care will help.

Parental education

Depending on circumstances, and whether the risk factor is short or long term, parents should be taught the risks and preventive care of pressure areas. They may also need instruction on the appropriate use of aids.

Equipment

The following guidelines may be helpful in deciding local policy (Southmead Health Services NHS Trust 1997, Waterlow 1997):

- In low risk cases use a standard mattress.
- In medium risk cases use a mattress or chair overlay or pad; there are many different varieties and makes. Local protection use padded bootees,

---

> **Box 29.1   The Stirling Pressure Sore Severity Scale (SPSSS)**
>
> **Stage 0:** No clinical evidence of a pressure sore. May be normal skin, or healed, scarred skin, or tissue is damaged but due to other causes.
>
> **Stage 1:** Discoloration of intact skin, light finger pressure to site does not alter discoloration. There may be some local heat.
>
> **Stage 2:** Partial thickness skin loss or damage involving dermis or epidermis. Blister, abrasion, shallow ulcer.
>
> **Stage 3:** Full-thickness skin loss, damage or necrosis of subcutaneous tissue not extending to underlying structures (bone, tendon, joint capsule).
>
> **Stage 4:** Full-thickness skin loss with extensive destruction and tissue necrosis extending to underlying structures.

silicone gel pads and silk or soft flannelette sheets. Use a soft, conforming theatre table top for theatre cases.

- In high risk cases use active pressure-relieving overlays such as Alpha Cell, Pegasus Biwave Plus, or a micro-air-loss system (e.g. Autoexcel); or dynamic flotation systems such as Nimbus, Pegasus Airwave.
- For patients who require care of difficult wounds, have multiple pressure sores, extensive skin loss, or whose care requires minimal handling use a Clinitron Airfluidised Therapy Bed and low flow therapy.

Wound management

Wound management should follow accepted principles of wound care (see Wound Care, p. 317).

Potential risks of inappropriate prevention and management of pressure sores

- To the child and family: pain, scarring and disfigurement, low self-esteem, risk of osteomyelitis, septicaemia, death.
- To the nurse: vulnerability to litigation for negligent practice; failure to meet professional code of conduct; decreased job satisfaction.
- To the organisation: cost of litigation cases; increased cost of patient care (e.g. dressings, equipment, inpatient bed days); poor quality service; damaged reputation.

COMMUNITY PERSPECTIVE

Children nursed at home with a variety of conditions may be at risk of developing pressure sores.

The responsibility of the CCN is to ensure that the carers are aware of potential problems. They will need to teach carers pressure-relieving techniques, including turning and positioning. Some families will require the loan of proprietary devices, which will need to be demonstrated. Sometimes household equipment can be adapted to meet a specific need.

The CCN will need a good knowledge of local resources to obtain appropriate pressure-relieving devices for use in the home. Often the Community Nursing Services have a good supply of such equipment. However, the CCN may need to be persistent in order to obtain the optimum equipment for a particular child.

Do and do not

- Do assess each child individually using the risk factors given above.
- Do assess the child's existing skin condition.
- Do not make the assumption that children do not get pressure sores.

References

Department of Health (DoH) 1993 Pressure sores. A key quality indicator. A guide for NHS purchasers and providers. DoH, Lancashire

Southmead Health Services NHS Trust 1997 Guidelines for the prevention and management of pressure sores. Southmead Health Services NHS Trust, Bristol

Waterlow J 1985 A risk assessment card. Nursing Times 81: 48–55

Waterlow J 1997 Pressure sore risk assessment in children. Paediatric Nursing 9(6): 21–24

Wienke V K 1987 Pressure sores: prevention is the challenge. Orthopaedic Nursing 6(4) 26–30

Further reading

Bergstrom N et al 1987 The Braden Scale for predicting pressure sore risk. Nursing Research 36(4): 205–210

Norton D et al 1979 An investigation of geriatric nursing problems in hospital. Churchill Livingstone, Edinburgh

Williams C 1993 Evaluation of the Medley Score. Part One: the study plan. In: Harlin K et al (ed) Proceedings of the 3rd European Conference in advances in wound management.

30

Radiography

Introduction

This section is written to help nurses understand their role in preparing children for radiological investigation and assisting the radiologist to perform radiological investigations in children. Some radiology departments may have a designated radiology nurse who is experienced in all aspects of the department and the procedures that occur. When this facility is not available, the role will often fall on the ward nurse who accompanies the child to the radiology department. The role of the escort nurse will be primarily that of patient's advocate but equally important will be the preparation of the child and carer based on a thorough assessment of the child and knowledge of the examination required. The nurse may be involved in the preparation of equipment prior to the examination and will also be required to support the child and her family. He may also assist the radiographer in ensuring that the child remains in the correct position.

Learning outcomes

By the end of this section the nurse should be able to:

- prepare a child and her family for X-ray examination
- describe the common types of radiological investigations.

Rationale

The need for an X-ray examination is primarily for diagnostic purposes but a child may also need to be supported during radiotherapy. Most children requiring X-rays will be seen in district general hospitals whose departments are mainly treating adults. The children's nurse will need to ensure that the child is adequately prepared, taking into account the size and unfamiliarity of the equipment.

Factors to note

- All X-ray examinations must be requested either by a medical practitioner, or in some specialist areas by, a nurse practitioner. The need for radiological

information that can aid in clinical diagnosis or treatment must be balanced against the potential hazards of the exposure to radiation.
- The X-ray examination is clinically directed by the radiologist or trained physicist.
- The radiographer normally directs and is responsible for the examination.
- All X-rays hold a potential risk.
  - It is important to remember that although the risk to the individual child is insignificant, it is general philosophy that the dose to the general public from medical use of ionising radiation should be reduced.
  - The dose to the child in diagnostic radiology varies from 0.1 to 10 millisieverts (mSv), equivalent to the natural background exposure of a few weeks to 4 years (2.5 mSv per year).
  - The net gain outweighs the risk.
  - Before any investigations are performed on any child the principles laid down in the Ionising Radiation Regulations must be adhered to.
  - Nurses should take responsibility and act as an advocate for the child.
- Nurses or mothers who are pregnant should not assist with X-ray examinations in order to protect the unborn child.

General principles

General environment

Many radiology departments are geared more to the adult patient, particularly in district general hospitals. It is important that consideration is given to the child in the environment of the X-ray department. The area should be child friendly with toys and games appropriate for different ages. Posters of current television favourites may be displayed. This helps to distract the child and may help in developing a relationship that will assist the radiographer. Children often feel that the X-ray room is a controlled environment where they can have no say or choice about whether the procedure is performed (Fegley 1988). Children can be encouraged to bring one of their favourite toys into the department with them so that they can be X-rayed together.

The X-ray room should be warm to avoid cooling of the child. Some clothing can be left in place, depending on the type of X-ray examination, and the nurse should check with the radiographer.

Full resuscitation equipment for all ages of children must be present within the department.

The stability of the child's condition must be assessed before considering a move to the radiography department. The use of portable X-ray machines within intensive care units is well established. Patients whose access to the department is difficult or whose condition might be compromised, e.g. patients in balanced traction or immune suppressed patients being reverse barrier nursed, should also be considered for a portable X-ray machine.

Preparation of the child and parent/carer

Preparation is one of the most important parts of any investigation in paediatric radiology. Parent participation is actively encouraged.

A full explanation of the procedure, equipment and process of events will help alleviate both the child's and the parent's anxiety. This explanation to the parents and the child should be performed before the patient enters the investigation room. The language and depth of the explanation should be appropriate to the patient's age and understanding and will include any activity expected of the child, e.g. drinking the medication or micturating during the procedure. If the investigation requires the insertion of a cannula or catheterisation, the child and family will need to be given an indication of how and when this is likely to occur.

The child and parents need to know and understand that it is important for the child to remain still during the X-ray examination. If analgesia or sedation is to be used, this needs to be discussed with the parents as part of the preparation. There should also be a discussion on the most fitting person to accompany the child to the department. This should be the person who is best fitted to comfort, calm, help restrain and offer reassurance to the child during the investigation.

An assessment of the child will be required as part of the admission process (see Assessment, p. 45). If the child is an outpatient, an explanation of what will happen and reinforcement of the events during the procedure are necessary. Heiney (1991) promotes the development of a care plan for a child who is undergoing any procedure, particularly if there may be discomfort or pain, e.g. cannulation.

There needs to be communication between the nurse and radiologist to arrange the most suitable time for the procedure and to enable analgesia and sedation to be administered at the most appropriate time for it to be effective.

The child should be weighed to enable the correct doses of drugs and radiopaque dye to be administered.

Always check the name and date of birth of the child prior to any investigation.

Preparation books

Books and leaflets written for children can help in explaining the type of equipment that will be used and the procedures involved. These will give a simple explanation of the process during the procedures and explain that the X-ray machines are large, can be mobile, i.e. move around the child during the procedure and may be frightening.

There are some very good inexpensive publications available that can be easily adapted by nursing and radiographic staff to the needs of their individual department (see Play, p. 329).

Some departments may have a photograph album with photographs of the various members of staff that the child and parents will meet and the various pieces of equipment they may encounter.

Play therapy

Some hospitals are fortunate in having a play therapy department. The play therapists are trained to help prepare the child for a variety of procedures, through play.

General care

Privacy

This is an important aspect of any procedure. All children should have their investigation in private and only people who are necessary for the investigation should remain in the X-ray room.

Protection

The nurse and/or parent must wear the lead covering apron if assisting with the X-ray examination. Local protection for the child may be required, for example ovary pads/gonad pads.

When X-rays are being taken on the ward using portable equipment, a safe zone should be established, ensuring that no unnecessary personnel are present in the area and that those who are required are wearing protective clothing.

The nurse may be asked to help if the mother is pregnant and is unable to hold the child herself.

Positioning

The correct positioning of the child and the maintenance of the position during the taking of the X-rays is one of the most important aspects of the care. The radiographer will assist the nurse and/or parent in achieving the position that is required. The difficulty in positioning is greater with a child up to the age of 5 (Gyll 1982) but does become easier as the child gets older. The radiographer may provide various adapted boxes or stools for the child to sit or lie on, to get the best exposure first time.

It is the nurse's role to ensure that the child is not restrained against her will or for any great length of time and that appropriate explanation and reassurance is given (RCN 1999).

In the cases of a wheelchair-bound or physically handicapped child it is always advisable to ask the child's usual carer how to lift the child without harming yourself or the child. It may not be possible to obtain particular X-rays on some physically handicapped children, because of their inability to move or maintain a particular position. The nurse should remember that he is the child's advocate on these occasions. Local lifting and handling policies must be adhered to (see Positioning, Handling and Exercises, p. 217).

Praise and reward

At the end of any X-ray examination the child must be praised for her cooperation and, if appropriate, a bravery certificate awarded.

Sedation and general anaesthetics

As technology improves and advances, the need to keep children absolutely still during some X-ray procedures, MRI and CT scans is increasing. This can only be achieved in younger children by using either sedation or general anaesthetics.

Invasive procedures require an appropriately trained nurse to remain with the patient, as any deterioration or distress may require intervention.

In very young babies, i.e. less than 6 weeks old, it is often worth feeding before any sedation is considered. By feeding the baby her normal feed, wrapping her well and allowing her to fall asleep, the need for sedation may be avoided.

The doctor will prescribe the sedation, and the type and method of administration should be adjusted according to the estimated length of the procedure. If children are attending as outpatients, sedation will normally be administered before they enter the fluoroscopy room. These children should be offered a day bed so that they can fully recover before going home.

Children who have been given sedation should arrive in the department already asleep or drowsy. Monitoring of these patients is the responsibility of the nurse present. A set of baseline observations should be taken, including colour, pulse, respiration and, if possible, presedation oxygen saturation.

During the investigation the patient should be constantly monitored for colour, O_2 saturation, pulse and respiration (see Assessment, p. 45).

The child should be sent back to the ward after the investigation with a full set of observations and a complete handover should be given to the ward staff.

A child who has any airway problem, raised intracranial pressure or difficult behavioural problems must receive a general anaesthetic, but most children if handled correctly could receive sedation. General anaesthesia will be administered by an anaesthetist who will be responsible for all patient monitoring during and immediately after the procedure.

The ward nurse should accompany the patient with the parents into the anaesthetic area and check the patient's name, hospital number and date of birth with the anaesthetic nurse. A consent form should also have been signed by the parents or carers prior to the investigation. In most anaesthetic areas one parent is usually allowed to stay with the child until she is asleep. Once the child is asleep the parent and ward nurse should leave the anaesthetic area unless the ward nurse is required to assist with the investigation (see Preoperative Care, p. 231).

Following the procedure and extubation, the nurse must stay with the child until she is able to guard her own airway and is rousable by speech (see Postoperative Care, p. 225). When a child is sedated or given a general anaesthetic to enable a procedure to be performed, appropriate resuscitation equipment must be available.

Investigations

Many of the practices used to administer radiopaque dye will use invasive procedures which are described elsewhere in this manual. Please refer to these prior to the practice occurring, e.g. catheterisation oenepuncture.

Some common investigations

Plain X-rays

These are X-rays usually of the chest, skeleton or abdomen. The radiographer should explain exactly what is to happen, before the child is positioned. The aim is to keep the child still and correctly positioned, e.g. not rotated for a chest X-ray, so that only the minimal number of exposures are taken. They are non-invasive and should not give any discomfort to the child.

Micturating cystogram

A micturating cystogram is one of the most common investigations performed on children with any indication of pelvic, ureteric or bladder obstruction or malformation and urinary reflux.

Radiopaque dye is instilled into the bladder via a catheter. In most hospitals the catheter is inserted by the radiologist but it may also be performed by the nurse if he is proficient in the practice. The child is then encouraged to micturate and X-rays are taken. As the bladder contracts, malformations or abnormalities of the bladder or ureter may be demonstrated.

Barium meal/contrast medium

Barium or contrast swallows, meals and follow-throughs are some of the most common upper gastrointestinal investigations performed in paediatric radiology. They are used to indicate the patency of the gastrointestinal tract and any abnormalities of anatomy or physiology within it.

According to the child's underlying condition, the choice of contrast medium will be at the discretion of the radiologist.

The child's age must be taken into account when selecting the vessel from which to drink the medium. A small baby can be given a bottle, but the hole in the teat has to be made slightly larger to allow the barium through. A toddler will normally take a drink from a beaker. It may be advisable to use the child's own beaker as the familiarity will help with the drinking of the barium. Older children can use a straw or ordinary cup. Flavouring the barium is also advised. This can be achieved with either milk shake flavourings or powders.

Barium swallow. This investigates the child's swallowing technique, the oropharynx, the oesophagus and the fundus of the stomach.

Barium meal. This follows on from the barium swallow and follows the gastrointestinal tract into the stomach, the duodenum and jejunum.

Barium meal and follow-through. This encompasses both of the above, but follows the entire intestinal tract to the terminal ileum and the ileocaecal junction.

Barium contrast enema. A contrast enema is used to investigate the large bowel, its patency and any abnormalities. The contrast is administered by a rectal tube via the anus and rectum.

In some sick children, the risks involved in contrast enemas are high and include perforation of the gut and respiratory distress in a child who is obstructed. The procedures should therefore not be undertaken lightly and must be under the direct supervision of a radiologist following a request from a surgical colleague. Full resuscitation equipment should be available and should include replacement fluids to counteract hypovolaemia should perforation of the gut occur.

Small intestinal biopsy

This investigation is undertaken if there is a provisional diagnosis of malabsorption. To obtain a biopsy of the small intestine a Crosby and Watson capsule is used, which incorporates a spring-loaded knife that fires on suction.

The biopsy is performed after a period of fasting as agreed by local policies and under sedation. The capsule is attached to tubing and is introduced through the mouth and the child encouraged to swallow the capsule. To aid the capsule in its descent to the proximal jejunum, the child is placed on her right side (Milner & Hull 1992). The passage of the capsule is checked by an image intensifier and, when in position, the tube and capsule are flushed with a small amount of water to remove any debris and then fired by suction of a 20 ml syringe attached to the end of the tubing. Once the biopsy is complete, the tube and capsule are gently removed and the child is returned to the ward. Complications of haemorrhage and perforation have been reported but are uncommon.

In many centres this type of investigation is now replaced by an endoscopy procedure.

Computed tomography (CT imaging)

A CT scan is a type of X-ray examination and refers to the way in which the equipment works.

X-rays, like radio waves, can pass through objects and be focused to create a picture. During an X-ray examination, the beam of rays goes through the body, where it is absorbed to differing degrees by tissues such as bone, muscle and by organs. When the rays emerge on the other side of the body, they create a pattern of light and dark on a film, the X-ray.

Because CT images are recorded electronically, only relatively low doses of X-rays need to be used.

The child has to lie on a table which moves slowly through the CT scanner. She is alone in the room while the X-ray pictures are taken, but can hear the radiographer speaking. If the child cannot be left on her own, a nurse may enter at the discretion of the radiographer, but must wear a lead apron and must not be pregnant.

The CT scan takes about 30 minutes. The preparation depends on the area of the body being scanned. Usually the child should not have anything to eat or drink for the 2 hours preceding the investigation.

It is often necessary for the child to have an injection of contrast dye into a vein in the arm via an intravenous cannula, which may have been inserted on the ward. This contrast allows better visualisation of some organs. It contains iodine which can cause an allergic reaction and the child may feel very warm whilst it is injected, but this feeling passes quickly and is quite normal. There are no long-term after-effects as the contrast passes quickly through the kidneys to the bladder.

Whilst the pictures are being taken, the child may sometimes be asked to breathe in and hold her breath. This should be practised beforehand. Children find it difficult to keep still, which is why a good explanation beforehand is vital.

When the scan is completed, the child can leave the department as there are no after-effects.

Ultrasound

This is a type of scan which takes place in the department, using sound waves not X-rays, and is therefore very safe. The sound waves pass through the body, giving back a signal and providing a black and white image which is produced on a television screen. This image is then interpreted by a radiographer or radiologist.

The preparation required will depend on the part of the body which is to be examined. When the abdomen is to be checked, it is important that the bladder is full as this provides a 'window' to look through and see the other organs in the pelvis.

The child lies on a couch and uncovers the part of the body which is to be examined. Gel is squirted on to the skin to give good contact between the machine and the skin. The transducer, which looks like a microphone, is then moved gently over the skin.

The examination does not hurt at all; it tickles. The child may be asked to breathe in and hold her breath whilst a clear picture is taken.

After the scan, the gel is wiped off and the child is free to go. As no X-rays are used, parents or nurses can accompany the child. The mother is often able to give the child a good explanation, as the procedure is similar to that used during pregnancy.

Magnetic resonance imaging (MRI)

MRI is a way of looking inside the body without using X-rays. MRI can produce two- or three-dimensional images using a very large magnet, radio waves and a computer. The magnet is large enough to surround a patient, which is why it is sometimes referred to as a tunnel. The magnetic fields used are not known to be harmful, which means that children can have someone with them, as long as they keep very still so that they do not disturb the magnet and radio waves.

There is no preparation required for an MRI scan, but everyone entering the magnetic area will be checked for metallic objects, which may not be taken into the room as they can damage the magnet or the patient if they become projectile. No patients with a pacemaker or aneurysm clip may enter the scan room.

Children do not have to undress as long as they are not wearing clothes with zips. They can come in pyjamas or zipless jogging suits.

The child has to keep very still during the scan, as one movement can spoil all the images, unlike X-rays. This is because the images are built up from information collected during the whole of the scanning time. A child who is not able to keep still for about 30 minutes may have to be sedated. The child will be asked to lie on the table, will be made as comfortable as possible and will then be moved into the scanner.

It can be frightening for a young child who may need sedation. Children over the age of 5 years may find it quite interesting. They can take a favourite toy in with them, as long as there is no metal in it.

Once the child is in the magnet, the machine starts to make a whirring and thumping noise which can get very loud and this continues for the whole of the scan. The child can talk to the radiographer whilst in the magnet and she also has a bell to press should she wish to stop. In practice, many children go to sleep and have to be woken up when the scan is finished.

Occasionally it is necessary to inject a small amount of contrast, which does not contain iodine, into the arm. Allergic reactions are therefore rare.

No special care is required following a scan, provided the child has not received sedation.

Note

All advice and the regulations concerning the administration and the protection of the children is contained in

The Protection of Patients Undergoing Medical Examination And Treatments Handbook, which should be available in every radiology department as it is the law. If not, the manual can be obtained from the National Radiation Protection Board or the Department of Health.

Do and do not

- Do ensure child and parents have received a full explanation of the procedure
- Do maintain child's privacy
- Do remove jewellery or any metal fastenings
- Do ensure resuscitation equipment for all ages of children is available
- Do observe child closely if any contrast medium containing iodine is used

- Do not allow pregnant mothers/carers or nurses to be exposed to X-rays.

References

Fegley B 1988 Preparing children for radiological procedures. Research in Nursing and Health 11: 3–9

Gyll C 1982 Investigations into and a comparative study of techniques for basic radiography in children's hospitals. Radiography 48(573): 175–184

Heiney S 1991 Painful procedures. American Journal of Nursing (Nov): 20–24

Milner A D, Hull D 1992 Hospital paediatrics, 2nd edn. Churchill Livingstone, Edinburgh

RCN 1999 Restraining, holding still and containing children. Guidance for good practice. RCN, London

31

Removal of Drains and Packs

Introduction
Removal of the drain or pack at a time specified by medical and nursing assessment will promote wound healing and therefore assist mobility, well-being and ultimately recovery.

Learning outcomes
By the end of this section you should:

- be aware of the different types of wound drains and packs
- be aware of their uses in wound healing
- following observation, be able to remove, or assist in the removal of wound drains or packs
- be aware of the initial follow-up care of the site.

Rationale
The aim of the drain or pack is to promote effective healing and therefore reduce the risk of complications. This in turn will lead to a quicker recovery and result in a shorter stay in hospital for the child.

Factors to note

Types of surgical wounds
- Clean wounds – where during surgery no infection is encountered and no organ is opened.
- Clean contaminated wounds – where during surgery an organ has been opened with little content leakage.
- Contaminated wounds – where during surgery an organ is opened and this is accompanied by extensive spillage of contents without pus. Also included in this category are fresh wounds occurring through trauma.
- Dirty wounds – where during surgery pus or perforation in an organ is found. Also included in this category are old wounds caused by trauma (i.e. > 4 hours old).

Types of healing
Wound healing is a complex process comprising four main phases: haemostasis, inflammation, proliferation and maturation. These phases occur concurrently, but the length of time taken in each phase can vary considerably. Factors which can affect the rate of wound healing include malnutrition (Pinchcofsky-Devin 1994), poor wound care, inquisitive fingers, and sleep disturbances (Adam & Oswald 1983).

Normal healing occurs by either primary or secondary intention, both of which involve all four stages outlined above.

Primary intention.   This occurs in wounds where there has been a clean cut or incision with little or no tissue loss. The edges can be brought together and held with sutures, tapes, etc. thus eliminating any space below the wound surface.

Secondary intention.   This occurs when there has been substantial tissue loss and it is not possible to bring the edges together. These wounds heal from the base upwards by the formation of granulation tissue and wound contraction. Owing to the large amount of tissue involved, these wounds take considerably longer to heal.

See also Wound Care, page 317.

Types of packs
Packs are used to fill a resultant cavity when healing by secondary intention is the intended and preferred healing process. They include:

- Wicks – an estimated length of ribbon gauze inserted into an open cavity after immersion in a suitable substance. Substances other than saline should be prescribed appropriately on the child's prescription sheet prior to use.
- Foam – a compound made from the mixing of a polymer and a base, which is poured into the cavity and expands to the contours of the wound, allowing for granulation, e.g. Cavi-Care.

Types of wound drains
Drains are used when healing by primary intention is the intended healing process. The aims of drains are:

- to drain intra-abdominal collections of pus
- to drain any postoperative collections
- to re-route body fluids from a new suture line.

Types of drains include:

- suction or sump drains – a vacuum is present to exert a low suction to remove any wound exudate from a cavity, e.g. Redivac drain, Monovac drain, Shirley Sump drain
- non-suction drains – these allow wound exudate to leave a cavity by a natural process, e.g. Penrose drain, Yates drain.

Note: The age and cooperation of the child should be taken into consideration by the surgeon when wound management is required.

All of these drains are removed when wound leakage has significantly reduced or stopped.

Analgesia

Effective analgesia and/or sedation must be taken into consideration and should be administered at least 30 minutes before the procedure is commenced to allow time for it to take effect. Children are naturally inquisitive and may be more cooperative if they are able to participate in their own care. However, the nurse must continually assess the situation, and involvement by the play specialist can provide useful distraction during procedures. Some ways in which the child can participate are by loosening or removing tape, holding tubing or counting down to the removal of the drain. Not all children will be able to cooperate owing to their age or inability to understand. In these instances it is helpful to have support from the parents to assist in providing comfort and security whilst the removal of the drain or pack is being carried out.

Equipment
- Dressing pack
- Sterile stitch cutter or scissors
- Cleansing agent
- Selection of sterile dressings to cover or re-dress the wound
- Sterile gloves, optional (these can be used in place of forceps)
- Wound swab (if required)
- Disposal bag

Note: It is preferable to overestimate your required equipment rather than having to stop the procedure to obtain more.

See also Wound Care, page 317.

Method for removing wound drains
1. Explain the procedure to the child and parents or carers as appropriate to facilitate understanding and cooperation.
2. Gather the required equipment and prepare your area for the procedure, i.e. the treatment room or bedside.
3. Wash your hands.
4. If applicable, uncover the wound to obtain access to the drain site. At this point, if the drain is of a suction type, release the vacuum. Sometimes the drain can rest against tissue inside the wound; by releasing the vacuum, any remaining fluid can be drained. Wash your hands.
5. Using aseptic technique (see Aseptic Non-touch Technique, p. 39), clean the wound if necessary to access sutures or clean away any exudate which may be a source of infection.
6. Remove any sutures by holding the knot with sterile forceps and gently raising it from skin level; then cut the shortest end of the suture as close to the skin as possible. This prevents any part of the suture which has been exposed externally from passing through the tissue, reducing the risk of infection. This should allow the drain to be released. *Note:* Only cut one end of the suture.
7. Remove the drain slowly by holding the tubing close to the patient and pulling gently, but firmly. If there is resistance which does not yield with firm pulling, stop the procedure and seek advice.
8. Cover the drain site with a sterile dressing. This will minimise infection entering the drain site whilst it heals.
9. Dispose of soiled equipment safely and record the amount of drainage in the appropriate nursing documentation.
10. Regularly check the wound site for any excessive drainage or swelling which could indicate an internal collection of fluid, i.e. 2- to 4-hourly with routine observations.
11. Further wound management will be as per unit protocol.

Method for shortening a wound drain
1–2. As for removal of wound drain.
3.   Wash your hands. Remove wound dressing and expose drain. This is likely to be a tube type of drain, e.g. Penrose or corrugated latex. These drains usually have a sterile safety pin or suture to maintain their position outside the wound.
4.   Wash your hands again and clean the wound if necessary.

5. Remove the suture by raising the knot from skin level and cutting the shortest end as close to the skin as possible. When the suture has been removed, grasp the end of the drain and pull gently. It is usually sufficient to shorten the drain by 2–4 cm unless instructed otherwise by the medical staff. If unsure, seek advice. Shortening the drain will ensure that it does not remain in contact with any single structure for any length of time or impede the healing process. It also enables the drain to continue its purpose throughout the depth of the wound. The excess tubing can be cut with sterile scissors.

6. Re-insert the safety pin just above wound level to prevent the drain slipping into it.

7. Re-dress the wound with an appropriate wound dressing. Copious amounts of drainage may be managed by placing a stoma bag over the drain site. This enables the bag to be emptied and prevents the frequent changing of dressings. This method of collection should be discussed with the child and carers before implementation as they may not feel comfortable with using a stoma bag.

8. Dispose of soiled equipment and measure or note the amount of drainage in the appropriate nursing documentation. This will aid further management of the drain.

Method for removing a ribbon gauze pack

1–2. As for removal of drain. Confirm the length of ribbon gauze (wick) in situ by either checking the operation notes or consulting the medical staff.

3. Wash your hands. Remove the outer dressing and assess the wound site.

4. Locate the end of the wick and gently ease it upwards out of the cavity. If there is any adherence, the wound and wick can be moistened with saline. Continue to ease the gauze from the cavity until no more is visible. (*Note:* Some wounds are managed by shortening the wick gradually over a period of time.)

5. Clean the wound as required.

6. Assess the wound bed for signs of healing and the possible need to insert a further wick. If a further wick is required, place an appropriate length in saline or a prescribed solution. (The wick is supplied as a tightly rolled coil in a sterile pack. Lengths are usually indicated on the packaging.)

7. Using two pairs of sterile forceps, one in each hand, grasp the wick with one pair whilst

keeping it submerged in the solution, and locate the loose end. Take hold of the end with the other forceps. Gradually unravel the wick and re-roll onto the second forceps ensuring that it is moistened throughout its length. The moistened wick can then be inserted into the wound from the bottom up. When the wound has been sufficiently packed, the wick can be cut with sterile scissors.

8. Dress the wound appropriately and dispose of soiled equipment.

9. Complete the nursing documentation and note the length of wick inserted.

10. If the wick has been removed, check the site for excessive leakage.

11. Further wound management will be as per local protocol.

Method for removing a foam pack

1–3. As for removal of ribbon gauze.

4. Grasp the edges of the pack with two pairs of sterile forceps and gently ease it from the wound cavity. Clean the wound if necessary.

5. Assess the wound healing to ascertain whether a further pack is required. If unsure, seek advice. If a pack is required, make up the foam preparation by following the manufacturer's instructions and pour it slowly into the cavity. Allow time for the expansion of the foam and, when it has solidified, cover the wound with an appropriate dressing. It may be necessary to secure the pack in position with tape, but this will depend upon the individual child and the location of the wound.

6. Dispose of soiled equipment and complete the nursing documentation.

COMMUNITY PERSPECTIVE

The removal of wound packs is frequently under-taken in the community, following conditions such as drainage of abscesses.

This procedure can be very frightening for the child and is potentially painful. The CCN must gain the trust of the child and family before undertaking the procedure and organise appropriate pain management (see Pain Management, p. 195). Analgesia should be timed to ensure maximum relief during the procedure. Older children may be able to use Entonox, but as this is self-administered, it is not suitable for the younger child. If the CCN feels that the pain cannot be adequately managed by drugs that can be given in the home, it may be necessary to request admission to hospital as a day case.

The CCN should be prepared to encounter less than adequate facilities for undertaking an aseptic non-touch technique in the home (see Aseptic Non-touch Technique, p. 39). It may be necessary to take additional equipment (sterile towels, plastic tray, hand-cleansing solutions).

Do and do not

- Do be honest with the child when explaining procedures.
- Do involve and inform the parents/carers.
- Do ensure that the child's safety and privacy are maintained at all times.
- Do involve the play specialist if available.
- Do ensure that adequate analgesia has been given before commencing procedures.
- Do not remove packs or drains without prior instruction.
- Do not assume that older children will cooperate or be brave.

References

Adam K, Oswald I 1983 Protein synthesis, body renewal and the sleep wake cycle. Science 165: 513–515

Pinchcofsky-Devin G 1994 Nutritional wound healing. Journal of Wound Care 3(5): 231–234

Further reading

Bale S, Jones V 1997 Wound care in the baby and young child. In: Wound care nursing – a patient centred approach. Baillière Tindall, London, pp 70–93

Brubacher L L 1982 To heal a draining wound. Registered Nurse 45(3): 30–35

Brunner L S, Suddarth D K 1982 Lippincott manual of surgical nursing. Harper & Row, London

Callery P, Smith L 1991 A study of role negotiation between nurses and parents of hospitalized children. Journal of Advanced Nursing 16(7): 772–781

Cruse P J E, Foord R 1980 The epidemiology of wound infection. Surgical Clinics of North America 60(1): 27–40

Flanagan M 1997 Wound management. Churchill Livingstone, Edinburgh

Holden P 1995 Psychosocial factors affecting a child's capacity to cope with surgery and recovery. Seminars in Perioperative Nurse 4(2): 75–79

Melforth N 1995 Strategies to reduce children's perception of pain. Nursing Times 91(2): 31–35

Neill S J 1996 Parent participation. 1: Literature review and methodology. British Journal of Nursing 23(2): 338–345

Whaley L F, Wong D L 1994 The essentials of paediatric nursing, 4th edn. Mosby, St Louis

32

Seizures

Introduction

Seizures are brief malfunctions of the brain's electrical system. Abnormal discharge of electrical activity within the brain can cause altered consciousness, loss of consciousness, involuntary movements and changes in perception, posture and behaviour (Wong 1995). Some children, particularly infants, can experience periods of apnoea when having a seizure. Seizures can be frightening and disturbing to observe. The nurse's role is to protect the child from injury, observe for obstruction of the airway, and administer anticonvulsant medication in some circumstances.

Learning outcomes

By the end of this section you should be able to:

- state the main causes of seizures in children
- describe how to nurse the child during a seizure
- state the possible complications of a seizure
- explain when and how anticonvulsant medication should be administered during a seizure.

Rationale for care of the child having a seizure

Seizures are the most commonly seen neurological disorder in children (Castledine 1993, Wong 1995). Between 2 and 4% of all children in Europe and the USA experience at least one seizure associated with a febrile illness in the first 5 years of life (Hauser 1994). Hardman (1990) states that 1 in 30 children will experience at least one febrile seizure in the first 5 years of life and Odeka & Brown (1992) that at least one-third of this group will have a recurrence. It is therefore important for paediatric nurses to know how to care for the child during a seizure and to be able to educate parents as to how to care for their child if she has a seizure.

Factors to note

Healthy children

Not every seizure is due to epilepsy. Febrile seizures are one of the most common neurological disorders of childhood (Campbell & Glasper 1995, Castledine 1993). A febrile seizure can be defined as a fit occurring in a child from 6 months to 5 years, precipitated by fever arising from infection outside the nervous system in a child who has no underlying neurological abnormality (Valman 1993). The fever usually is above 38°C and mostly is over 38.8°C to precipitate a seizure. A febrile seizure is one that is of short duration < 20 minutes (Valman 1993), <15 minutes (Odeka & Brown 1992), and having a febrile seizure does not mean that the child has developed epilepsy. The vast majority (95–98%) recover completely even if they have more than one febrile seizure (Wong 1995). However, around 2–4% of children will develop epilepsy after febrile seizures (Hull & Johnston 1993). The children most at risk of developing problems are those who experience more prolonged febrile seizures of over 20 minutes duration with focal features of the seizure (see Types of epileptic seizure, below). Febrile seizures have a familial tendency (Campbell & Glasper 1995, Hull & Johnston 1993, Valman 1993).

Sick infants under 2 years

Seizures are more common in the first 2 years of life than at any other time in childhood (Wong 1995). Other than febrile seizures, causes of seizures include acute infections which may be acquired prenatally, e.g. toxoplasmosis, herpes simplex, and postnatally, e.g. meningitis, urinary tract infection and otitis media. Birth trauma, e.g. intracranial haemorrhage and anoxic brain damage, can cause seizures, as can a head injury due to abuse. Idiopathic seizures (of unknown cause) can be seen in infants, as can seizures due to congenital defects such as tuberous sclerosis. Biochemical disorders, e.g. hypoglycaemia, hypocalcaemia, hyponatraemia and hypernatraemia, can induce seizures. These events may be due to a single illness (e.g. dehydration with diarrhoea and vomiting) or an underlying metabolic disorder (e.g. phenylketonuria, adrenocortical insufficiency).

Children over 2 years of age

Although febrile seizures continue to be seen until about 5 years of age (Valman 1993, Visentin 1989), most have discontinued by 3 years (Campbell & Glasper 1995, Castledine 1993). Wong (1995) says that recurrent seizures in children over 3 years are most commonly due to epilepsy.

Epilepsy itself is a chronic disorder with recurrent and unprovoked seizures (Wong 1995). It can take many weeks of careful adjustment of anticonvulsant medication to control the seizures. Children with epilepsy must have careful monitoring of their growth and development. This is to ensure that their anticonvulsant medication is adjusted appropriately to achieve effective seizure control as they grow.

Adolescents

Adolescents who have epilepsy may find that the onset of puberty and its accompanying hormonal changes can lead to further seizures. This may occur, even though they were previously well controlled on medication. This can be particularly distressing, especially if they had been free of seizures for some time. In addition to the distress of seizures recurring, the adolescent in particular may be extremely sensitive about involuntary loss of control of bladder and bowel which can occur with some seizures.

Types of epileptic seizures (Campbell & Glasper 1995, Hull & Johnston 1993; Box 32.1)

Primary generalised seizures

Simple absences.   Consciousness is impaired briefly; the child looks vacant for a few seconds, then continues with whatever she was doing as if nothing has happened.

Complex absences.   Impaired consciousness lasts longer than in simple absences. There may be involuntary movements, e.g. chewing, myoclonic jerks, loss of postural tone, semi-purposeful movements and peculiar sensations. It is difficult to distinguish clinically between these and partial complex seizures.

Myoclonic.   Sudden shock-like jerks occur affecting one part or the whole of the body. If the whole body is involved, the jerkiness is usually bilateral, symmetrical and mostly flexor or extensor jerks. If mild, the head may drop but if more severe, the child may be thrown suddenly forwards or backwards. Frequently they are associated with learning disability or abnormal neurological physiology. Infantile spasms are a type of myoclonic seizure with a poor prognosis for the development of an affected infant.

Tonic–clonic.   There is sudden loss of consciousness and an initial tonic phase lasting about 10–20 seconds in which limbs are extended symmetrically, the back is arched and breathing stops. This leads into the clonic phase when there is generalised jerking. Micturition, defecation and salivation may occur. Respiration is usually irregular during the clonic phase.

Partial seizures

Simple partial.   There is twitching or jerking of one side of the face, one arm or leg with consciousness only slightly impaired, if at all. Sometimes the jerkiness will start in one part of the face or limb and spread across or up the rest of the face or limb (the Jacksonian march).

Box 32.1   International classification of seizures (after Hull & Johnston 1993)

Primary generalised seizures
The abnormal electrical activity appears to arise in the reticular formation with initial involvement from both hemispheres of the brain.

- Simple absences
- Complex absences
- Myoclonic
- Tonic–clonic

Partial seizures
Abnormal electrical activity discharges from a focal point in one cerebral hemisphere and spreads to a more or less specific area of the cerebral cortex.

- Simple partial
- Complex partial
- Partial with secondary generalisation

Temporary weakness of the affected part of the body is common after a simple, partial seizure.

Complex partial.   Altered or impaired consciousness is common. Disturbance of sensation occurs and may affect auditory, olfactory (smell), gustatory (taste) or emotional senses. Complex semi-purposeful movements may be seen, e.g. getting up and walking about. The attack commonly lasts a few minutes and the child has little recollection of it afterwards.

Partial with secondary generalisation.   A partial seizure starts from a focus in one cortex of the brain, but the electrical activity then spreads to both hemispheres simultaneously producing a generalised tonic–clonic seizure.

Guidelines

Parental involvement is vital when a child has recurrent seizures. A large part of the nurse's role is to provide support and education. This may be to teach about managing their child's fever, as in the case of febrile seizure. In a child who has recurrent seizures, it is likely to be necessary to teach the family how to administer rectal anticonvulsants in an emergency. As with any chronic condition, it is important for the nurse to provide support as well as education in order to help the child and family adjust to the diagnosis and realities of living with a chronic disease

Equipment

Very little equipment is required to actually care for a child during a seizure. If any is required, the unpredictable nature of seizures is such that it will most probably have to be gathered as the child is experiencing the seizure. When a child is known to be affected with recurrent seizures, it may be possible to have appropriate equipment available at all times. For example, if she is known to have problems maintaining adequate oxygenation during a seizure, a resuscitator bag and mask are kept near at hand.

- Pillows/blankets
- Record of seizures chart
- Watch from which minute and second recordings can be easily read

The following may be needed if the child is unable to maintain adequate oxygenation:

- Oxygen supply (portable if piped supply not available)
- Oxygen tubing
- Resuscitator bag and mask which will fit snugly over the patient's mouth and nose.

The following may be needed if the seizure does not stop spontaneously after about 5 minutes:

- Prescription chart
- Rectal diazepam or paraldehyde and 0.9% saline or olive oil
- Filling quill – to enable rectal administration of paraldehyde
- Non-sterile rubber gloves
- Lubricating jelly.

If paraldehyde is to be given you will also need a syringe big enough to take the dose of paraldehyde and the same volume again of saline or olive oil.

A glass syringe should be used, if available. Paraldehyde reacts with plastic and rubber.

However, if no glass syringe is available, mixing the drug with olive oil is acceptable.

The olive oil should be drawn up first into the plastic syringe; then immediately prior to administration the paraldehyde should be drawn up and mixed with the olive oil. If it is drawn up and remains in the syringe for more than a few seconds, it reacts with the plastic and the syringe plunger will stick and cannot be depressed.

Paraldehyde should be prepared in a well-ventilated room using a protective mask and goggles (Merck 1995).

Method

1. If the nurse realises that the seizure is about to occur and the child is standing or sitting, she should be lowered gently to the ground and put on her side if possible. If the infant is sitting, she should also be placed on the ground or her cot on her side. Do not attempt to restrain her in any way or try to put anything into her mouth.
2. Be prepared to call for help. A child should not be left unattended whilst she is having a seizure and a second nurse may be required to fetch equipment/drugs.
3. Note the exact time that the seizure started and continue to observe the passage of time.
4. Remove any objects in the immediate area on which the child might hurt herself if the seizure causes her to jerk in a particular direction. It may be necessary to pad a rigid surface temporarily with a pillow to prevent the child hitting a limb.
5. If possible, ensure privacy – draw curtains, ask onlookers to move away.
6. Observe the child/infant for signs of cyanosis. Be prepared to administer oxygen if her colour does

not improve quickly. If she is in repeated spasm for any length of time, it may be necessary to use a resuscitator bag to instil oxygen if she is unable to inspire for herself.

7. If relatives are present, try to reassure them about what is happening. It can help to reassure them that the child is unaware of what is happening during most seizures, so that even if it looks painful, the child is not actually in pain.

8. Be aware of how long the seizure has been in progress. Determine from the child's prescription sheet when action may need to be taken to administer anticonvulsant drugs. For example, a child is often prescribed rectal diazepam for a seizure lasting longer than 5 minutes (see Administration of Medicines p. 37).

9. If necessary, administer rectal anticonvulsant drugs as prescribed, in accordance with local drug policy, noting their effect.

10. If the seizure does not resolve within 10 minutes of administration of these drugs, be prepared to seek medical assistance as intravenous drugs may be required.

11. Once the seizure has finished, place the child in the recovery position to prevent a hypotonic tongue from blocking her airway (Campbell & Glasper 1995).

12. If the child has been incontinent, she may need a clean nappy or change of clothing.

13. If it was a febrile seizure, due to high temperature, take measures to cool the child down. Assess whether she is able to be given an antipyretic such as paracetamol. This may have to be given rectally if she is not sufficiently awake to take it safely, orally. Remove excess clothing and ensure that the room is not hot and stuffy, but comfortable and well ventilated.

14. Record the seizure and describe it in detail (see Observations and complications, below). Record the precise duration of the seizure and whether or not intervention was required, such as oxygen, assistance with breathing or administration of drugs.

Observations and complications

Observation is especially important when caring for a child having a seizure. It can be important both in aiding diagnosis and in helping to achieve effective control. Carefully observe all aspects of the seizure. How did it start? Which part of the body was affected first? Was more than one area of the body affected at one time? What kind of movements occurred? Did the movements

change? Was there more than one phase of the seizure: did it start with spasm and then progress to jerkiness? Did the movements affect more than one part of the body as the seizure progressed? Did the child appear to have any prior warning of any kind? What was the child doing before the seizure occurred? Did she cry out? Can she describe any 'odd' sensations prior to the seizure? Observe the child carefully for signs of cyanosis. If it does not improve spontaneously, be prepared to provide assistance with breathing if necessary. Be aware that if the child has had diazepam, it may depress her respiration, particularly in the infant. Carefully note the duration of the seizure. If it has lasted for over 5 minutes, prepare to seek assistance and give rectal diazepam or paraldehyde. If the seizure is still in progress 10 minutes after administration of rectal drugs, she may be going into status epilepticus.

There are three main complications of a seizure:

- the risk of respiratory difficulty, as described above
- the risk of injury as a result of falling or hitting something during the seizure
- status epilepticus.

Status epilepticus is defined as a continuous seizure lasting more than 30 minutes or a series of repeated seizures between which the child does not fully regain consciousness. It is an emergency situation in which the child is at risk of permanent brain damage due to anoxia. It is important to support the child's vital functions: maintain an adequate airway and adequate oxygenation and ensure she has hydration. She will then be treated with intravenous anticonvulsant drugs. Sometimes these children require mechanical ventilation support.

COMMUNITY PERSPECTIVE

One of the most frightening occurrences for parents is to witness their child having a seizure. Much reassurance is required and in some circumstances discussions in their home environment with a CCN may help the parents to adapt to living with a child who has seizures.

The CCN will be able to support the family by allowing time for them to talk about their anxieties and help to educate them about the seizures and any treatment required, as well as monitoring the child's progress. The parents may feel guilt and humiliation and may be concerned that the seizures will affect their child's mental capacity and her future (Whaley & Wong 1993).

The CCN will be able to:

- Assess how much information the family have understood prior to discharge. Parents may need help to supplement their understanding once they have been discharged home (Bailey & Caldwell 1997).
- Reinforce the education given in hospital, stressing the importance of drug compliance and the potential complications from sudden drug withdrawal (Kempthorne 1994).
- Ensure that parents know how long to wait before seeking medical help if their child has a seizure:
  – 10 minutes for the first seizure, or
  – 2 minutes longer than the usual length of seizure, or
  – when a second fit occurs without the child regaining consciousness (British Epilepsy Association 1991).
- Discuss with the family the information that should be given to playgroup, nursery or school staff and any other adults who may take responsibility for caring for the child. If rectal diazepam is to be used, staff will need to be taught how to administer the drug either by the CCN or the school nurse; it is advisable to agree a protocol.
- Ensure that parents are aware that their children can undertake sports, although they should not be allowed to swim alone (Joint Epilepsy Council of the UK and Ireland 1995) and restrictions may need to be placed on where they cycle. The wearing of a protective helmet may need to be considered if the child's seizures cause regular falls resulting in injury. Parents may find this difficult to accept as it is an outward sign of their child's seizures.

Most importantly, the family should be encouraged to take a positive attitude and encourage the child to take part in normal activities.

Do and do not

- Do position the child on her side if possible.
- Do observe carefully and thoroughly.
- Do be prepared to provide assistance with breathing.
- Do try to protect the child from injury.
- Do be prepared to administer rectal anticonvulsant drugs if the seizure does not stop spontaneously within 5 minutes.
- Do not attempt to restrain the child in any way.
- Do not attempt to put anything into the child's mouth; you may get your finger badly bitten and push her tongue backwards, causing a blocked airway.

References

Bailey R, Caldwell C 1997 Preparing parents for going home. Paediatric Nursing 9(4): 15–17

British Epilepsy Association 1991 The modern management of epilepsy. Yorkshire Television/Chevron Communications, p G19

Campbell S, Glasper E A (eds) 1995 Whaley and Wong's children's nursing. Mosby, London, ch 31, pp 674–679

Castledine G 1993 Neurological emergencies 2: nurse-aid management of fits. British Journal of Nursing 2(6): 336–337

Hardman M 1990 Febrile seizures. Paediatric Nursing 2(4): 12–13

Hauser W A 1994 The prevalence and incidence of convulsive disorders in children. Epilepsia 35(suppl 2): S1–S6

Hull D, Johnston D I 1993 Essential paediatrics. 3rd edn. Churchill Livingstone, Edinburgh, ch 18, pp 279–284

Joint Epilepsy Council of the UK and Ireland 1995 New horizons: a guide for young people with epilepsy p 16

Kempthorne A 1994 Epilepsy in childhood. Paediatric Nursing 6(4): 30–33

Merck 1995 Safety data sheet for paraldehyde GPR ID NO 2944800. Merck, Poole

Odeka E B, Brown R 1992 Educating parents about febrile convulsions. Maternal and Child Health (May): 143–146

Valman H B 1993 ABC of one to seven: febrile seizures. British Medical Journal 306: 1743–1745

Visentin L C 1989 What are febrile seizures? Professional Nurse 4(11): 557–559

Whaley L F, Wong D 1993 Essentials of paediatric nursing, 4th edn. Mosby, St Louis p. 973

Wong D L (ed) 1995 Whaley and Wong's nursing care of infants and children, 5th edn. Mosby Year Book, St. Louis, ch 37, pp 1713–1729

33

Skin Care

Introduction

The skin is the largest organ of the body and has many functions, the most important being:

- thermoregulation
- protection: from physical and mechanical injury
- waterproofing
- synthesis of vitamin D
- transmission of sensation.

In the absence of disease it is important to maintain the skin in good condition to minimise infection and dry skin. In many cultures this can be achieved through regular bathing and drying (Denyer & Turnbull 1996).

Often underestimated in their effects on general health and well-being, childhood skin disorders may reduce quality of life through pain and irritation. Although rare, some skin conditions can prove to be life-threatening.

Appropriate skin care is essential in those with healthy or diseased skin in order to maintain the functions of the skin as far as possible.

Learning outcomes

By the end of this section the nurse will be able to:

- maintain good skin care in the presence of health and disease
- develop an understanding of children who require additional skin care
- apply topical treatments as prescribed in the correct way
- adapt such treatments to the individual child.

Rationale

Children's nurses are frequently involved in care of children with many skin conditions, including atopic eczema, in general wards when the child is admitted for another condition, in outpatient departments and in the dermatology ward.

The healthy child may suffer from dry skin conditions or infections. The majority of dermatological conditions are exacerbated by the dry hot atmosphere of the hospital. A hospital admission, whether for management of the skin condition or for another reason, provides an ideal opportunity for intensive skin care and for parental education.

Painful and irritated skin has a profound effect on the child's self-image, mood and peer acceptance. Those who will require additional skin care over and above routine cleansing include:

- infants with cradle cap and dry skin
- infants with nappy rash
- children with skin infections
- children with eczema or psoriasis
- the preterm infant whose skin is thin and delicate
- children with serious inherited skin disorders.

Factors to note

- Children can develop a range of skin conditions, many of which are transient, e.g. contact dermatitis, and cause few ill-effects, whilst others can develop into more persistent serious conditions.
- Dry skin is a common problem and its management can be incorporated into the regime of daily hygiene.
- Children enjoy bubble baths but these may have a drying effect and may necessitate restriction. After bathing the skin should be checked for any signs of dryness or irritation and moisturisers applied as necessary.
- Children's skin is often sensitive and an unscented preparation should be chosen.
- Use of coconut and olive oils features in Asian and Afro-Caribbean cultures as a part of daily skin care. Caution must be exercised in using nut oils in view of the increasing awareness of the risk of anaphylaxis in response to such products.
- Treatments must be specific to the child's needs.
- Where possible, the child and parents should be encouraged to participate in the care. Children may be afraid or fractious and adolescents may rebel against lifelong daily treatments.

- It should be remembered that treatments are often time-consuming and monotonous.
- Preparations can stain all clothing and soft furnishings, and can make carers reluctant to pick up or cuddle the child.

Equipment
- Plastic aprons to protect clothing/uniform
- Gloves, for use when applying medicated creams/ointments or when dealing with children whose skin is infected
- Bath situated in a warm private environment
- Soft towels
- Prescribed bath additive
- Soap substitute
- Prescribed cream/ointment
- Emollient
- Foil bowls and spatula (for decanting creams/ointments not in pump dispensers)
- Selection of toys for distraction
- Clothing
- Nappies if required

Guidelines for performing skin care
Cradle cap

Cradle cap is a common condition caused by dryness of the scalp and exacerbated by failure to rinse out shampoos or bath additives adequately.

Olive oil or similar should be applied and gently massaged to loosen the scales and encourage them to separate. Temptation to remove adherent scales must be resisted as hair loss may result (Stewart 1990).

Nappy rash

Nappy rash often results from infrequent changes of napkins and failure to cleanse the skin at each change, allowing build-up of ammonia on the skin.

Use of commercial products, and such as barrier creams, lotions, and exposure of the excoriated skin will help minimise nappy rash. The carer must be educated on prevention of nappy rash by frequent changing and cleansing followed by application of barrier cream/ointments.

When there is no improvement using simple measures, secondary infection such as with candida (thrush) should be suspected and a swab obtained for culture before commencing prescribed treatments.

Children suffering from gastroenteritis or malabsorption syndromes frequently pass watery stools which may be acidic and cause damage to the nappy area. These children require more frequent nappy changes and application of occlusive ointments such as petroleum jelly; this can reduce contact with irritants.

Eczema herpeticum

This is caused by the herpes simplex virus (HSV) and many eczematous children have an abnormal response to HSV which can result in dissemination of the herpes and subsequent toxaemia (Harper 1990).

It is recognised as small clusters of clear fluid-filled vesicles, which in turn become filled with pus.

All parents should be alerted to this condition and advised to keep the child away from those with cold sores. Health care workers with cold sores should not care for the child with eczema and should refrain from work until clear.

Impetigo

This is a highly infectious disorder caused by *Staphylococcus aureus* and/or group A streptococci. It is characterised by small blisters that burst easily releasing a yellow exudate which in turn forms a pale honey-coloured crust (Atherton 1994, Harper 1990).

The infectious nature of this condition necessitates the child being kept off school or nursery. Sites around the nose and mouth are most commonly affected.

The use of systemic antibiotics is indicated and they should be prescribed immediately and not withheld until microbiology results are available.

Topical antibiotics are only of use if the infection is identified early enough; however, one must be aware that in some instances such as eczema the possibility of multiresistant strains should be a consideration.

Crusts can be removed by the use of warm saline soaks or a weak solution of potassium permanganate.

Do and do not
- Do isolate the child from others. If in hospital, universal precautions are indicated against infection. At home, the child should have his own towel and avoid using a flannel. Bed linen such as pillow cases will be changed daily to minimise reinfection.
- Do cut the child's fingernails to minimise damage if the skin is scratched. The wearing of mittens/gloves will minimise skin damage.

- Do introduce distraction methods to stop the child scratching or picking at crusts and so spreading the infection.

Atopic eczema

Eczema is a chronic inflammatory disorder of the skin. The condition is erratic and varies somewhat in severity. It presents in infancy from age 3 months and there is often a genetic predisposition, i.e. family history of asthma, eczema, allergy. Any area of the body can be affected and education on factors that may exacerbate the condition is crucial in order to give optimum care to the child and promote an adequate quality of life.

Factors to note
- Eczema results in intense pruritus (itching) which makes the child irritable and fretful; this in turn results in sleep disturbance and can result in alterations in behaviour.
- The skin becomes red (erythematous) and small blisters (vesicles) occur which when scratched result in weeping, bleeding areas of skin.
- There is no cure and the aim is to control the condition and minimise exacerbations. A basic regime may be enough to maintain control of the skin.
- The ultimate aim of treatments is to replace moisture and reduce inflammation.
- If frequent exacerbations are common, one should establish who does the skin care and how it is carried out. It may be necessary to re-educate the carer and where appropriate the child and together negotiate achievable goals.
- One must constantly assess and reassess the child's progress and treatment and alter the treatment accordingly. Attention to the following may serve to improve the child's eczema:
  - Avoid any known aggravating factors.
  - Wear 100% cotton clothing, wool will irritate the skin.
  - Sleep in a well-ventilated room.
  - Use special mattress covers to minimise harbouring of the house dust mite (HDM).
  - Daily vacuuming of the house and mattress, and damp dusting of the room will also reduce HDM.
  - Avoid all hairy/furry animals.
  - Keep finger- and toenails short to minimise damage caused by scratching.
  - Encourage the child to rub on the skin instead of scratching it.
  - Develop distraction techniques and help parents to develop these to minimise anger and frustration.

- Swimming – where possible, the child should not be excluded. A thin smearing of Vaseline or similar will serve to protect the skin. The child must shower thoroughly afterwards, using emollients and soap substitute.
- To ensure adequate rest and sleep administer prescribed sedative antihistamine early enough to allow a good 10-hour period before the child is due to rise.

Method
- Bathing in warm/tepid water at least once daily with added emollient oil and use of a soap substitute such as Aqueous or Diprobase cream will serve to remove surface debris and hydrate the skin.
- To minimise irritation use a soft towel and pat, not rub, dry.
- Prescribed topical steroids should be applied twice daily after bathing (unless medical advice differs) to all areas of eczema; there should be enough to show a fine visible film.
- To avoid dilution of the topical steroid, the prescribed emollient should be applied 30 minutes later and then regularly as necessary throughout the day. Emollients should be applied liberally and in a downward direction to minimise plugging of hair follicles which could result in infection (Atherton 1994). The use of regular emollients serves to soften the skin and therefore reduce pruritus and the need for more potent topical steroids (Harper 1990).

If it is not possible to control the child's eczema with this basic regime, it may be necessary to use more potent steroid preparations under wet wraps for a short time. These increase steroid absorption as well as cooling the skin and reducing pruritus (Turnbull & Atherton 1994). Wet wraps must be used under the direction of the dermatologist. Wet wraps are lengths of tubegauze or tubefast cut to make a full body suit with normal clothing worn on top. They are relatively time-consuming to apply and should be seen not as a maintenance treatment but as a means of regaining control of the child's eczema. Wet wraps can also be used for the short-term treatment of acute erythrodermic eczema (Goodyear et al 1991). The length of time wraps are required will depend on the child's response to treatment; once control is achieved, then the strength of topical steroids should be reduced to achieve maintenance.

Lichenification is a thickening of the skin as a result of repeated damage through scratching and is visible behind the knees and elbows. Limbs may respond to application of icthopaste bandages overnight, but the bandages can be left in situ for up to 3 days. They are useful to soften the skin as well as producing a cooling effect.

A low-potency topical steroid can be applied under the bandages if need be; the icthopaste is then covered with Coban elasticated dressing.

Observations and complications

The skin of most children with eczema will be colonised with *Staphylococcus aureus*. Infection should be considered when there is a deterioration in the skin. Symptoms may include:

- weeping/wet areas of eczema
- areas of crusting
- enlarged lymph nodes
- pyrexia
- irritability.

Streptococcal infection should be considered if there is family history of sore throats.

Do and do not

- Do educate parents in the management and treatment of the condition and regularly assess and reassess their techniques.
- Do be aware of the side-effects of prolonged or incorrect use of topical steroids. Preparations used in children tend to be mild and should not cause problems. Misuse of stronger steroids can result in thinning of the skin.
- Do monitor growth, as prolonged use of topical steroids, especially moderate and potent types, can inhibit normal growth. Growth should be monitored at each clinic appointment by measuring the child's height and weight and recording the results on a growth chart.
- Do ensure that the school receives education on the child's eczema and conditions that may aggravate the skin, i.e.:
  - Avoid sitting in the centre of the room or next to radiators.
  - Use a soap substitute at all times.
  - Identify an area where the child can apply emollients.
- Do not bath in hot water as heat causes vasodilatation and will increase irritation.
- Do not use scented bath oils, creams, laundry powders, fabric softeners as they include fragrance which will irritate the skin.
- Do not dip fingers into pots of cream or ointments as this will increase the risk of contamination and cause infection. The preparation should be decanted onto a saucer each time it is used.
- Do not sit in hot, dry environments.

Psoriasis

There are various types of psoriasis affecting people in different ways; therefore, treatments are tailored to meet individual needs. Psoriasis can affect any age but is uncommon in children and rarely seen before 3 years of age (Harper 1990).

Factors to note

Psoriasis is a chronic relapsing non-infectious inflammatory disease, the cause of which is not yet understood. There are many factors that can trigger or exacerbate the disease process:

- trauma – lesions appear at sight of injury
- infection – beta haemolytic streptococcal tonsillitis
- stress/emotional upset
- sunlight – the majority will improve but a small percentage will become worse.

Treatments for psoriasis are mainly topical and can only be used when the disease process is active and not as preventive measures.

Method of treatment

Coal tar preparations: the exact mode of action is unclear but they are known to inhibit DNA synthesis, therefore reducing cell proliferation and inhibiting the psoriatic process.

Keratolytic agents is the name given to creams and ointments that reduce scaling by reducing thick plaques.

Bathing daily in a prescribed tar-based preparation and application of the keratolytic cream or ointment to affected areas may help to regain control of the disease process. The application of emollients regularly throughout the day will promote skin softening and so reduce scaling and flaking of skin.

Care of the scalp

- Cocois or olive oil is massaged into the scalp and left in situ for the prescribed length of time; the hair is then combed out to remove loosened plaques.
- Shampoo using tar-based solution.
- Comb again to remove plaques and then allow hair to dry naturally.
- The procedure should be performed separately from the bath to minimise irritation to the skin of the body.

Dos and do nots

- Do remove the preparation immediately and notify medical staff, if irritation during treatment occurs.

- Do inform the parent and child that many preparations are messy and will stain clothing and sometimes skin. It should be stressed that any skin discoloration from treatments will fade.
- Do encourage the wearing of pale clothing to minimise the visibility of shed skin scales.
- Avoid stressful situations.
- Inform the child's school and arrange to chat with teachers, which will help reduce teasing; it is also crucial to refer the child to someone who will help him develop coping mechanisms.
- Do not allow the child to see this as a handicap but try to promote positive aspects of body image.
- Do not omit any prescribed treatments or use products prescribed for other people as treatment for psoriasis is individualised.

The preterm infant

The skin of the preterm infant is thin and there is absence of subcutaneous fat.

Often, preterm infants receive intensive therapy which involves the use of intravenous cannulae and monitoring with sticky equipment such as cardiac electrodes. Endotracheal tubes are sometimes secured with sticky tapes. Wherever possible, use of such tapes should be avoided and silicone or hydrocolloid dressings used in their place. Where use of adhesive tape is essential, care must be taken on removal to ensure no tearing of the skin results. Petroleum jelly or liquid paraffin may be used to destroy the adhesive properties of the tape prior to removal.

The child with fragile skin

Skin fragility may be a feature of prematurity or a genetic defect such as epidermolysis bullosa. Epidermolysis bullosa is a rare genetically determined skin disorder occurring in 1:50 000 live births in the UK. Affected children often require multidisciplinary care at a specialised centre, but day-to-day care is carried out at home with support of the community nurses. Its aim are:

- to maintain skin integrity
- to minimise damage.

Bathing

This is a clean, rather than a sterile procedure. Prescribed analgesia must be given and replacement dressings prepared.

Prior to bathing the nurse must consider whether it is an appropriate procedure, or if the child is very sore and bathing is likely to cause added distress. Washing of unaffected areas may be a more suitable alternative (Lin & Carter 1992).

Observation should be made of the site, size and condition of any wounds and the general condition of the skin. Observations should be recorded and photographs taken as necessary in order to monitor progress or deterioration.

Method
- Line a baby bath with a towelling sling or soft towel to prevent skin damage from the base or sides of the bath by avoiding shearing forces from a hard surface.
- Add prescribed emollients.
- Use a second person if necessary to assist and minimise trauma.
- Pat rather than rub the child dry using a soft non-shedding towel to avoid leaving fibres in the wound which may result in overgranulation.
- Apply prescribed non-adherent dressings to promote a warm moist environment in order to encourage wound healing.

Note: Avoid prolonged bathing which may result in a fall of temperature and result in delayed wound healing.

General care of child with fragile skin
- Ensure that all those who are in contact with the child are aware of the skin fragility and appropriate method of handling.
- Avoid use of plastic namebands which could rub and cause skin damage.
- Avoid use of adhesive tapes.
- Use alternative fabrics to secure intravenous cannulae and electrodes, such as silicone dressings or hydrocolloids.
- Choose soft cotton clothing. Turn underclothes inside out to avoid seams rubbing.
- Use glass rather than Tempa DOT thermometers which may stick to the skin and cause tearing.
- Educate theatre and anaesthetic staff prior to any procedures.

COMMUNITY PERSPECTIVE
The health visitor is likely to be the first community health care professional to become aware of skin problems in the younger child. Depending on her level of knowledge of dermatology, she may be con-

fident to manage conditions such as atopic eczema in partnership with the general practitioner. If the eczema is severe, the child should be referred to a consultant dermatologist.

The amount of involvement CCNs have with families of children with eczema will vary according to local policies.

When a child has been admitted to hospital with infected eczema or a severe exacerbation, home visits to check the child's progress and assist the family with the time-consuming treatments have been shown to be beneficial.

Families may find it easier to understand the important aspects of eczema management in their own homes, than in a busy outpatient department. Home visits also enable the CCN to identify factors which may be exacer-bating the eczema, e.g. pets in the bedrooms or high levels of house dust mite. She will also gain insights into the nature of the condition at its most severe and how exhausted the families may become.

The CCN is in an ideal position to liaise with schools concerning the care of pupils with eczema, thus giving the teachers additional insight into problems which may occur.

Currently, families who give a high input of care to their child with eczema are entitled to a disability living allowance. The CCN may be asked to assist in filling in the application forms.

A multidisciplinary approach to the care of children with eczema has been proved to work well (Masini et al, unpublished work, 1997). Health visitors, CCNs, dermatology nurses together with their medical colleagues can develop a service to support the many families who struggle to cope with the demands of a badly affected child.

Useful addresses

Dystrophic Epidermolysis Bullosa Research Association (DEBRA)

DEBRA House
Wellington Business Park
Dukes Ride
Crowthorne
Berkshire RG11 6LS
National Eczema Society
Eversholt Street
London

Psoriasis Association
Milton House
7 Milton Street
Northampton NN2 7JG

References

Atherton D J 1994 Eczema in childhood: the facts. Oxford University Press, Oxford

Denyer J, Turnbull R 1996 The skin. In: McQuaid L, Huband S, Parker E (eds) Children's nursing. Churchill Livingstone, Edinburgh, ch 17

Goodyear H, Spowart K, Harper J 1991 Wet wrap dressing for the treatment of atopic eczema in children. British Journal of Dermatology 604: 125

Harper J 1990 Handbook of paediatric dermatology. Butterworth-Heinemann, London

Lin A N, Carter D M (eds) 1992 Epidermolysis bullosa: basic and clinical aspects. Springer-Verlag, New York

Stewart M 1990 Cradle cap. Nursing Times 86

Turnbull R, Atherton D 1994 Use of wet wraps in atopic eczema. Paediatric Nursing 2(6): 22–26

Further reading and viewing

Bridgeman A (undated) Wet wraps, a professional's guide. Seton Healthcare, National Eczema Society Publications, London

Donald S 1995 Atopic eczema: management and control. Paediatric Nursing 7(2): 29–31, 33–35

Dystrophic Epidermolysis Bullosa Research Association (DEBRA) Publications, available from: DEBRA House, Wellington Business Park, Dukes Ride, Crowthorne, Berkshire RG11 6LS

National Eczema Society Publications, Eversholt Street, London

Spowart K 1995 Childhood skin disorders. Paediatric Nursing 8(7): 29–33

Williams R et al 1991 Guidelines for management of patients with psoriasis. BMJ 303: 829–835

Video on Wet Wrap Treatment for Childhood Eczema, Seton Healthcare, Great Ormond Street, London

34

Specimen Collection

Introduction

Nurses often have responsibility for the collection and safe transportation of samples to the laboratory. The validity of test results largely depends on their good practice in the pre-test stage. Improved technology has seen the introduction of tests being performed by the bedside or 'near patient' testing, and nurses are involved in documentation and sometimes interpretation of results (Higgins 1994). Although the principles of specimen collection are the same, local variation may occur.

Learning outcomes

By the end of this section the nurse should:

- be aware of the psychosocial implications to the child and family when collecting specimens
- know how to collect appropriate specimens and transport them safely to the laboratory
- be aware of the need to record the investigation
- be aware of his responsibilities in obtaining specimens, interpreting and communicating results in conjunction with medical staff and the family
- be aware of any complications that may arise from specimen collection.

Rationale

Specimen collection is undertaken when laboratory investigation is required for the examination of tissue or body fluid to aid diagnosis.

Factors to note

- Always explain the procedure to the child and parent and the reasons for taking the specimen. Ask permission from the child and parent if specimens are obtained for research purposes. They have a right to refuse without any obligation (Ethics Advisory Committee 1992).
- Hands should be washed before and after specimen collection. Gloves should be worn when collecting or handling specimens to avoid skin contamination.
- Contamination of the specimen must be avoided as

this may produce misleading results and delay in appropriate treatment.

- When collecting the specimen, avoid infecting the child. For example there is an increased risk of infection if an aseptic technique is not used when collecting a catheter urine specimen or during the collection of cerebrospinal fluid.
- All pathological specimens must be treated as potentially infectious and local written laboratory protocols should be followed for the safe handling and transportation of specimens (Health Services Advisory Committee 1986). Specimens should be collected in sterile containers with close-fitting lids to avoid contamination and spillage. All specimen containers must be transported in a double-sided, self-sealing polythene bag with one compartment containing the laboratory request form and the other the specimen.
- All specimens must be clearly labelled to identify their source. A laboratory request form with the following information must accompany the specimen. This aids interpretation of results and reduces mistakes.
  - Patient's name, age, ward/department and hospital number
  - Type of specimen
  - Date and time collected
  - Diagnosis with history and relevant clinical signs and symptoms such as returning from abroad (specify country) with diarrhoea and vomiting, rash, pyrexia, catheters in situ or invasive devices used, or surgical details regarding postoperative wound infection
  - Any antimicrobial drug's given
  - Consultant's name and cost code
  - Name of the doctor who ordered the investigation, as it may be necessary to telephone preliminary results and discuss treatment before the typed report is dispatched
  - Biohazard label, if appropriate.
- Ideally, microbiological specimens should be collected before beginning any treatment such as

administering antibiotics or using antiseptics. However, treatment must not be delayed in serious sepsis.

- When collecting pus specimens, obtain as much material as possible as this increases the chance of isolating microorganisms which may be difficult to grow or are minimal in number, e.g. in tuberculosis.
- Transport medium is used to preserve microorganisms during transportation. Charcoal medium, used for bacteria, neutralises toxic substances such as naturally occurring fatty acids found on the skin. Because many viruses do not survive well outside the body, special viral transport medium is used.
- Specimens sent through the postal system must be packed and labelled according to the post office guidelines. The specimen must be wrapped in a plastic bag, encased in an absorbent material within another plastic bag, placed in a rigid cardboard container and firmly taped. A warning 'Pathological Sample' along with the sender's name and address must be visible on the outside.
- In children suspected of suffering from viral haemorrhagic fevers such as Lassa fever, Marburg or Ebola virus, the infection control team must be consulted before any specimens are taken (Advisory Committee on Dangerous Pathogens 1990, 1994, 1996).
- Chlorine-releasing granules or a hypochlorite solution (10 000 ppm of available chlorine) must be available for decontamination of any spillages. Care must be taken, as release of chlorine fumes has occurred when chlorine-releasing agents were mixed with urine (SAB 1990).

Equipment

This will vary according to the specimen required but must include:

- Disposable gloves – sterile for blood cultures
- A protective tray
- A sterile container for the specimen
- Appropriate transport medium, if required
- Laboratory specimen form
- A polythene transportation bag
- Biohazard label, if required.

Eye swab

- Where possible ask the child to look upwards; then gently pull the lower lid down or gently part the eyelids.
- Use a sterile cotton wool swab and gently roll the swab over the conjunctival sac inside the lower lid.

Hold the swab parallel to the cornea to avoid injury if the child moves.
- Place the swab in the transport medium.
- For suspected chlamydia infection:
  - Clean the eye first with sterile normal saline to obtain a clear view of the conjunctiva
  - Use a pernasal wire swab, part the eyelids and gently rub the conjunctival sac of the lower lid to obtain epithelial cells; identification of the organism is by fluorescent monoclonal antibodies
  - Wipe the swab over the marked area on the glass slide and allow to dry
  - Place the glass slide into a slide holder or Petri dish to protect the specimen.

Nose swab

- If the nose is dry, moisten the swab in sterile saline beforehand.
- Insert the swab into the anterior nares and direct it up into the tip of the nose and gently rotate. Both nares should be cultured using the same swab to obtain adequate material.
- Place in transport medium.
- For viral investigation, moisten the swab in the viral transport medium prior to taking the swab.
- The outside of the nostrils may be rubbed after the procedure to alleviate the unpleasant sensation of swabbing.

Pernasal swab

This investigation is used to diagnose whooping cough (*Bordetella pertussis*). When obtaining this specimen, the nurse must be proficient in the procedure and ensure that suction, oxygen and resuscitation equipment are easily available. The child should be held securely and observed carefully as the procedure may produce paroxysmal coughing and/or vomiting.

- Place the child in a good light to facilitate observation.
- Use a special soft-wired sterile swab to minimise trauma to the nasal tissue.
- Holding the child's head upwards, pass the swab along the floor of the nasal cavity to the posterior wall of the nasopharynx.
- Gently rotate and withdraw the swab and place it in special transport medium or dispatch the swab in its container immediately to the laboratory to ensure maximum enhancement of growth of the organism.

Sputum

- Encourage the child to cough, especially after sleep, and expectorate into a container. Alternatively, nasopharyngeal/tracheal suction using a sputum trap can be undertaken.

- Physiotherapy may help to facilitate expectoration.
- Ensure that the material obtained is sputum and not saliva.

Throat swab

- Place the child in a position with a good light source. This will ensure maximum visibility of the tonsillar bed.
- Either depress the tongue with a spatula or ask the child to say 'aahh'. The procedure is likely to cause gagging and the tongue will move to the roof of the mouth and prevent accurate sampling.
- Quickly, but gently, rub the swab over the tonsillar bed or area where there is exudate or a lesion.
- Place the sample into transport medium.

Ear swab

- No antibiotics or other therapeutic agents should have been in the aural region for about 3 hours prior to sampling the area as this may inhibit the growth of organisms.
- If there is purulent discharge, this should be sampled.
- Place a sterile swab into the outer ear and gently rotate to collect the secretions.
- Place the swab in transport medium.
- For deeper ear swabbing, a speculum should be used. This procedure should be undertaken by experienced medical staff as damage to the eardrum may occur.

Wound swab

Interpretation of results must be in conjunction with clinical signs. In the absence of clinical signs of infection, wound swabs will not provide any useful information and normal colonisation may be confused with infection (Gilchrist 1996).

- Obtain the specimen prior to any dressing or cleaning procedure of the wound. This will maximise the material obtained and prevent killing of the organism by the use of antiseptics.
- Use a sterile swab; gently rotate it on the area to collect exudate from the wound and place into transport medium. Where there is ample pus, collect as much as possible in a sterile syringe or sterile container and send to the laboratory.
- For detection of *Mycobacterium tuberculosis*, a calcium alginate swab can be used. The swab gradually dissolves, maximising the isolation of the organism as its numbers are usually small.

Faeces

- A faecal specimen is more suitable than a rectal swab.
- A specimen can be obtained from a nappy or clean potty.
- Using a scoop, place faecal material into a container.
- Where diarrhoea is present, a small piece of non-absorbent material lining the nappy can be used to prevent material soaking into the nappy.
- Examine the sample for consistency, odour or blood and record observations to monitor changes.
- If segments of tapeworm are seen, send them to the laboratory. Tapeworm segments can vary from the size of rice grains to a ribbon shape, 1 inch long.
- For the identification of *Enterobius vermicularis* (threadworm/pinworm), material should be obtained first thing in the morning on awakening by using a Sellotape slide. Place the sticky side of a strip of Sellotape over the anal region to obtain the material and stick the Sellotape smoothly onto a glass slide. The eggs of the worm can then be identified under the microscope. Threadworms lay their eggs on the perianal skin at night and therefore they will not be seen in a faecal specimen.
- Where amoebic dysentery is suspected, the specimen of stool must be freshly dispatched to the laboratory. The parasite causing amoebic dysentery exists in a free-living motile form and in the form of non-motile cysts. Both forms are characteristic in their fresh state but difficult to identify when dead.

Urine

Bedside urine testing for the presence of blood, protein, ketones and other analytes is usually undertaken with reagent strips, the results of which are indicative of further laboratory investigation (Cook 1995).

Urine samples should be dispatched to the laboratory as soon as possible, or after no more than 2 hours if kept at room temperature or up to 24 hours if kept at 4°C, to avoid multiplication of organisms and misleading results (Griffiths 1995, Higgins 1995a).

Some laboratories request the specimen to be put into a sterile specimen bottle containing boric acid which inhibits multiplication of most bacteria. However, the growth of some bacteria such as *Enterococcus faecalis* is inhibited by boric acid and therefore it is not always used.

Where laboratory access is limited or rapid testing is required, a commercial dip slide, which consists of a plastic tongue coated with suitable culture medium, can be dipped into the urine immediately after collection, a colour change noted and results obtained in 2 minutes. It tests for leucocyte esterase and nitrites, two indicators of infection. However, these are not 100% accurate and some organisms such as enterococci do not produce nitrites. Enterococci may therefore be missed where there is a real possibility of infection, such as in children with complex renal problems (Griffiths & Woodward 1993).

Urine collection from disposable nappies for microscopy, culture and biochemical analysis has been described (Ahmed et al 1991, Roberts & Lucas 1985, Vernon 1995). This procedure is not yet widely used and requires further evaluation.

Normal social hygiene such as washing the genitalia with soap and water and drying thoroughly is considered sufficient to minimise contamination from the skin prior to collection of the specimen. Assess the clinical and psychosocial needs of the child as to whether cleaning the genitalia is necessary. The nurse must be sensitive to the cultural issues surrounding touching intimate parts of the body.

Collection of urine by a suprapubic stab should only be considered in an emergency as this is a painful procedure.

Midstream specimen

This is the most reliable non-invasive urine specimen collection method but may not be possible in the very young child. In the female, encourage separation of the labia to prevent perianal contamination whilst passing urine. In the male encourage retraction of the prepuce, if appropriate.

- The first part of the urine stream is passed into the toilet to exclude meatal contamination.
- The middle part of the urine stream is collected into a clean container.
- The remaining urine is passed into the toilet.
- Pour the urine into a sterile container.
- For viral investigation pour the urine into viral transport medium.

Clean-catch or bag specimen

- Select the correct size of sterile urine bag to avoid leakage or contamination with faeces.
- Remove the protective seal:
  - for the female, place the bag over the vulva, starting from the perineum and working upwards, sticking the bag to the skin
  - for the male, place the bag over the penis.
- Observe the bag frequently until urine is passed, to avoid leakage.

- Remove the bag and pour the urine into a sterile container.
- For viral investigation pour the urine into viral transport medium.
- Wash the genitalia after the procedure to prevent soreness of the skin.

Catheter specimen

This is collected from the self-sealing bung of the urinary drainage tubing in a child who is already catheterised. Do not disconnect the closed drainage system as infection may be introduced, nor take the sample from the urinary drainage bag as the specimen may be contaminated.

- Using an aseptic technique, clean the bung with an alcohol swab and allow to dry.
- Using a sterile syringe and needle insert the needle into the bung at an angle of 45 degrees. This will minimise penetration of the wall of the tubing and subsequent needlestick injury.
- Gently withdraw the urine into the syringe.
- Remove the needle and syringe, wipe the area with the alcohol swab and allow to dry. The rubber bung will self-seal.
- Place the urine in a sterile container.
- Discard the needle and syringe into a sharps container.

Obtaining urine from a Mitroffanof stoma

The specimen should be obtained by a nurse who is familiar with the mitroffanof operation and the specific anatomy of the area on the child.

- The specimen should ideally be taken in conjunction with normal bladder emptying.
- A new sterile catheter of the child's normal catheter size should be used.
- Clean the stoma with soap and water and dry.
- Gently insert the lubricated sterile catheter into the stoma and collect the urine into a sterile container. A water-soluble lubricant should be used.
- Ensure that the bladder is completely empty before withdrawing the catheter.
- Wipe the area dry with a tissue.

Vaginal swab

The taking of this specimen in children should be avoided where possible because of its invasive nature.

- In the case of suspected or actual sexual abuse do not clean the area. Identification of semen or sexually transmitted diseases may be required for evidence.

- Expose the vaginal area and part the labia.
- Gently insert a cotton wool swab into the outer entrance of the vagina. Care must be taken not to tear the hymen.
- Place the swab into transport medium.
- For suspected chlamydia infection:
  – Obtain special transport medium
  – Use a pernasal swab and gently rotate the swab in the vaginal orifice
  – Place in transport medium.

Blood samples

Venepuncture or capillary blood sampling may be performed by a nurse who is trained in the procedure. As there are many haematological (Higgins 1995b, Higgins 1997), biochemical (Higgins 1996), immunological and microbiological blood tests, the nurse should seek local information as to the appropriate laboratory containers required for specific tests and the amount of blood required. Protective clothing such as gloves, aprons and facial protection as appropriate should be used along with an aseptic technique (see also Venepuncture and Cannulation, p. 311).

Blood culture

Isolation of a causative organism is enhanced by careful collection of the blood, using a sterile technique to avoid skin contamination (Higgins 1995c). Sterile gloves should be used, and if possible avoid palpating the vein after cleansing the skin. The specimen should preferably be taken during pyrexial episodes as the organism may be there in greater numbers.

- Use blood culture bottles according to local policy.
- The skin must be decontaminated with an alcohol-based antiseptic agent and allowed to dry.
- After withdrawing the blood, insert the blood into the container with a new sterile needle. There is a risk of contamination of skin organisms on the needle used to withdraw the blood.
- Place as much blood as possible (up to 3–5 ml) in the bottles.
- Inoculation of the blood into the blood culture bottles should be performed first before inserting blood into other bottles as many of these other bottles are not sterile and accidental contamination may occur.
- In children in whom line sepsis is suspected, blood for culture may be taken from a peripheral vein stab and also from the appropriate intravascular lines to enable identification of colonisation of the line. In cases of suspected bacterial endocarditis more than one blood culture (three where possible) should be

taken to ensure isolation of organisms which may be low in number.
- Blood culture bottles should be placed into an incubator at 37°C to enhance growth of the organism.

Analysis of antibiotic levels

The relationship between drug dose, drug concentration in biological fluid and the individual child's metabolic process must be understood for interpreting results. The results may be affected by the route of administration, the age of the child and the disease process, such as liver and renal disease. The analysis involves testing levels in blood serum in direct relationship to drug administration.

- For intravenous antibiotic bolus administration, the first blood sample (trough) is taken just before the dose is given. The second sample (peak) is taken 30–60 minutes after the dose is given. The time may vary according to local policy and the drug given.
- Record on the laboratory form the drug, dose and mode of administration, the time the drug is given and whether the sample is a peak or trough level.
- Levels of antibiotics given other than intravenously must be discussed locally with the microbiologist because interpretation of the results will differ for drugs given by other routes.
- Blood for antibiotic assay must not be taken through the same catheter which has been used to give the antibiotic at any time. Antibiotics bind to plastic and the drug may release intermittently, giving false results. The same principle applies for some other drugs such as glucose.

Vesicular fluid for electron microscopy

Explain to the child that the procedure is usually pain-free as the needle only penetrates the vesicle not the skin.

Virus particles can be seen under electron microscopy and combined with the clinical presentation this may aid rapid diagnosis. The vesicular fluid should also be cultured in order to confirm the clinical diagnosis such as varicella-zoster (chickenpox or shingles) or herpes simplex.

- Obtain a glass slide with a marked area for the specimen, holder, sterile syringe and needle, sterile swab and viral transport medium.
- Pierce the top of the vesicle with a sterile needle and if there is sufficient fluid draw up the exudate into a

syringe. Keep the needle flush to the skin to prevent accidental stabbing if the child moves. Remove the needle and seal the end of the syringe with a sterile cap. Dispose of the needle in a sharps bin.

- If there is minimal fluid, place the marked area of the glass slide over the vesicular fluid to allow the fluid to attach to the slide. Let it dry.
- Place the syringe in a safe container or place the glass slide in a slide holder.
- Dip the sterile swab into the transport medium then rotate it gently over the vesicle fluid on the skin. Place the swab into the transport medium.
- Place a sterile dressing over the vesicle until dry.

Fungal samples of hair, nail and skin
Special containers may be obtained locally from the microbiology department.

- Samples of infected hair should be removed by plucking the hair with forceps or gloves. The root of the hair is infected, not the shaft.
- Samples of the whole thickness of the nail or deep scrapings should be obtained.
- The skin should be cleaned with an alcohol swab. Epidermal scales scraped from the active edge of a lesion or the roof of any vesicle should be obtained.

Gastric washings
Swallowed sputum containing tubercle bacilli may be obtained through gastric washings. Children generally do not produce sufficient sputum, therefore gastric washings are obtained for laboratory analysis to aid diagnosis of pulmonary *Mycobacterium tuberculosis*. If alcohol–acid-fast bacilli are seen under the microscope, further tests are performed to aid the provisional diagnosis. Culture of the organism may take between 6–12 weeks to confirm diagnosis. Three consecutive early morning specimens should be obtained. There are usually only small numbers of organisms present so as much material as possible should be obtained. As alcohol–acid-fast bacilli are often found in tap water, sterile water must be used.

- Fast the child for at least 6 hours overnight.
- Pass a nasogastric tube (see Enteral Feeding p. 119).
- Aspirate the stomach contents and place in a sterile container.
- Instil at least 30 ml of sterile water down the tube to obtain as much stomach content as possible.
- Aspirate the contents back and place in the same container.
- Remove the tube, if appropriate.

Biopsy material
Specimens such as skin, muscle, kidney, liver, jejunal, tissue or brain biopsies are generally obtained by medical staff either under general or local anaesthetic according to the site. A sterile technique is required for all these procedures. All biopsy specimens must be discussed with the relevant laboratory personnel in order that:

- the most appropriate specimen and laboratory tests are undertaken to aid diagnosis; selection of tests may be necessary if the specimen is small
- a fixative such as formalin is not used for microbiological investigation.

Cerebrospinal fluid
Cerebrospinal fluid (CSF) is commonly obtained via a lumbar puncture performed by medical staff (See Lumbar Puncture, p. 167). A sterile technique is required as there is a risk of introducing infection, causing meningitis. Specimens of CSF should be dispatched to the laboratory immediately. Do not store the specimen in a refrigerator as this causes the cells to lyse and deteriorate rapidly, thus giving rise to false results.

COMMUNITY PERSPECTIVE
The types of specimen that can be taken in the home are limited. These may include routine specimens of:

- blood, urine and stools
- swabs from wounds, skin, throat, eyes, etc.

Consideration must be given to the transportation of such specimens to the laboratory. It would not be appropriate for specimens to be carried around in a hot car for several hours, so visits will need to be planned. It is worth considering the use of a cool bag.

Some specimens, e.g. stools and urine samples, can be taken to the GP's surgery, from where they are collected and taken to the local hospital. This may help the family and the CCN by diminishing the need for hospital visits.

Do and do not
- Always explain the procedure to the child and parent and the reasons for taking the specimen.
- Ensure that the specimen and laboratory form contain all the correct information.
- Dispatch specimens with the laboratory form in the protected polythene bags to the laboratory as quickly as possible.

- Ensure that results are communicated to the child and parent as appropriate.
- Seek help from the laboratory staff and infection control team as necessary.
- Always document the type of specimen, the time and date it was taken and any abnormalities noted.
- Wash your hands before and after handling specimens.
- Do not send unprotected needles to the laboratory as this increases the risk of injury.
- Do not contaminate the outside of the container with blood or body fluids.
- Do not leave specimens lying around at room temperature as organisms multiply rapidly and false results may occur.
- Do not put anything in your mouth whilst collecting or handling specimens nor put the containers on surfaces where food may be served, such as locker tops. This increases the risk of ingestion of pathogenic organisms.
- Do not place blood cultures in the refrigerator as this may kill any organisms you are wanting to culture for diagnosis.
- Do not repeat specimens unnecessarily as this is not cost-effective.
- Do not catheterise a child just to obtain a urine specimen as this may introduce infection.
- Do not use an antiseptic solution to clean the genitalia prior to obtaining a midstream or bag specimen of urine. This is unnecessary and may inhibit growth of organisms.

References

Advisory Committee on Dangerous Pathogens 1990 Categorisation of pathogens according to hazard and categories of containment, 2nd edn. HMSO, London

Advisory Committee on Dangerous Pathogens 1994 Precautions for work with human and animal transmissible spongiform encephalopathies. HMSO, London

Advisory Committee on Dangerous Pathogens 1996 Management and control of viral haemorrhagic fevers. HMSO, London

Ahmed T, Vickers D, Campbell S, Coultard M G, Pedler S 1991 Urine collection from disposable nappies. Lancet 338: 674–676

Department of Health 1990 Spills of urine: potential risk of misuse of chlorine-releasing disinfecting agents. Safety Action Bulletin SAB(90)41. DoH, London

Cook R 1995 Urinalysis. Nursing Standard, Continual Education Article 343 9(28): 32–37

Ethics Advisory Committee 1992 Guidelines for the ethical conduct of medical research involving children. British Paediatric Association, London

Gilchrist B 1996 Wound infection – sampling bacterial flora: a review of the literature. Journal of Wound Care 5(8): 386–388

Griffiths C 1995 Microbiological examination in urinary tract infection. Nursing Times 91(11): 33–35

Griffiths D M, Woodward M N 1993 Use of dipsticks for routine analysis of urine from children with acute abdominal pain. British Medical Journal 306: 1512–1513

Health Services Advisory Committee 1986 Guidance on the labelling, transport and reception of specimens. Health and Safety Commission, London

Higgins C 1994 An introduction to the examination of specimens. Nursing Times 90(47): 29–32

Higgins C 1995a Microbiological examination of urine in urinary tract infection. Nursing Times 91(11): 33–35

Higgins C 1995b Full blood count (RBC, Hb, PCV, MCV, MCH and reticulocytes). Nursing Times 91(7): 38–40

Higgins C 1995c Microbiological examination of blood for septicaemia. Nursing Times 91(16): 34–35

Higgins C 1996 Laboratory measurement of sodium and potassium. Nursing Times 92(12): 40–42

Higgins C 1997 Erythrocyte sedimentation test as an aid to diagnosis. Nursing Times 93(6): 60–61

Roberts S B, Lucas A 1985 A nappy collection method for measuring urinary constituents and 24 hour urine output in infants. Archives of Disease in Childhood 60: 1018–1020

Vernon S 1995 Urine collection from infants: a reliable method. Paediatric Nursing 7(6): 26–27

Further reading

Ayton M 1982 Microbiological investigation. Nursing 2(8): 226–232

Expert Advisory Group on AIDS 1990 Guidance for clinical health care workers: protection against infection with HIV and hepatitis viruses. HMSO, London

Holton J, Prince M 1986 Blood contamination during venepuncture and laboratory manipulations of specimen tubes. Journal of Hospital Infection 8: 178–183

35

Stoma Care

Introduction

A stoma nurse, if employed in a hospital where surgery is performed, should be involved in the care of all children requiring stoma surgery. If there is no specialist nurse within the hospital, attempts must be made to refer the family to a stoma nurse within the family's community. Most areas of the UK have stoma care nursing support (Health Services Development 1978).

Stoma formation in childhood is generally a temporary measure in the surgical correction of congenital abnormalities. Conditions that may require stoma formation include:

- imperforate anus
- Hirschsprung's disease
- necrotising enterocolitis
- cloacal extrophy
- ulcerative colitis
- Crohn's disease
- familial polyposis coli
- bladder tumours.

There are three main types of stoma:

- Ileostomy: a portion of the ileum is brought through the abdominal wall and is normally sited in the right iliac fossa.
- Colostomy: a portion of the colon is brought through the abdominal wall and is normally sited in the left iliac fossa (in children the transverse colon, descending colon or sigmoid colon may be used).
- Urinary diversion:
  – vesicostomy: the neck of the bladder is brought through the abdominal wall low down at the pelvis.
  – ureterostomy: one or two of the ureters can be brought out to the abdominal wall, either side by side or at either side of the abdomen.
  – ileal conduit: a small segment of the ileum is isolated to act as a reservoir and the ureters implanted into it. This stoma can be sited either in the left or right iliac fossa.

Learning outcomes

The aim of this section is for the nurse to be able to:

- identify different types of stomas
- recognise potential problems with stomas
- identify recurring or continuing problems with management of the stoma
- change a stoma appliance efficiently and effectively
- help maintain a healthy stoma and peristomal skin integrity
- be aware of how to dispose of a used appliance
- be aware of how families obtain stoma appliances in the community
- be aware of any dietary implications following stoma formation.

Rationale

Children undergoing stoma surgery and their families will need to be taught how to care for a stoma and be aware of the implications of stoma surgery. Support is needed through what can at times be a traumatic experience.

Factors to note

Neonates and babies

- A large number of babies who have undergone surgery on the small intestine will have a temporary intolerance to lactose. Their ileostomy output will be extremely loose and test positive to sugar. These babies will be given special formula milks such as Pregestaimil or Peptijunior (Blackwell 1993).
- If an infant is taking a special formula milk, the parents should follow dietetic advice when weaning. It is usual for infants to take a milk-free diet until the ileostomy is closed. Babies with colostomies who take regular formula milks can have a normal weaning diet.
- Sodium depletion is a common problem for children with ileostomies. Regular urinary sodium levels need to be taken and, if low, sodium supplements should be given.
- Dehydration can occur very quickly; if the stools are very loose and adequate oral intake cannot be taken, intravenous therapy will be needed.

Children with special needs

Siting the position of a stoma in the child confined to a wheelchair needs careful consideration. If any appliances such as callipers or a spinal brace are worn, they should be put on for the siting procedure. Often the stoma needs to be higher on the abdomen than is usual, to enable the child to be self-caring.

Adolescents

- Privacy should be maintained at all times.
- Any complaints of cramp from children with ileostomies should be noted and urinary sodium levels checked. If low, children should be encouraged to take more salt in their diet. Oral salt supplements can be given if necessary.
- Older children with ileostomies should be encouraged to take plenty of fluids in hot weather to avoid dehydration.
- Patients and their parents need to be aware of the problems that can be caused by some foods. Some examples are: popcorn or dried fruits if eaten in large amounts can swell in the gastrointestinal tract and cause a small bowel obstruction; some foods can produce more odorous stools, e.g. onions, fish, eggs and cheese; flatus can be increased by beans, greens, onions and fizzy drinks. However, it must be remembered that the children need a well-balanced diet and they should be allowed to eat what they want in moderation.
- Children with urinary diversions may benefit from eating foods with a high vitamin C content, which helps to keep urine acid. By doing this and drinking plenty of fluids, especially in hot weather, the urine is prevented from becoming concentrated, and urinary infections may be reduced.
- Older children with colostomies may wish to manage their colostomy by some other means than a pouch. Colostomy irrigation has been used by individuals successfully for many years. More recently, a colostomy plug has been produced which can be used by older children.
- Some children may need extra psychological support in coming to terms with an altered body image.
- Some discussion at the adolescent's school may be required, e.g. about using a school nurse's or staff toilet to empty or change a pouch. Communal showers also generate enormous stress for the young person with a stoma. If discussion with the school takes place, many worries can be alleviated (Forest-Lalande 1995).

Guidelines

The carers of the child should be taught all aspects of stoma care prior to discharge into the community. Children can be involved in this to varying degrees according to their age and development.

To change a bag

Equipment

- Disposable gloves (for hospital staff)
- Bowl of warm water
- Gauze or cleansing wipes
- New pouch
- Bag to dispose of used pouch and cleaning materials
- Scissors
- Template or measuring device

Before changing the pouch make sure you have everything to hand. If the colostomy/ileostomy is long-standing, the new pouch can be prepared beforehand.

Stoma pouches. There are many different pouches produced by a number of manufacturers. However, there are basically two designs of pouch. A one-piece pouch has an adhesive flange with a pouch bonded onto it. A two-piece pouch has an adhesive faceplate or flange and a separate pouch that attaches to the flange. Both the one-piece pouch and the two-piece pouch can be either a closed pouch (for formed stool) or an open-ended (drainable) pouch for loose stool. In the early postoperative period it is advisable to use a transparent, one-piece, drainable pouch. This ensures that the stoma can be observed easily, is more comfortable for the patient when being applied and can be drained rather than changed frequently.

Method

- Position the child – babies lying down, older children lying or standing.
- If a drainable pouch is worn, its contents need to be emptied before removing it. In the immediate postoperative period the stoma output may require measuring, therefore the pouch will be emptied into a measuring jug, which can then be emptied into the toilet. Before children go home, they and their carers will need to be taught how to empty the pouch directly into the toilet.
- Remove the old pouch by carefully peeling off the pouch from top to bottom with one hand, whilst supporting the skin with the other. If the child has a closed pouch, the end of the pouch should be cut and the contents emptied into the toilet. Once emptied, both the drainable and closed pouches can then be put into a disposal bag and discarded in a clinical waste bin. At home, the used pouch can

either be put in a nappy sack or wrapped in newspaper, put into a plastic bag and then disposed of in the dustbin. In some areas people are offered a used-dressing disposal service, whereby they are given clinical waste sacks which are collected separately from household rubbish. Used pouches should never be put down the toilet (unless they are biodegradable, of which there are only two types available), neither should they be burnt in an open fire.

- Clean the peristomal skin with warm water and gauze. If some residue of paste or pouch adhesive is left on the skin, then remove this first with a dry piece of gauze. Do not use cotton wool as this can deposit strands that will stick to the stoma. Prepare the new pouch if not already done. The aperture should be cut to fit snugly around the stoma with no peristomal skin exposed. Put on the new pouch. If a one-piece pouch is being used, fold the adhesive in half, placing the pouch on the underside of the stoma first, then flip the adhesive over the stoma and secure all around. If a two-piece appliance is being used, secure first the base plate and then attach the pouch.
- If a drainable pouch is being used, ensure that the clip is secured correctly at the bottom of the pouch.

Observations and complications

- In the immediate postoperative period the stoma should be observed to determine if there is a good blood supply. Sometimes stomas can look dark in the early postoperative period, but will become more pink later on. The normal colour of a healthy stoma is pink or red.
- Medical staff will want to know if bowel sounds are returning; any wind passed will inflate the stoma pouch. Always use a one-piece, transparent, drainable pouch for the first few postoperative days.
- When first formed, the stoma will be oedematous. Over a period of about 6 weeks the stoma will shrink in size. It is important to check the size before fitting a new pouch to ensure that no peristomal skin will be exposed. The size of the stoma can be checked by using a template; the adhesive release paper of the previous pouch can be used if it was saved.
- Check for any peristomal skin soreness; this can be caused by stoma effluent being in contact with the skin as a result of incorrect fitting of the pouch, or the pouch adhesive not being cut accurately. Avoid applying any creams as this will prevent pouch adhesion. Plaster removal preparations can dry the skin, sting and cause increased soreness.

- There are specific stoma barrier cream preparations available to protect the skin around the stoma. They come in pastes, powders, sprays, etc. All have instructions for use and these should be studied carefully. Remember that babies have sensitive skin and alcohol-based preparations can have a very drying effect.
- Surface bleeding. This can happen if the cleaning routine is too vigorous, or the stoma is knocked, or the child scratches it. Unless the bleeding is prolonged it should cause no alarm. If the bleeding comes from inside the stoma, it should be reported to a doctor.
- It is not uncommon in children for the stoma to prolapse. This usually occurs after a period of crying or coughing or following strenuous exercise. Generally the stoma will settle back at rest. If the stoma does not settle back, becomes tense or darker in colour, medical advice must be sought.
- If the stoma becomes retracted, it can cause problems with pouch leakage. This can be remedied in some cases by using a pouch with a convex flange. If this cannot solve the problem, the stoma may need refashioning.
- Some children may experience a rectal discharge. Usually it is only mucus which continues to be produced in the rectal stump. If the child cannot pass it into the toilet or nappy, or it becomes copious in amount, a gentle rectal washout may be required.
- Children with stomas can get gastroenteritis like any other child. If a child's stoma output becomes loose, he should be encouraged to drink plenty of fluids and seek medical advice. Dehydration can occur very quickly, especially in the child with an ileostomy.
- Children with urinary diversions can still be susceptible to urinary infection. If the urine smells or is cloudy, and the child is unwell, a specimen of urine should be examined. It is very important for a child with a urinary stoma to drink plenty of fluids.

On discharge

On discharge, the family need to be given 2 weeks' supply of the type of pouch the child is using. The order numbers of the pouch along with the manufacturer's name should be written down and given to the parents. This is to ensure that the GP knows what to prescribe. Once the family have the prescription they can either get their appliances from the local chemist or they can send off their prescription to a dispensing service. If a dispensing service is being used, the parents need to ensure that no medication is on the prescription as medicines are not dispensed by these services. One of the benefits of such services is that if a template is sent with the prescription the pouches will be cut to size; also they dispense gauze squares and nappy sacks free of charge. Children up to the age of 16 are exempt from prescription charges; those between the ages of 16 and 60 are exempt from prescription charges if they have a permanent stoma. An exemption certificate must be signed by a doctor or a stoma care nurse.

Every attempt must be made to refer these families to a stoma nurse within the community.

Facilities can be available at school such as a welfare assistant to help the child when emptying or changing the pouch. The parents need to inform the school beforehand as this may take a while to arrange. For older children, arrangements can be made to use staff toilets or the school nurse's room to empty or change their pouch. Adolescents also, understandably, worry about changing or showering with other youngsters and alternative arrangements can be made if discussed with the relevant teacher.

COMMUNITY PERSPECTIVE

In areas where there is no stoma care nurse in post, the CCN may need to undertake the role of supporting the family during the period of adaptation to coping with a stoma. Some families will need continuing support.

The CCN can act as liaison between school nurses, education staff and the referring hospital.

Families should have details of the National Advisory Service for Parents of Children with a Stoma (NASPCS, John Malcolm (Chairman), 51 Anderson Drive, Valley View Park, Darvel, Ayrshire KA17 0DE).

The collection and disposal of clinical waste at home will need to be organised.

Do and do not

- Do refer any child who has had stoma surgery to a stoma care nurse.
- Do cut a template the size of the stoma out of a piece of card. This will make preparing new pouches easier. The template will need to be altered as the stoma shrinks postoperatively.
- Do not use cotton wool to clean the stoma. It deposits strands, can hinder pouch application and will be more time-consuming.
- Do not cut the pouch adhesive bigger than the stoma as the peristomal skin will get sore.
- Do not cut the pouch adhesive smaller than the stoma as the pouch will leak.
- Do not put creams on the skin if it gets sore; the pouch will not stick to greasy skin and the result will be that the skin soreness will worsen. Many babies get thrush around the stoma, usually as a result of antibiotics postoperatively. Doctors should prescribe oral nystatin rather than cream.

References

Blackwell T Y D 1993 Food and food additives intolerance in childhood. Scientific Publications, pp 33–34

Forest-Lalande L 1995 Ostomies in adolescence: a challenge for the enterostomal therapy nurse. WCET Journal 15(Jan/March): 16–17

Health Services Development 1978 The provision of stoma care. DHSS publication HC78. Department of Health and Social Security, London

Further reading

Fitzpatrick G 1996 The child with a stoma. In: Myers C (ed) Stoma care nursing – a patient centered approach. Arnold, London, pp 184–201

36

Suctioning

Introduction and rationale

Normally, children and babies will keep their airway clear by coughing, sneezing, blowing their noses, and by the protective mechanism of the gag reflex. The use of careful positioning can also help clear airways. Suction is a traumatic process, and therefore should be used with care to help sick or disabled children where less invasive treatments are ineffective.

Though suction is most often used in intensive care areas, it is important for any trained nurse to understand the principles and techniques, as it forms a vital element of resuscitation, and of basic care for disabled and sick children.

Suction may be performed by nurse, physiotherapist, doctor or parent. For this reason it is important that procedures are agreed at a multidisciplinary level.

Learning outcomes

After reading this chapter you should be able to demonstrate that you:

- understand the indications and contraindications for suctioning
- understand the common techniques used for suctioning
- understand the problems associated with suctioning.

Factors to note

Healthy children

Children who are healthy do not normally need suction.

Babies and toddlers

Babies and toddlers do not always have the necessary ability to clear their airways, especially when they have an upper or lower airway infection causing overproduction of mucus and secretions. It can be helpful to give suction prior to a feed.

Disabled children

Disabled children may also not have learned the coordination skills needed to keep their airways clear. Severely disabled children may also lack the gag or cough reflex which prevents food being inhaled into the lungs.

Sick children

There are some childhood conditions which can cause overproduction of mucus, or a difficulty in combining swallowing and breathing. Examples include cystic fibrosis, tracheo-oesophageal fistulae prior to surgical repair, some laryngeal disorders, and tracheostomy.

Surgery

After some surgery the child may bleed postoperatively, threatening inhalation of blood and a blocked airway (e.g. after tonsillectomy). Depending on the child's level of consciousness, it may be appropriate to suck the blood out, but it is important not to cause further trauma. Some ENT surgeons encourage regular suctioning of newly formed tracheostomies (see Tracheostomy Care, p. 281).

Emergencies

If the child has stopped breathing, assess whether the airway is compromised, and if so, clear it. Suction is the most effective way of doing this. If the child is inhaling vomit, suction is needed.

Indications

Equipment

- Suction catheter: select size according to age of child, size of nostril or airway, amount of secretions, condition of mucosa. If suctioning orally, a larger size of catheter can be used. A catheter with an in-built Y connector will make control of suction less traumatic (Young 1984). A smaller-sized Yankauer catheter can be very effective, but should be used with care.
- Endotracheal catheters: size should be approximately twice the French gauge of the endotracheal tube (e.g. for a size 3.5 Fg tube use a size 6–8 Fg suction catheter).
- Disposable gloves. There is some controversy over the use of powdered gloves in suctioning, because, if

the powder enters the airways, it can cause some allergic response. This is unproven, but the sensible approach would be to select non-powdered gloves.

- Suction tubing
- Collection device: (e.g. disposable bag and container, special suction specimen container)
- Piped suction or suction machine
- Tap water
- Sterile normal saline (endotracheal suction only)
- Emergency equipment including oxygen and Ambu bag (if the child's condition is unstable)

Indications

If the child is able to clear his secretions independently, this is always more pleasant than suction. Physiotherapy techniques for clearing secretions should be considered, for example percussion, postural drainage (Parker 1990). Discussion with physiotherapists and medical staff may assist in planning effective care.

- Suction should be considered if the child's respiration is compromised by excessive secretions; this can be assessed visually or aurally. The child may be visibly frothing or bubbling from nose or mouth, or wet crackles may be heard when listening to the child's chest with or without a stethoscope.
- If the child's oxygen saturation is low and his respiratory rate and effort high, his breathing may be obstructed and he may need suction. His colour may be poor: pale, blue or grey.

The following points should be considered:

- Great care should be taken if epiglottitis is suspected, as suction can cause laryngeal spasm which may exacerbate the condition.
- If the child is intubated, suction should be performed only when required, not on an unquestioning hourly basis (Ackerman 1985, Knox 1993, Redding 1979).
- If secretions are dry and sticky, techniques for loosening them should be used, e.g. humidification, physiotherapy.
- Laboratory analysis of nasopharyngeal or endotracheal secretions can aid diagnosis (e.g. in respiratory syncytial virus bronchiolitis) (see Specimen Collection, p. 261).

Beware: Suction can be very unpleasant for the child, and cause serious side-effects (see below): use with care.

Method

Preparation

- Explain to the child and family what is about to occur.

- Preset suction to between 60–120 mmHg (higher levels of negative pressure can cause mucosal damage (Carroll 1989)).
- Connect all equipment and check function.
- Place the child in a comfortable, secure position. If necessary, ask for assistance.
- If oxygen therapy is required, giving the child a short amount of increased oxygen to prevent desaturation, either by increasing the oxygen flow or ventilator rate, may be of benefit; this should always be discussed with medical staff. Remember to turn the oxygen down afterwards (Shorten 1989).
- Put on gloves. The glove which is in contact with the suction catheter should be kept clean, and glove and catheter should be changed every time suction is performed.
- If nasal passages are dry, lubricate the catheter with some tap water or gel prior to carrying out the procedure.

Positioning

If the child is conscious, the best position is lateral, to prevent inhalation of vomit, preferably on a parent's or carer's lap for comfort and reassurance. However, a child who can see what is happening will feel more in control, and an upright position is acceptable for a child who is used to suctioning. If the child is unconscious the procedure can occur in any position, either lateral or supine. There may be situations in which sedation is appropriate (e.g. intensive care).

Technique

There are three main techniques for suctioning, which will be considered separately:

- oro- and nasopharyngeal suction
- endotracheal suction
- tracheostomy suction (see also Tracheostomy Care, p. 281).

Oro- and nasopharyngeal suction

- Gently insert the suction catheter, not yet applying suction, upwards and backwards into the child's nostril or mouth:
  - If the child has a gag reflex, the child will cough.
  - If the child does not have a gag reflex, measure the catheter from nose or mouth to the suprasternal notch to estimate length (see Fig. 36.1), then insert the catheter as above.
- Gently withdrawing the catheter, apply intermittent suction.

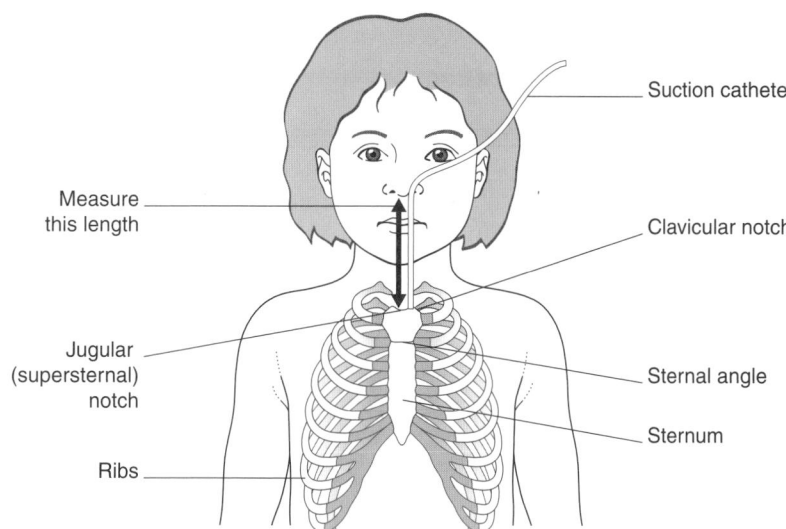

Figure 36.1
Measuring the suction catheter in a child with no gag reflex.

Where a mechanical suction source is not available, the nurse or midwife may use a mucus extractor to suck mucus from a baby's nose and mouth to clear the airways, thus assisting breathing and preventing aspiration (for example at a birth when meconium is present). Modern mucus extractors have a safety trap and valve to prevent secretions passing to the operator.

Endotracheal suction
- If an ET tube is in place, and secretions are dry, common practice is to instil a small amount of sterile normal saline (0.5–2 ml depending on size of child and dryness of secretions) to lubricate secretions. There is debate as to the effectiveness of saline in preventing blocked tubes; however, the practice is widely used and unlikely to cause problems (Ackerman 1985, Redding et al 1979, Shorten 1989). Humidification at body temperature is effective in preventing secretions drying.
- An in-built port, designed so that the endotracheal tube does not need disconnection, is advantageous. It has been shown that each time a child is disconnected from the tube, hypoxia occurs. This hypoxia can be alleviated with the integral system (Fiorentini 1992).
- Gently insert the catheter into the endotracheal tube, with no suction applied.
- Insert the catheter to 0.5 cm beyond the end of the endotracheal tube. It is recommended to pre-measure the catheter. In traditional practice the resistance technique was used, in which the nurse

would withdraw the catheter when she felt resistance; this has, however, been shown to traumatise the mucosa (Kleiber et al 1988).
- Apply suction continuously, and gently withdraw the catheter. In some centres the practice is to twist the catheter as it is withdrawn, though this has not been shown to add any benefit.

Tracheostomy suction
The technique is as for endotracheal suction, but insert the catheter to the tip of the tracheostomy tube, not beyond it (see Tracheostomy Care, p. 281).

General
- Ensure that the catheter is withdrawn within 15 seconds to reduce hypoxia (Carroll 1988, Young 1984).
- Flush the suction tubing with tap water to clean it.
- Ensure that the child is left in a comfortable position, has recovered from the procedure, and her condition is stable (see below).
- Dispose of waste and change equipment as per local procedures (see Control of Infection, p. 13).

Observations
- Observe the child's colour. If the child's condition is unstable, observe oxygen saturation, respiration rate and effort, and heart rate.
- Inspect the colour, viscosity and amount of secretions.

- Record care in nursing notes.

Summary of possible complications

(Knox 1993, Shorten 1989)

- Increased intracranial pressure, caused by raised blood pressure (see below).
- Hypoxia: during suction the child receives less oxygen than normal, especially if the procedure is prolonged and the child has pre-existing lung disease.
- Laryngospasm caused by traumatic stimulation of the larynx.
- Mucosal trauma from the same source.
- Microatelectasis, related to trauma and negative pressure.
- Pneumothorax: traumatic suction may perforate the lung.
- Discomfort/pain: described by some children as 'gagging, suffocating'.
- Overstimulation of secretions, often from too frequent suction.
- Sepsis, due to poor infection control techniques and a child already possibly more vulnerable to infection.
- Hypo/hypertension: caused by indirect vagal stimulation through hypoxaemia, as well as direct stimulation of the vagal nerve by the suction catheter.
- Tachy/bradycardia in neonates, due to direct and indirect vagal stimulation, and hypoxaemia.

Dos and do nots

- Do perform and repeat the process *only* if necessary.
- Do not ever reuse the catheter.

References

Ackerman M H 1985 The use of bolus normal saline: useful or necessary? Heart and Lung 14(8): 505–506

Carroll P F 1988 Lowering the risks of endotracheal suctioning. Nursing 18(5): 46–50

Carroll P F 1989 Safe suctioning. Nursing 19: 48–51

Fiorentini A 1992 Potential hazards of tracheobronchial suctioning. Intensive and Critical Care Nursing 8: 217–226

Kleiber C, Kutzfeld N, Rose E F 1988 Acute histological changes in the tracheobronchial tree associated with different suction insertion techniques. Heart and Lung 17(1): 10–14

Knox A M 1993 Performing endotracheal suction on children: a literature review, and implications for nursing practice. Intensive and Critical Care Nursing 9(1): 48–54

Parker A 1990 Expert handling. Nursing Times 86(12): 35–37

Redding G J, Fan L, Cotton E K, Brooks J G 1979 Partial obstruction of endotracheal tube in children. Critical Care Medicine 7(15): 227

Shorten D 1989 Effects of tracheal suction on neonates: a review of the literature. Intensive Care Nursing 5: 167–170

Young C S 1984 Recommended guidelines for suction. Physiotherapy 70(3): 106–108

COMMUNITY PERSPECTIVE

Some babies and children may be discharged home still requiring suctioning. Parents who are willing can undertake this after appropriate instruction.

The families will require both electric and portable suction apparatuses so that they are not confined to the house.

An ongoing and adequate supply of suction catheters must be organised prior to discharge.

Equipment will need regular servicing and families need to know how to seek help in the event of equipment failure.

The family are likely to need support from the CCN until they feel competent and comfortable in undertaking the procedure. Most families will need ongoing support, depending on the condition of the child who requires suctioning.

37

Temperature Control

Introduction

Despite wide fluctuations in environmental temperature the human body, through homeostatic mechanisms, can maintain the internal temperature at 37°C ± 1°C (Donahue 1983, Tortora & Grabowski 1996). This internal temperature is referred to as the core temperature or set point.

The production of heat and the promotion of heat loss is maintained by a delicate balance of physiological mechanisms. Heat loss is increased by vasodilatation and sweating, while heat production and conservation are stimulated by shivering and vasoconstriction (Gildea 1992). The balance between heat production and heat loss is controlled by a group of specialised neurons located in the anterior portion of the hypothalamus.

If the blood temperature rises these neurons fire nerve impulses more rapidly; if the temperature decreases the opposite occurs (Tortora & Grabowski 1996). These impulses are sent to other portions of the hypothalamus, which stimulate either a temperature increase or decrease. Thus these cells serve as an internal thermostat.

An increase in body temperature is one of the most common symptoms of illness in children and may be caused either by an infection or by a head injury in which the temperature control centre of the hypothalamus has been affected.

Learning outcomes

On completion of this section the nurse should be able to:

- identify the child at risk of pyrexia
- initiate appropriate action to reduce or maintain a child's body temperature
- understand the use of antipyretic medication and environmental interventions to reduce temperature in the fevered child
- appreciate the problems of maintaining temperature in the term and preterm neonate (see Incubator Care, p. 139).

Rationale

The primary aim of reducing an ill child's temperature is to promote comfort by relieving the discomfort caused by the fever.

Factors to note

Research has indicated that fever has a therapeutic purpose (Smith & Their 1985). Fever is caused by the raising of the set point as a result of the initial infection. The raising of the set point is thought to be stimulated by the action of protein-like substances, produced by phagocytic white blood cells, on the cells of the hypothalamus. This action causes a release of prostaglandins, which resets the set point or core temperature at a higher level. The resetting of the core temperature may induce shivering and vasoconstriction to enable the body to reach the new temperature even if the body temperature is recorded at a higher than normal level. This will occur until the new set point has been reached (Tortora & Grabowski 1996).

The rise in body temperature decreases the level of free serum iron, required for bacterial/viral growth, as well as damaging the cell membranes of the microorganisms (Gildea 1992).

Under normal conditions body temperature fluctuates throughout the day. The temperature of a child is higher in the late afternoon and early evening.

Because they have a higher metabolic rate, children tend to have higher body temperatures.

An increase in temperature caused by bacterial or viral infection renders the child more prone to febrile convulsion. This occurs in approximately 4% of children (Campbell & Glasper 1995, Johnson 1996).

In the infant, overheating has been identified as a risk factor for sudden infant death syndrome (Brooks 1993).

Infants and young children are highly susceptible to alterations and fluctuations in temperature. Their body temperature is altered not only by the environmental temperature, but also by crying, playing and emotional upset. Body proportions of infants and young children are different from those of the older child or adult, with the head of the infant or young child being larger in proportion to the rest of the body. Consequently, a greater amount of heat can be lost via the head (Wong 1997) (see Incubator Care, p. 139).

Equipment
- Thermometer
- Cotton sheets/blankets
- Cool fan
- Medicine cup/spoon for antipyretic medication

Guidelines
The main reason for treating a fever is to relieve discomfort.

Measures taken to reduce the temperature include pharmacological and environmental intervention.

The most effective intervention is the use of antipyretic medication.

Pharmacological intervention
- Reduction of the set point is achieved by the use of antipyretic medicine, although the use of such medication in children is controversial. Paracetamol is the main drug of choice; however, more recently ibuprofen is being used for older children. Both of these medicines act by inhibiting the synthesis of the prostaglandins secreted by the hypothalamus, as described previously.
- The antipyretic of choice will be given at the prescribed amount.

Environmental intervention
Environmental measures may be used, if tolerated by the child and if they do not induce shivering. They should be used in conjunction with pharmacological measures to help reduce a temperature and may be used to promote comfort in a child with persistent pyrexia, as long as they do not induce shivering and are used at least 1 hour after the antipyretic has been given, so that the set point is lowered.

- Reduce the amount of clothing.
- Use loose-fitting cotton clothing.
- Reduce the amount of bedding. Preferably use sheets and blankets rather than quilts.
- Reduce the room temperature by opening windows, using a cool fan (directed away from the child).
- Encourage cool oral fluids.

Avoid chilling as this will cause the child to shiver and subsequently raise the set point.

Observations and complications
- Check the child's temperature after an antipyretic has been given to assess its effect. This will normally be done around 30 minutes to 1 hour after the dose. There is no need for continued frequent monitoring.
- The child should be observed to ensure that he is gaining some comfort from the antipyretic, i.e. becoming more settled, reduction in flushing.
- The child should be observed for seizure activity.

COMMUNITY PERSPECTIVE
Temperature taking by the CCN is usually only required for children who:

- have malignant disease
- are prone to febrile seizures
- are particularly vulnerable to infection.

It is usually sufficient to assess whether the child is pyrexial and needs his temperature taken by feeling the forehead.

Routine temperature taking can heighten the parents' anxiety.

Digital thermometers appear to be accurate to one decimal point and are popular with parents who need to monitor the temperature accurately.

Do and do not
- Do ensure that the child's temperature is monitored regularly.
- Do ensure that the parents are provided with information related to febrile seizures. This helps relieve anxiety.
- Do ensure that parents are provided with both verbal and written information on discharge.
- Do not use environmental measures to reduce the temperature in the febrile child before the use of antipyretics. They may induce shivering, which will cause a further rise in the temperature.
- Do not use cool moist compresses on the skin before the use of antipyretics.
- Do not use aspirin for fever in children under 12 years of age, because of its identified correlation with Reye's syndrome (Campbell & Glasper 1995).

References
Brooks J G 1993 Unravelling the mysteries of sudden infant death syndrome. Current Opinion in Pediatrics 5: 266–272

Campbell S, Glasper E A (eds) 1995 Whaley and Wong's children's nursing. Mosby, London

Donahue A M 1983 Tepid sponging. Journal of Emergency Nursing 9(2): 78–82

Gildea J H 1992 When fever becomes an enemy. Pediatric Nursing 18(2): 165–167

Johnson W 1996 Childhood fevers: advising parents on management. Community Nurse 2(2): 20, 22–23

Smith L H, Their S O 1985 Pathophysiology: the biological principles of disease, 2nd edn. W B Saunders, Philadelphia

Tortora G J, Grabowski S R 1996 Principles of anatomy and physiology, 8th edn. HarperCollins College Publishers, New York

Wong D 1997 Whaley and Wong's essentials of pediatric nursing, 5th edn. Mosby, St Louis

Further reading

Bartlett E M 1996 Temperature measurement why and how in intensive care. Intensive and Critical Care Nursing 12: 50–54

Braun S K, Preston P, Smith R N 1998 Getting a better read on thermometry. RN 61(3): 57–60

Mahar A F, Allen S J, Milligan P et al 1994 Tepid sponging to reduce temperature in febrile children in a tropical climate. Clinical Pediatrics 33(4): 227–231

O'Toole S 1997 Alternatives to Mercury thermometers. Professional Nurse 12(11): 783–786

Soud T 1993 Pediatric update: the febrile child in the emergency department. Journal of Emergency Nursing 19: 355–358

Thibodeau G A, Patton K T 1993 Anatomy and physiology, 2nd edn. Mosby, St Louis

Thomas V, Riegel B, Andrea J, Murray P, Gerhart A, Gocka I 1994 National survey of pediatric fever management strategies among emergency department nurses. Journal of Emergency Nursing 20(6): 505–510

Whybrew K, Murray M, Morley C 1998 Diagnosing fever by touch. BMJ 317(8): 321

38

Tracheostomy Care

Introduction

A tracheostomy is an artificial opening into the trachea via the neck (Fig. 38.1), providing a channel for effective respiration and for the removal of tracheobronchial secretions when circumstances make breathing impossible via the mouth and nose.

Indications for tracheostomy include:

- congenital abnormalities: laryngeal papilloma, laryngeal haemangioma, laryngeal webbing, vocal cord paralysis, choanal atresia, upper tracheal stenosis, tracheo-oesophageal anomalies and micrognathia (underdevelopment of the mandible as in Pierre Robin syndrome and Treacher–Collins syndrome)
- trauma: subglottic stenosis, children requiring long-term ventilation, children with facial or neck tumours, emergency situations, e.g. road traffic accidents
- infections: acute epiglottitis and laryngotracheobronchitis

- a foreign body may totally occlude the upper airway resulting in the need for an emergency tracheostomy.

It is therefore essential that paediatric nurses are aware of the signs and symptoms of airway obstruction:

- Stridor – a high-pitched sound produced by narrowing within the more rigid confines of the larynx or trachea. In laryngeal obstruction the stridor is inspiratory; in tracheal lesions it is usually both inspiratory and expiratory (Bull 1996).
- Use of accessory muscles of respiration resulting in intercostal and sternal recession (Fig. 38.2).
- Pallor, sweating and restlessness.
- Tachycardia (limits vary according to age).
- Cyanosis – the lips will show a subtle dusky coloration.
- Exhaustion – a late stage. The child makes less effort to breathe, stridor and recession become less pronounced and apnoea will follow. Bradycardia is a dangerous sign indicating severe oxygen

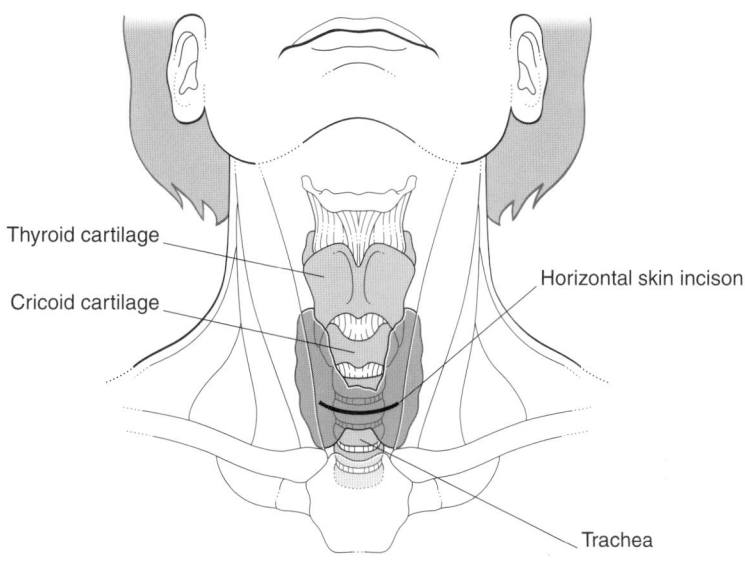

Figure 38.1
Tracheostomy showing the landmarks of the neck and the incision site.

Thyroid cartilage

Cricoid cartilage

Horizontal skin incison

Trachea

deprivation which is incompatible with life – hypoxia. The circulation is slow and the blood pressure low with profound vasoconstriction but little cyanosis. Lack of immediate treatment will result in death (Bull 1996).

Learning outcomes

By the end of this section you should:

- be able to identify the conditions which more commonly necessitate the formation of a tracheostomy
- understand the rationale behind the various procedures required to maintain a patent airway in a child with a tracheostomy
- be able to list the various pieces of equipment required to perform certain necessary procedures
- understand the rationale of when these different procedures are required
- be able to list the skills that staff and the child's carers need to acquire to care for a child with a tracheostomy
- be able to list the equipment required at home prior to the child's discharge.

Rationale for tracheostomy care

Children requiring tracheostomies may initially be in intensive care units in a critical condition. Some children may require long term tracheostomies and will be cared for in general children's wards or at home. The main aim when caring for a child with a tracheostomy is to main-tain patency of the tube, so ensuring a clear airway at all times. Tracheal suction must be applied to achieve this. The frequency of suction varies from child to child, and is dependent upon the age of the child and the viscosity and amount of secretions. The child may need extra humidity to help keep the secretions thin and easily removable (Clarke 1995). This is because the normal mechanism (passage through the nose) is bypassed when a tracheostomy is formed (Allan 1987). If necessary, humidity is administered, e.g. via an East Blower Humidifier connected to a tracheostomy mask or headbox. Other methods of humidification may be used in other hospitals and set up according to manufacturer's instructions.

Guidelines

Parents should be encouraged to learn the necessary skills to enable them to care for their child at home as soon after the formation of the tracheostomy as possible (Wilson & Malley 1990). These include: suction, irrigation, cleaning the stoma site, changing the tapes and changing the tracheostomy tube. Theoretical knowledge includes what to do if there are changes in secretions, signs of infection, signs of aspiration, signs of a mucus plug or blocked tracheostomy tube, and cardiopulmonary resuscitation (CPR). In addition, nursing staff should understand and be competent in the anatomy of children's airways, predisposing factors which may lead to the formation of a tracheostomy, operative procedures, preparation of bedside equipment, immediate postoperative care (including the treatment of potential

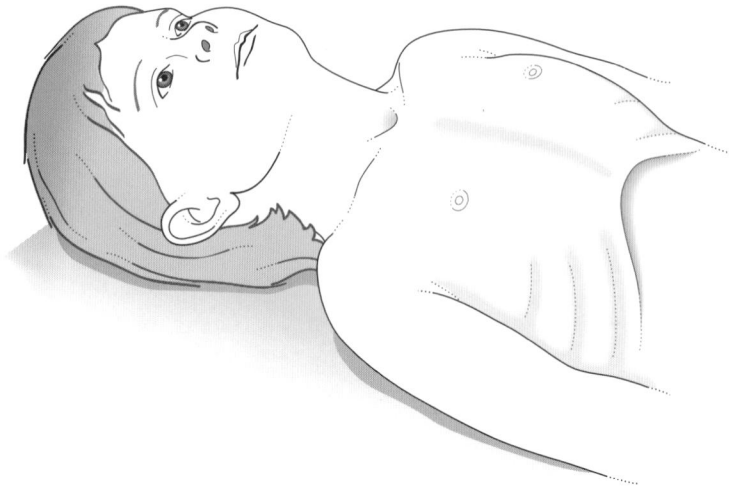

Figure 38.2
Sternal and intercostal recession.

complications), care of a child following decannulation, care of an East Blower Humidifier, discharge planning, education of parents and relatives, and allowance entitlements. They should also have an awareness of current research (Allan 1987).

Equipment required at the child's bedside

The following are required at the bedside of all children with a tracheostomy, both in hospital and at home, so that accidental displacement of the tracheostomy tube can be dealt with immediately and tracheal suction and irrigation can be performed when necessary (Gibson 1983).

- Oxygen point and tracheostomy mask (not required at home unless the child is oxygen dependent)
- Suction apparatus with tubing and a box of suction catheters of appropriate size; one catheter attached to the suction tubing
- Box of 5 ml ampoules of 0.9% normal saline
- 2 ml syringes, several of which have 0.5 ml of 0.9% normal saline already drawn up (to save time in an emergency)
- Sachets of sterile 0.9% normal saline
- Sterile gallipots
- Disposa-gloves (unsterile, unpowdered)
- Sterile bowl with water
- Disposal bag for hazardous waste
- Spare tracheostomy tube (same size as the child has in situ)

- Spare tracheostomy tube (one size smaller)
- Tracheal dilators
- Ambu bag – fits directly into plastic Shiley tubes
- Blue endotracheal connector to fit Ambu bag for silver tubes

Points to note

Gloves are only worn when the child is suspected of or has infected secretions, to prevent the spread of infection. Unpowdered gloves are used to prevent the introduction of powder into the trachea. Unsterile, unpowdered gloves are used because tracheostomy care does not need to be carried out using a sterile procedure. A clean technique, i.e. thorough handwashing and not touching the part of the suction catheter which goes inside the tracheostomy, is sufficient.

Examples of tracheostomy tubes

Shiley Tracheostomy tube.   This is a plastic tube with an introducer (Fig. 38.3). Sizes are 00, 0, 1 and 2, available for both paediatric and neonatal use. This make of tube tends to be used most frequently in infants (up to the age of about 2 years) and in newly formed tracheostomies. This type of tube needs to be changed approximately every 3–4 weeks unless it becomes blocked.

Sheffield tracheostomy tube.   This is a silver tube with an introducer, two inner tubes (one being a spare), a speaking tube and a blocker (Fig. 38.4). The inner tube

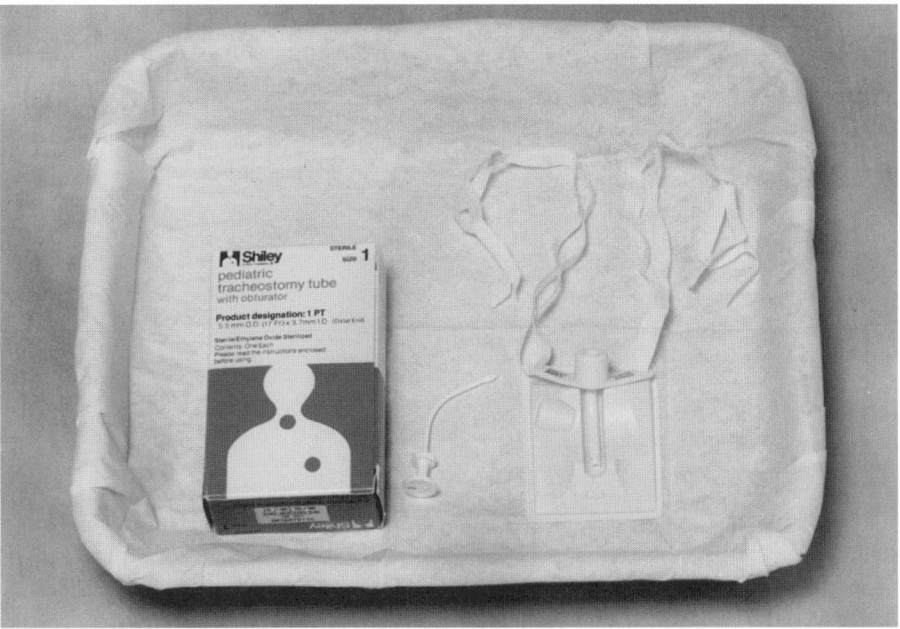

Figure 38.3
Shiley tracheostomy tubes: box (left); introducer (centre); spare tracheal tube with tapes attached (right).

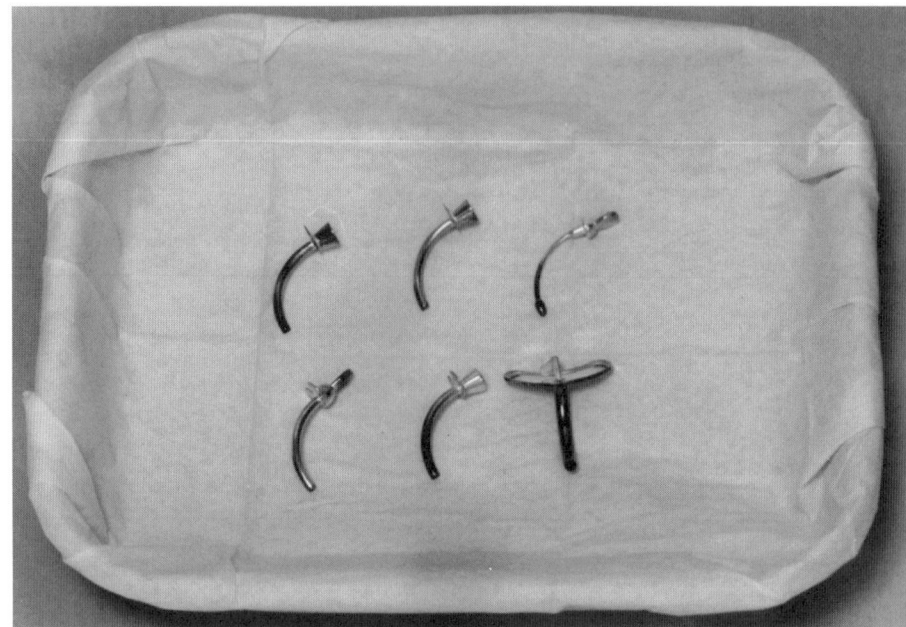

Figure 38.4
Sheffield tracheostomy tubes: (i) tracheostomy tube; (ii) and (iii) inner tubes; (iv) speaking tube; (v) introducer; (vi) blocker.

can safely be removed and cleaned without disturbing the outer tube. Therefore, this and the variety of inner tubes makes it the preferable one to use (Bull 1996). The Sheffield tube is used for children who require long-term airway management, i.e. for subglottic stenosis (Bull 1996).

There are other types of tube available and their use will vary according to surgeon preference and paediatric care.

Tracheostomy suction and irrigation

Rationale
Indicators that irrigation of the tube prior to suction may be necessary include thick tenacious secretions, inability to pass a suction catheter or a child experiencing breathing difficulties. In such instances instil 0.5 ml normal saline into the tube prior to inserting the suction catheter and apply suction immediately. Repeat if necessary. As stated by Clarke (1995), this is a potentially hazardous procedure and must be undertaken with care.

Points to note
- Saline – 0.9% normal saline must always be in plastic ampoules as it is possible that minute fragments of glass may contaminate the saline and be instilled accidentally into the child's tracheostomy (Kempen et al 1989).

- Suction catheters – it is important to use the correct size of suction catheter. A catheter that is too small will not aspirate the secretions efficiently, and a catheter that is too large will block off too much of the airway during suction.
- Suction – it is important to apply only enough suction to remove secretions. Suction that is too vigorous can damage the tracheal mucosa. Suction that is too gentle is inefficient at removing secretions and may mean that the procedure has to be repeated. Research has shown that suctioning at a negative pressure of 100 mmHg is effective in most clinical situations, whilst causing minimal tracheal damage.

Equipment
- Suction equipment (either wall or portable)
- Appropriate size of suction catheters
- A box of disposable gloves (unsterile, unpowdered)
- Disposal bag for hazardous waste
- Sterile bowl filled with tap water
- 2 ml syringes filled with 0.5 ml 0.9% normal saline

Method
1. To prevent trauma during the procedure, check that the suction equipment is set to a low setting (50–100 mmHg) and that there is a suction catheter of the correct size attached to the suction tubing.

2. In order to gain the child's/parents' cooperation, allow the child to perform her own suction if this is usual for her. If not, explain the procedure.
3. To reduce the risk of infection, wash hands thoroughly.
4. To minimise the risk of cross-infection put on gloves and withdraw the suction catheter from the sleeve. Do not touch the part of the catheter that will be introduced into the tracheostomy.
5. To prevent damage to the tracheal mucosa, which can lead to trauma and respiratory infection, turn the suction equipment on, do not apply suction, but gently introduce the catheter to the length of the tracheostomy tube + 0.5 cm (*no further*). Measure the length against a spare tube.
6. To minimise irritation of the mucous membranes, apply suction as the catheter is gently withdrawn; at the same time rotate the catheter. Do not apply suction for more than 15 seconds at a time, as prolonged suction can damage mucous membranes. The child cannot breathe effectively when the suction catheter is partially occluding the tracheostomy tube.
7. Repeat the procedure if necessary, using both a fresh suction catheter and glove.
8. To prevent a build-up of secretions in the suction tube, discard the catheter and glove and rinse the tubing. Apply a fresh suction catheter to the tubing to ensure that suction can be rapidly applied when necessary.
9. Ensure that the child is comfortable and able to continue with the activity she was involved with prior to suction (Kleiber & Krutzfield 1988).

Observations

If the secretions are particularly copious, which often occurs routinely when a child first wakes up after sleeping, unusually tenacious (thick) or have changed in any way record this information in the nursing documentation and liaise with medical staff. This ensures that any evidence of infection or other problems are detected as early as possible. If tenacious secretions persist for longer than 1 hour, humidified air will be required for a few days until the secretions return to their usual consistency.

Cleaning the tracheostomy stoma site

This is a socially clean technique which usually requires performing once or twice a day.

Equipment
- Gallipot

- Cotton buds
- Cool boiled water or a sachet of 0.9% normal saline

Method
1. Wash your hands.
2. Explain the procedure to the child and parent.
3. Empty 10 ml normal saline or cooled boiled water into the gallipot.
4. Dip the end of the cotton bud into the solution and wipe in one direction underneath the flange of the tracheostomy tube.
5. Dispose of that cotton bud and repeat the procedure as many times as necessary, i.e. until the area is clean.
6. Finally, dry under the flange with a cotton bud.

Observations
Observe, record and report to medical staff:

- any offensive smell which may indicate an infection
- any bleeding which may indicate an excessive growth of new skin around the stoma (granulation) (Fig. 38.5).

Cleaning a silver tracheostomy inner tube

This is a socially clean procedure and needs to be performed 3- to 4-hourly or more or less frequently as the child's condition dictates. The aim of this procedure is to maintain a clear airway at all times; therefore the frequency depends upon the consistency and amount of secretions produced.

Equipment
- 2 gallipots, one labelled 'clean' and one labelled 'dirty'
- Disposable gloves
- Pipe cleaners
- Sodium bicarbonate

Method
1. To prevent cross-infection keep gallipots in their bags and label one 'clean' and the other 'dirty'. Also write the date and time that the bag was opened. These should be replaced every 24 hours.
2. To protect yourself and prevent cross-infection, wash your hands and put on a pair of gloves prior to starting this procedure.
3. To prevent cross-infection, keep the pair of gloves on and remove the dirty inner tube. Place in the 'dirty' gallipot.

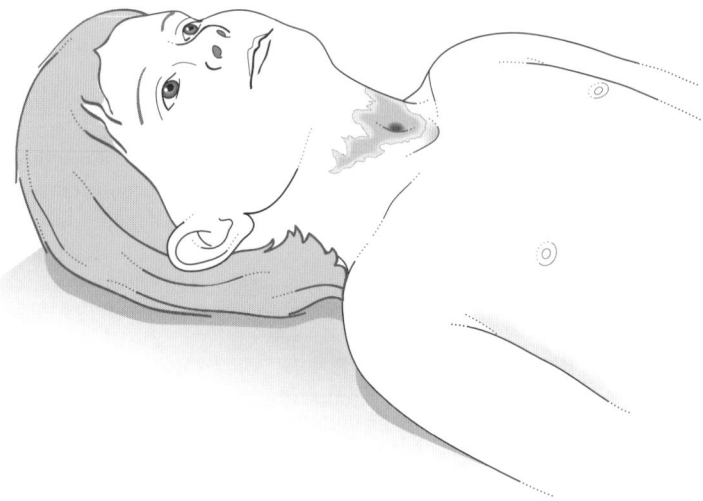

Figure 38.5
Excoriated skin with granulation.

4. Take the 'clean' gallipot and the 'dirty' gallipot containing the inner tube to the sink.
5. To ensure that the inner tube is free from secretions, place some sodium bicarbonate and water into the 'dirty' gallipot and clean the inner tube by passing pipe cleaners through it until all the secretions have been removed. Finally rinse the inner tube with tap water to remove any pipe cleaner fibres.
6. Place the clean tube in the 'clean' gallipot. Take the equipment back to the child's bedside and replace the clean tube into child's tracheostomy.

Observations
Record in the nursing documentation any increased amount of secretions, or tenacious secretions, and inform medical staff if the tracheostomy tube requires changing more frequently than is usual for each individual child.

Points to note
- Some silver tubes have a spare inner tube, e.g. Sheffield tubes. In this case, the clean tube should be kept in the 'clean' gallipot and, once the dirty tube has been removed, the clean tube can be immediately placed into the child's tracheostomy site. The dirty tube can then be taken away for cleaning as described earlier.

- Do not place silver tubes in Milton as this turns them black not shiny. The caustic nature of Milton will cause trauma to the trachea.
- Shiley (plastic) tubes are meant for once-only use. They should not be cleaned and replaced.

Changing the tracheostomy tube tape

This is a socially clean procedure (i.e. thorough hand-washing) which protects the skin underneath the tape from soreness caused by secretions and wet tapes. This procedure is performed at least once a day, more frequently if the tapes become wet (McGee 1990).

Equipment
- Two equal lengths of tracheostomy tape
- Pair of clean scissors

Method
1. To minimise anxiety and gain the child's and parents' cooperation, explain the procedure.
2. Wash your hands.
3. Thread a piece of tape through the flange on each side of the tracheostomy tube.
4. To ensure that the tracheostomy tube does not fall

out *always* secure the new tapes by tying a reef knot (right over left and left over right) on one side of the neck before cutting the old tapes. Alternate the sides daily to prevent soreness. On young babies *never* fasten the tapes behind, as this may become confused with the ties on a bib. Fasten them on alternate sides.

5. To ensure that the tapes are not too tight (which leads to sores) or too loose (which may allow the tube to fall out) check the tightness of the new tapes by inserting the tip of your little finger under the new tapes.

6. Carefully remove the old tapes.

Observations

Observe and report immediately to medical staff any redness or excoriation around the child's neck.

Points to note

- If the tracheostomy is new, the child's neck may be swollen, making it difficult to insert the clean tapes. This is made easier by wrapping a small amount of Sellotape around the end of the tracheostomy tape, like the ends of a shoe lace.
- *Never* remove the old tapes before securing the new ones as the tracheostomy tube may fall out.

Changing a tracheostomy tube

This is a socially clean procedure. Normally, tracheostomy tubes are changed by consultant ENT staff, senior registrars, parents or competent nursing staff. It is recommended that two people perform this procedure when possible, one to support the child. In an emergency situation, i.e. when the child is experiencing respiratory distress and irrigation and suction have failed to clear the tube, this procedure may be performed without the presence of medical ENT staff, although following the tube change ENT medical staff must be informed. It is recommended that a tube change should be avoided in newly formed tracheostomies for at least 4–5 days to allow swelling to subside.

Equipment

- KY jelly
- Sterile dressing towel
- Sterile tracheostomy tube (appropriate size)
- Sterile tracheostomy tube one size smaller
- Tracheal dilators

- Scissors
- Hand towel (used as a roll to extend the child's neck)
- Suction apparatus with the appropriate size of suction catheter connected
- Oxygen with the appropriate size of endotracheal connector.

Method

1. To promote a safe procedure prepare the correct equipment.
2. To minimise anxiety and gain cooperation explain the procedure to the child and parent.
3. Wash your hands.
4. Prior to starting the procedure ensure that the inner tube fits correctly inside the main tube, thus avoiding the need for a second tube change.
5. To prevent trauma to the trachea, insert the introducer into the main tracheostomy tube and apply a small amount of KY jelly to the tip.
6. In order that the new tracheostomy tube can be secured immediately, insert the new tapes into the flanges of the new tracheostomy tube prior to performing the tube change (Fig. 38.6).
7. To promote easy insertion of the tube place a rolled towel under the child's head and ensure that the neck is extended and the child held securely.
8. Cut the old tapes, remove the old tube and immediately insert the new tube (Figs 38.7–38.11). *Immediately* remove the introducer as the airway is occluded whilst this is in situ. The child may cough following this procedure, so perform suction immediately and secure the tapes.
9. Dispose of the dirty tracheostomy tube appropriately – plastic tubes are disposable; silver tubes are re-sterilised.

Observations

Observe and report to medical staff any inflammation or excessive granulation around the stoma site.

Points to note

- If the tracheostomy tube is changed in an emergency situation (i.e. the tube has totally blocked), the child will need oxygen therapy and suction until her condition stabilises.
- If the new tube is difficult to insert, i.e. the tracheostomy is newly formed, try a smaller size. Ensure that the appropriate ENT surgeon is informed immediately of the problem.

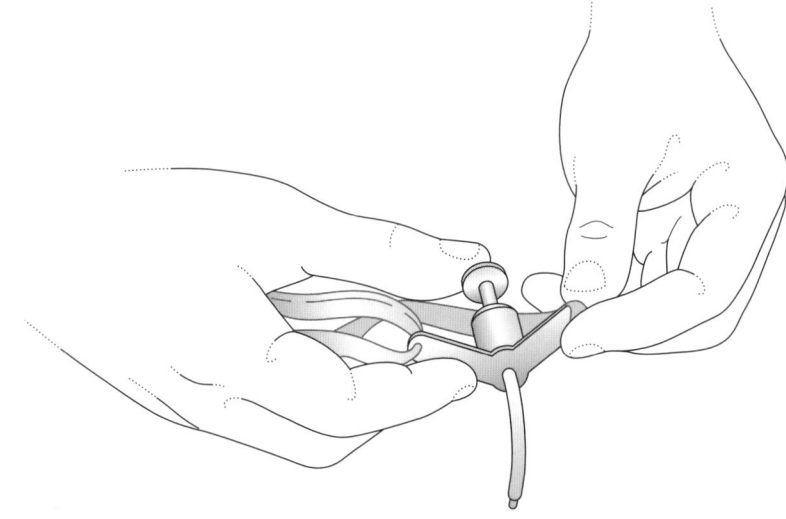

Figure 38.6
Tracheostomy tube is prepared for insertion: tapes are threaded and introducer is inserted.

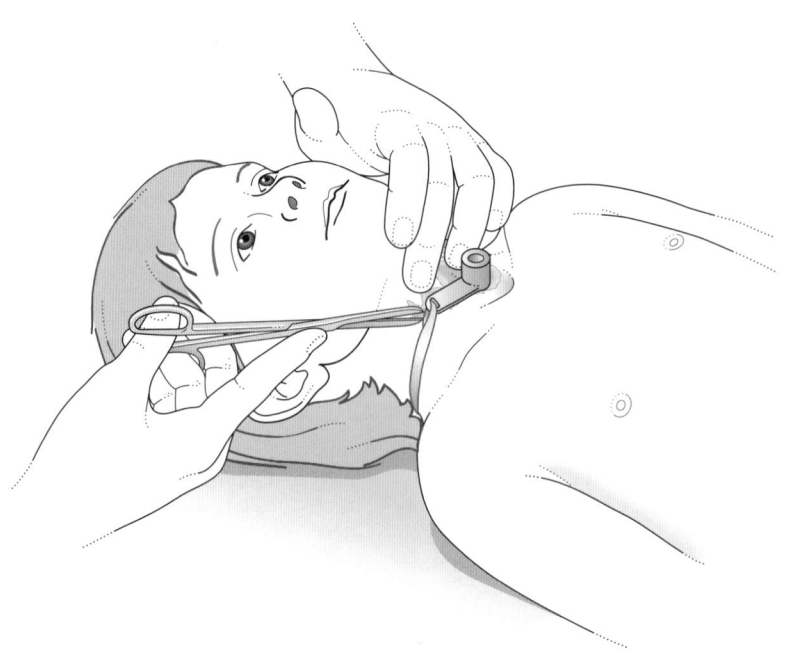

Figure 38.7
Existing tracheostomy tape is cut.

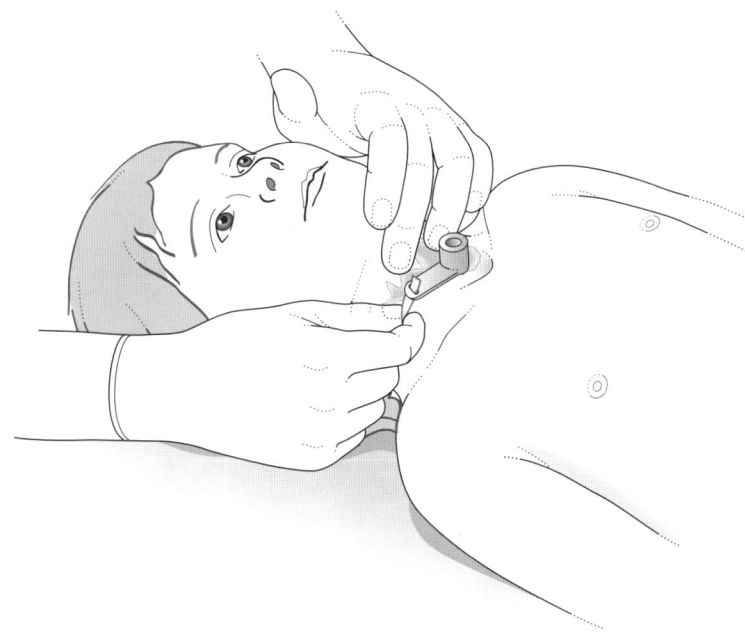

Figure 38.8
*Existing tracheostomy
tape is unthreaded.*

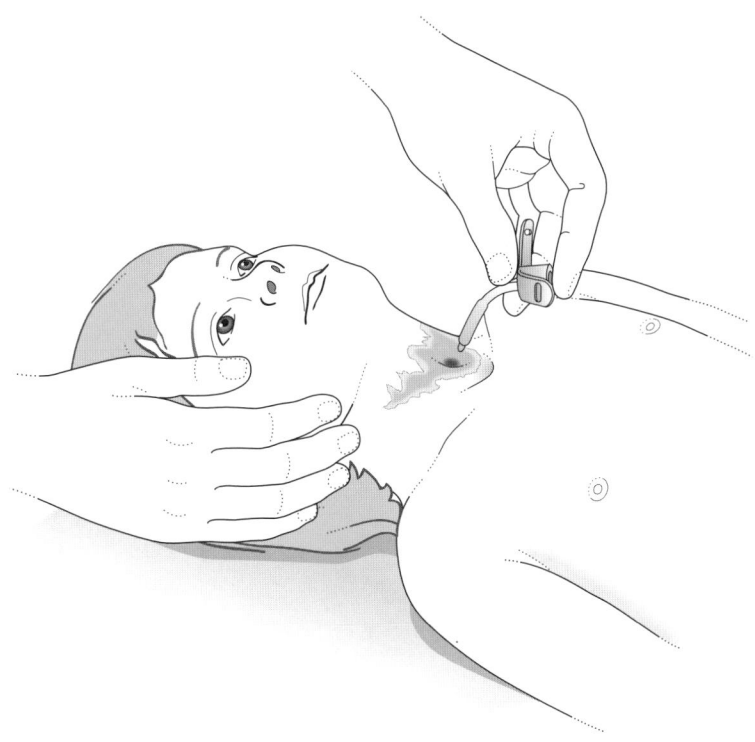

Figure 38.9
*Tracheostomy tube is
removed.*

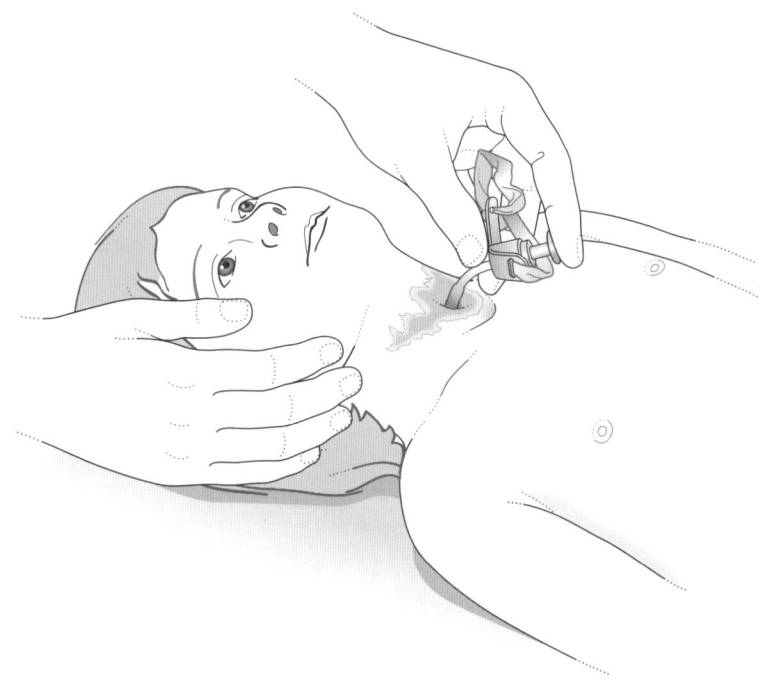

Figure 38.10
*New tracheostomy tube
is reinserted and
introducer removed
immediately.*

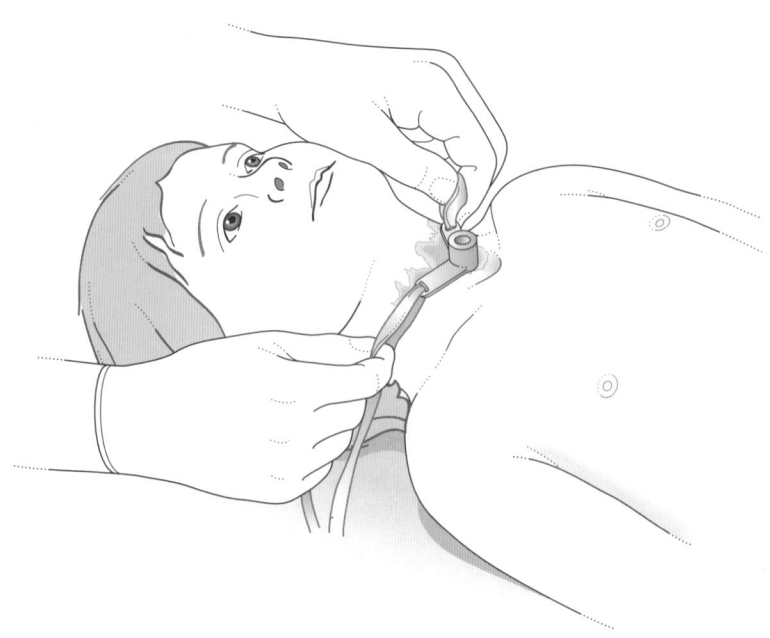

Figure 38.11
*Tracheostomy tapes
are secured.*

COMMUNITY PERSPECTIVE

Safety dictates that parents/carers caring for children with a tracheostomy will have been fully trained in the necessary care and management and assessed as competent in that care prior to planned discharge from hospital.

The family and/or child will need to be able to take full responsibility for routine tracheostomy care.

The specific details of tracheostomy care will depend on the child's individual needs, the type of tracheostomy device and the types of ancillary equipment being used.

The CCN must be familiar with these variables before accepting a child for home care.

All children discharged home with a tracheostomy must have both a mains and a portable suction machine. A maintenance schedule must be agreed and cleaning instructions given.

Responsibility for the supply of essential equipment such as tracheostomy tubes and suction catheters should be agreed before discharge.

Direct humidification, e.g. via an East Blower, should only be supported in the home at the direction of the referring paediatrician and then only if home conditions are appropriate and safe. Warm air delivered by a humidifier to a tracheostomy mask can be dangerous in the home environment as the child can suffer burns or scalds, or condensation can enter the tracheostomy tube. The hot humidifier containing boiling water is a danger to the child and others. The close supervision that is required if this equipment is to be used in the home, may be impossible.

A sick child with a tracheostomy is likely to be extremely dependent and this can affect the freedom and mobility of the whole family. Discharge planning should include a bid being made for continuing care monies so that respite care can be provided in the home.

It is sensible to notify electrical and telephone companies in writing so that the home can be given priority for restoration of power in the event of a failure.

Support group

ACT – Aid For Children With Tracheostomies
Terence Foster
14a Catterick Drive
Little Lever
Bolton BL3 1EL

References

Allan D 1987 Making sense of tracheostomy. Nursing Times 83(45): 34–38

Bull P D 1996 Diseases of the ear, nose and throat. Blackwell Science, Oxford

Clarke L 1995 A critical event in tracheostomy care. British Journal of Nursing 4(12): 676, 678–681

Gibson I M 1983 Tracheostomy management. Nursing 2(18): 538–540

Kempen P M, Sulkowski E, Sawyer R A 1989 Glass ampules and associated hazards. Critical Care Medicine 17(8): 812–813

Kleiber C, Krutzfield N 1988 Acute histologic changes in tracheobronchial tree associated with different suction catheter insertion techniques. Heart and Lung 17: 10–14

McGee L 1990 Case study: maintaining skin integrity during the use of tracheostomy ties. Osteotomy Wound Management 30: 37–40

Wilson E B, Malley N 1990 Discharge planning for the patient with a new tracheostomy. Critical Care Nurse 10(7): 73–74, 76–79

Further reading

Bostick J, Tarrant Wendelglass S 1987 Normal saline instillation as part of the suctioning procedure: effects on PaO_2 and amount of secretions. Heart and Lung 16(5): 532–537

Dougherty J M et al 1995 Part 1: developing a competency-based curriculum for tracheostomy and ventilator care. Pediatric Nursing: 21(6): 581–584

Lichtenstein M S 1986 Pediatric home tracheostomy care: a parent's guide. Pediatric Nursing 12 (1): 41–48, 69

Sacker M 1979 Pathogenesis and prevention of tracheobronchial damage with suction pressures. Chest 76: 283

Wellitz P B, Dettenmeier P A 1994 Test your knowledge of tracheostomy tubes. American Journal of Nursing 94(2): 46–50

Wilson F 1976 Tracheostomy for the nurse. Edward Arnold, London

Young C 1988 Airway suctioning: a study of paediatric physiotherapy practice. Physiotherapy 74(1): 13–15

39

Traction

Introduction

Traction is a pulling force. In orthopaedics traction therapy is used as a conservative intervention. It is used to reduce and maintain alignment of fractures, to immobilise inflamed or injured joints, relieve pain, correct mild deformities and reduce muscle spasm.

Learning outcomes

By the end of this section you should:

- understand why traction is used
- be able to identify the different types of traction
- recognise the methods of applying traction
- be able to care for a child on traction
- recognise the common complications that may occur as a result of the use of traction.

Rationale

Traction, in all its many guises, is extensively used in orthopaedic practice, especially in paediatrics. Like many aspects of orthopaedic therapy, it does not remain constant and therefore requires a high degree of nursing input.

Factors to note

Effects of hospitalisation on the family

Traction is often indicated following trauma such as a road traffic accident. The parents often feel shocked, guilty or angry about the trauma and find the application of traction very stressful at an already difficult time. An emergency admission, however routine for nursing staff, or a planned admission, is a time of great stress for both the parents and child. It is essential that explanations of all that is happening and why are given to the child and his parents. When appropriate, the child and his parents should be encouraged to participate in care of the traction when they feel able to do so. It is important that they feel confident and happy with this and do not undertake it out of a sense of duty to do so. Traction equipment can be daunting to a nurse unfamiliar in its use and may be very frightening to a parent. Traction is often used for prolonged periods of time. This can be disruptive to family life. Parents should feel welcomed onto the ward and be able to stay with their child if they wish, though this may be difficult if there are siblings at home.

Equipment

Traction equipment and terminology can be confusing and anxiety provoking to nurses who do not fully understand the components and how each attaches to the other. The type and method of traction used is indicated by the type and position of the fracture, the age of the child and the desired outcome. Other factors such as trauma, surgeon's preference and availability of equipment will be considered.

Nurses caring for patients on traction need a working knowledge of each of the various types of traction along with its rationale, correct set up and maintenance (Styrcula 1994). Davis (1989) states that there are many variations in practice, all of which fulfil the same purpose. What is essential is that a uniform approach is used once the traction is established. There are many types of traction and the names may vary from centre to centre. There may also be variations and alterations to accommodate individual needs.

Types of traction

Traction is either fixed or balanced:

- Fixed traction is achieved by exerting a pulling force on the point splinted between two fixed points.
- Balanced traction exerts a pulling force on the part held between two mobile points, and works by using the patient's weight against the applied load (Heywood-Jones 1990).

Both skin and skeletal traction are used in paediatrics.

Skin traction. This is the first choice of treatment and involves applying adhesive strips of material to either side of the affected limb. The limb is then bandaged, taking care to leave the knee free. The skin traction kits include cords to allow a pull to be exerted on the strips which is transmitted from the material and skin to the underlying tissues and bone. Only a moderate amount of pull can be exerted using weights and the bed end is then elevated.

Skeletal traction. This is used at the surgeon's preference if the alignment of the fracture is difficult to achieve and maintain and internal fixation is not possible. This involves the insertion of a sterile pin through an area of strong bone such as the femoral condyles, tibial tuberosity or calcaneum. This is performed under general anaesthetic using aseptic conditions. A metal stirrup is then attached to the pin ends and cord fastened to it. Weights are then attached to the stirrup and hang over a pulley; they are then left free hanging over the elevated bed end. Skeletal traction is also used following trauma, such as when the integrity of the skin is damaged and the application of skin traction would be difficult. Skeletal traction allows for easier access to wounds, dressings or any other injuries.

The following types of traction are most commonly used in paediatrics:

- Dunlop traction: used for contractures of the elbow and immobilisation of supracondylar fractures of the elbow – this can be skin or skeletal and is balanced (Fig. 39.1).
- Simple leg traction or Buck's extensions: used for pre- and postoperative positioning and immobilisation, rest for inflammatory disorders such as irritable hip syndrome – this is either fixed or balanced, and is usually skin traction.
- Gallows or Bryant's traction: used in infants usually under 1 year of age for femoral fractures and preoperative positioning prior to hip surgery – this traction is always bilateral and is fixed (Fig. 39.2).
- Burns frame, Japanese frame or hoop traction: used in infants to correct congenital dislocation of the hip – fixed skin traction.

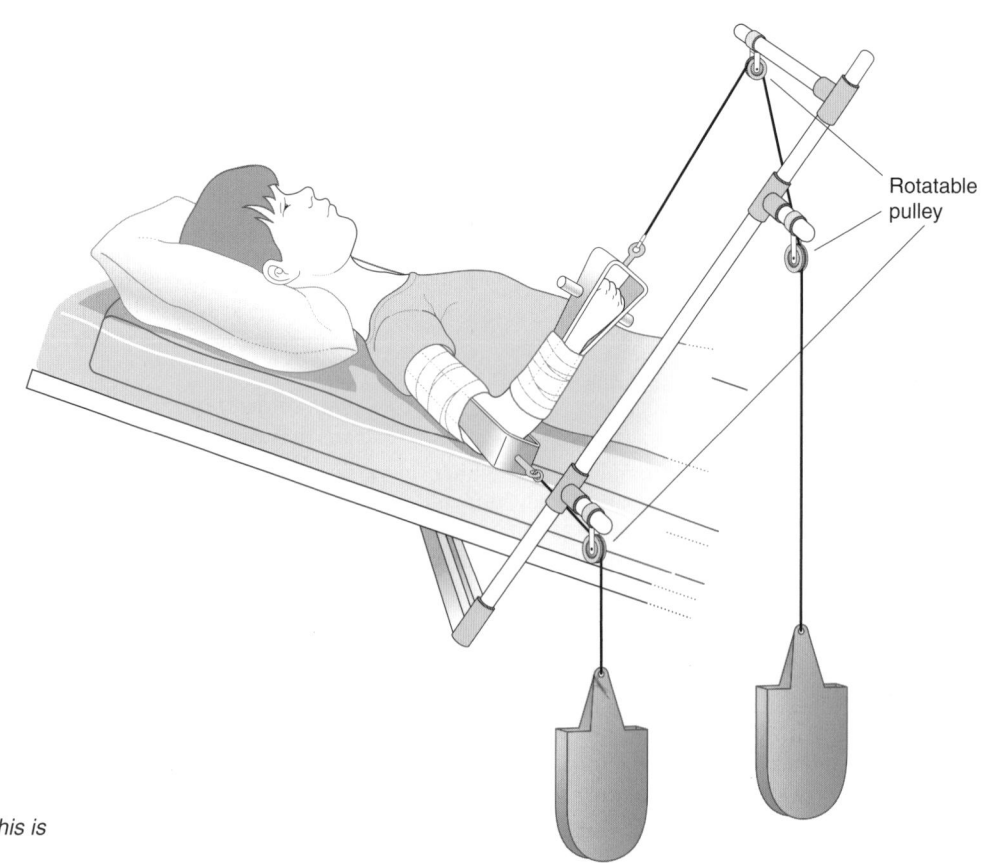

Rotatable pulley

Figure 39.1
Dunlop traction. This is balanced traction.

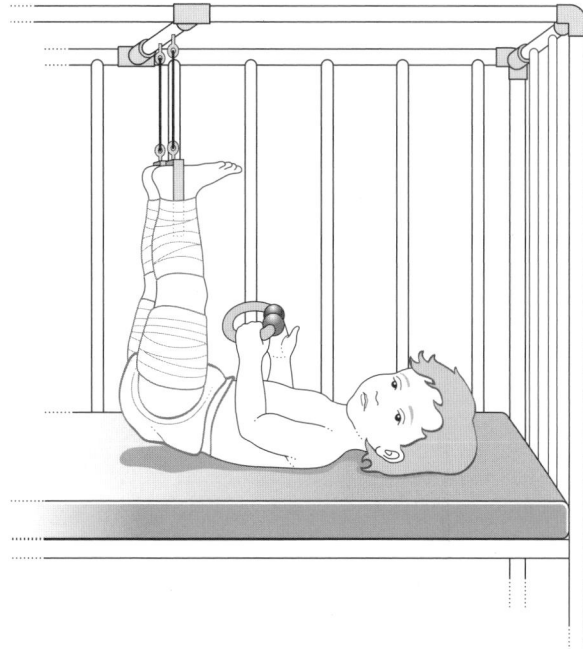

Figure 39.2
Gallows traction. This is fixed traction.

- Thomas splint traction: used for femoral fractures – this can be either skin or skeletal, fixed or balanced (Fig. 39.3).
- 90–90 traction: used for displaced femoral fractures – balanced (Fig. 39.4).
- Pelvic sling traction: used for low back pain – fixed or balanced (rarely used now in paediatrics).
- Halter neck traction: used for torticollis, cervical injuries or disease processes – balanced (Fig. 39.5).
- Halo traction: used for cervical injuries – this is skeletal and fixed.
- Hamilton–Russell or modified Hamilton–Russell traction: used for immobilisation of fractured femur, postoperatively following hip surgery, treatment of hip dislocation. It combines balanced traction with suspension – skin or skeletal (rarely used in paediatrics) (Fig. 39.6).

Guidelines

Developmental issues

Traction is used for all age groups from the newborn in gallows traction, to the adolescent on Thomas splint traction. It is an immobilising device and therefore restricts independence and the freedom to move. Consideration should be given to the environment and where these children are to be nursed.

Infants and young children should have their developmental needs met whilst in hospital. An open ward and the company of other children may provide a stimulating environment, but equal consideration must be given to parents who wish to be resident and will require a degree of privacy.

Young children often regress in their development, for example a child who is toilet trained may start to wet the bed. This can be upsetting for both the child and parent, but it is common and only temporary, so reassurance and support must be given.

Adolescents sometimes wish to be with their peer group, as they are often in for prolonged periods. However, some find it difficult to adjust to the loss of control over their environment and will prefer to be on their own.

All children and parents need to know what is expected of them, they need explanation of procedures and routine and they should be given choices (Houston 1996).

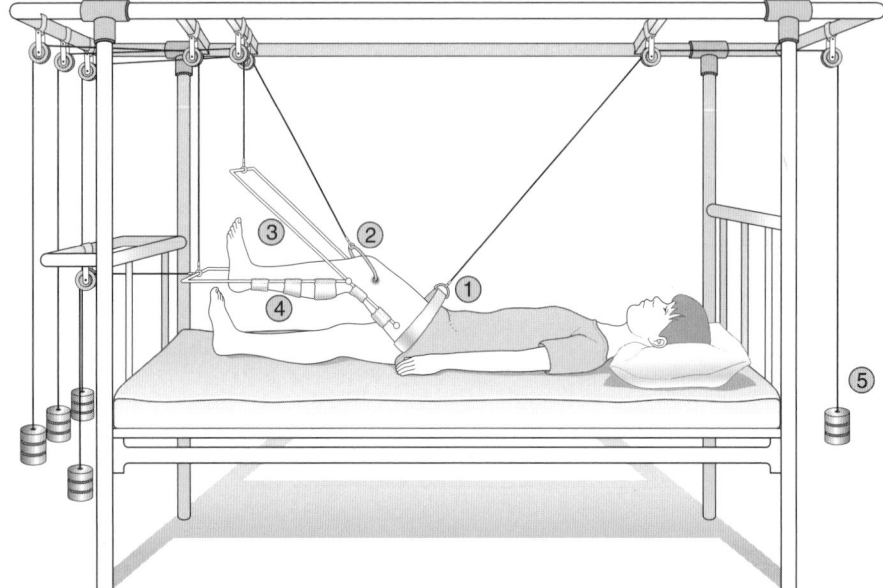

Figure 39.3
Thomas splint. The figure shows complex traction: (1) use of Thomas splint; (2) skeletal traction; (3) skin traction (below the knee); (4) Pearson knee piece; (5) counterbalance traction. This is balanced traction.

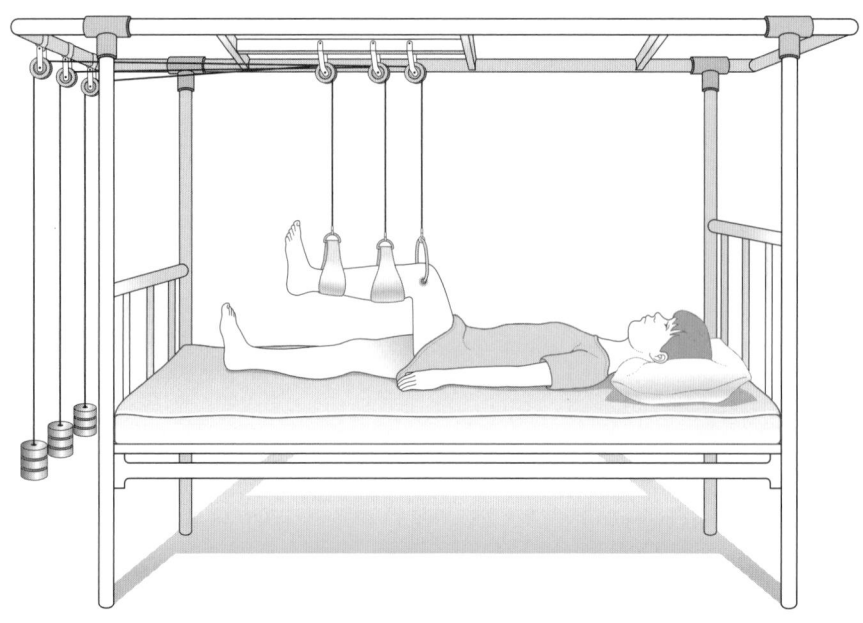

Figure 39.4
90–90 traction. This is balanced traction.

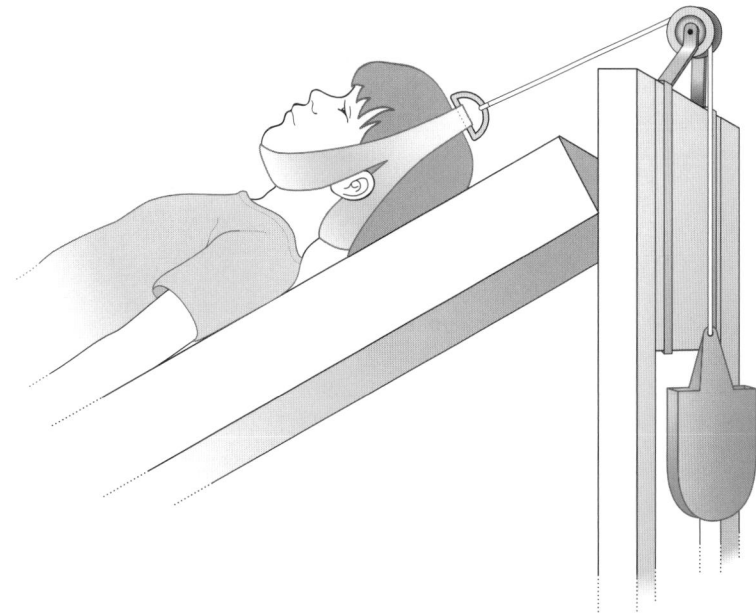

Figure 39.5
Halter neck traction.
This is balanced
traction.

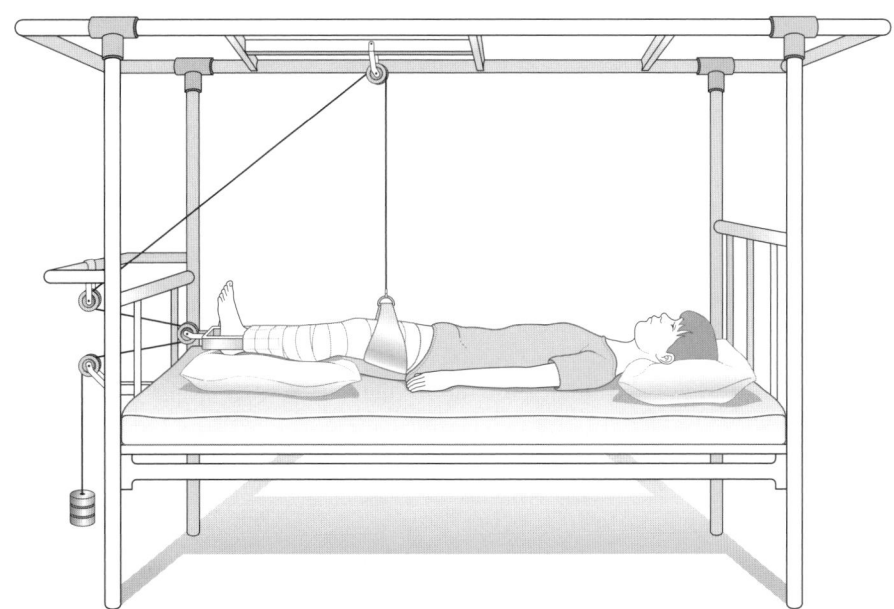

Figure 39.6
Hamilton–Russell
traction – using skin
traction.

The multidisciplinary team

Children requiring traction have input from many members of the team during their stay in hospital.

Physiotherapists.   Their role can be vital to the overall outcome of the traction. Their aim is to prevent complications of joint stiffness, muscle wasting and deformities by using exercises which are taught and supervised. Early intervention is required to prevent complications arising and should be within 24 hours of the application of traction.

Occupational therapists. If splints or slings are required as a result of complications such as foot drop or toe/finger deformities, the occupational therapist will assess the child's needs and organise the necessary equipment.

Play specialists. A child experiencing regressive behaviour may benefit from play therapy (Le Vieux-Anglin & Sawyers 1993). Play specialists provide activities not only to prevent boredom but also to support staff in carrying out painful procedures with the use of distraction therapy. Physiotherapy and exercise can often be disguised as play and can be quite imaginative and developmentally stimulating (see Play p. 329).

Ward-based schoolteacher. Traction is often a prolonged therapy and may cause long absences from school. *Services for Children and Young People* (DoH 1996) states: 'Your child has a right to receive suitable education while in hospital for a long time.' Liaison often takes place with the child's school to ensure continuity of education needs, and home education can be arranged if necessary.

Parental participation

'Ultimately it is the patient who requires the care, not the traction system.' (Davis 1989).

Once the traction has been established and is no longer daunting to the parents, they can often participate in their child's care. This is usually with the activities of daily living, but particular activities relating to the care of the traction, such as care of splints and greasing Thomas splint rings, can also be undertaken. Supervision of exercises as taught by the physiotherapists can be done by the parent and child together, though parents must be willing participants and must not feel that they have to undertake these roles.

When administering care, the nurse should be constantly thinking of ways to help the child 'do for himself', and ways to reward the child for any accomplishments (Houston 1996).

Equipment

For all skin traction
- Commercial skin traction kits, either adhesive or non-adhesive foam backed
- Bandages and securing tape
- Traction cord
- Traction beams and frames

Other equipment that may be used for all traction
- Wooden blocks (for fixed traction, used to keep the heel off the bed)

- Weights and pulleys (for balanced traction)
- Balkan beams on four-poster frame
- Splints, e.g. Thomas splint
- Slings, e.g. pelvic or halter neck
- Padding – gauze or cotton wool
- Monkey poles or trapeze

Equipment used specifically for skeletal traction
- Skeletal pins, e.g. Steinmann or Denham
- Stirrups, e.g. Bohler
- Knee piece, e.g. Pearson

Application of skin traction

A full nursing assessment needs to have been completed prior to the application of traction to obtain baseline information upon which all plans of care are based (see Assessment, p. 45).

1. Prepare the child and parent for the procedure with careful explanation of the plan of care.
2. Ensure that the child has had adequate analgesia prior to the procedure. Application of traction can be stressful and sedation may be required in addition to analgesia. If manipulation of the fracture is required, a general anaesthetic will be given.
3. Maintain privacy.
4. Clean the skin prior to the application of traction.
5. Leave the ankle free. This allows for movement of the joint and prevents stiffness.
6. Bony prominences, especially of the malleoli and head of fibula, should be left free from pressure. Padding may be applied to these areas.
7. Strapping must be firm but not tight or constricting (Heywood-Jones 1990, Pritchard & David 1990), and must be applied wrinkle-free to prevent sores developing.
8. Two people are required to apply traction safely, one to do the application and one to support the affected limb.
9. If weights are to be used, pulleys and cord cut to the appropriate length will be required. The amount of weight to be used will often be indicated by the medical staff. Too much can result in the child being pulled down the bed, and not enough will be ineffectual in providing any form of traction. When using weights, the bed end should be slightly elevated.

Nursing care of the child in traction

Having applied the traction, the nursing care is then based on the care of the immobilised child, with additional factors implied by the traction.

Pain and discomfort

Once traction has been applied the child is usually more comfortable. Pain needs to be assessed and analgesia given. One of the most common causes of discomfort is muscle spasm; this is resolved with antispasmodics but does settle after a short time on traction.

Positioning

Traction often demands the patient to be nursed in an unnatural position, such as lying flat, head down (e.g. gallows traction). This often affects the usual activities of daily living in the early stages but children quickly adapt.

Skin care

The skin on the injured limb needs to be checked at least daily. It is important to look for signs of allergic reaction to traction kits and adhesive tapes. Following trauma, damaged skin must be monitored and dressings applied as directed and necessary. Skin care also extends to washing and pressure area care as the child is immobile. Frequent change in position if possible, or relief of pressure on bony prominences such as sacrum, elbows and heels are extremely important.

When skeletal traction is in use, care of the pin sites is essential. The aim is to prevent infection, which if undetected or untreated can develop into osteomyelitis. There may be variations in the care of pin sites; usually the dressings applied in theatre are left intact for the first 48 hours, then a regime of daily cleaning with normal saline is established. The sites are then left exposed. Observe for redness and swelling or presence of any exudate and report any changes to the medical staff.

Elimination

Changes in the child's usual bowel and bladder activities are common. Constipation frequently occurs owing to decreased gastrointestinal motility. A high-fibre diet and increased fluid intake can help. Bowel movements should be monitored. Urinary tract infections can also be an initial problem owing to awkward positioning and fear of using bedpans. Bed wetting due to regression in younger children is common.

Eating and drinking

This can be difficult because of the position of the patient, and reduced appetite can be expected. Frequent small meals should be encouraged and these can be in the form of milky drinks or milk shakes to include high calcium intake. Fluid balance should be recorded.

Small children on gallows traction should always have their meal times supervised to prevent the dangers of choking.

Specific nursing care may be required dependent on the child's condition, e.g. postoperative care if the child has been to theatre for application of skeletal traction.

Observations and complications

Trauma and constriction of a limb due to traction can cause disturbance to the circulatory system, the muscles and the nerve supply.

Neurovascular observations will monitor the following:

The circulatory system. Circulatory problems are indicated by the change in colour of the injured limb usually to a pale or blue colour, temperature change from warm to cool and the absence of a distal limb pulse. Regular monitoring following the application of traction, usually for the first 24–48 hours, is vital. Medical attention needs to be sought if problems arise.

The muscles. Damage to muscles can occur after injury or surgery to a limb. Muscle damage is known as acute compartment syndrome or Volkmann's ischaemic contracture. Early detection of damage to the muscle is critical as muscle, once infarcted, can never recover.

The signs and symptoms are:

- Pain – often disproportionate to the injury
- Pallor – a mottled, bluish or pale colour
- Paraesthesia – tingling or altered sensation
- Paralysis – inability to move the limb
- Pulselessness – absence of a distal pulse.

These are known as the five Ps. Not all symptoms are present at the same time. As with changes in the circulatory system, any change must be reported immediately.

Observation and monitoring of the above are undertaken for at least 24–48 hours at a frequency of half- to 1-hourly intervals according to the condition.

Joints. Joint stiffness can result from bad positioning and inactivity. Passive and active exercise taught by the physiotherapist can prevent this. Excessive traction force or over-distraction (more than 1 inch of buttock off the mattress), especially in gallows traction, must be avoided as this can cause damage to infants' hips.

Nerves. Nerve damage is indicated by numbness, pins and needles or altered sensation. Prolonged nerve damage can cause foot drop.

Osteomyelitis. Infection of the bone is a potential but serious hazard of skeletal traction. Observation for signs of infection around pin sites and regular cleansing are necessary.

COMMUNITY PERSPECTIVE

In some areas, orthopaedic surgeons are in favour of children with femoral fractures or congenital hip dislocation being nursed at home on traction for part of the treatment (Clayton 1997, Orr et al 1994). A child nursed on gallows traction or with a Thomas splint can be considered for home traction.

Prior to discharge

The child should be well established on traction and fractures should be stable.

Pain should be well controlled with oral analgesia.

Parents/carers must understand the principles of the traction, be familiar with the equipment and be able to recognise any problems.

The suitability of the home to accommodate the equipment must be assessed by the CCN. This includes measuring the doorways to ensure that frames will go through and that there is sufficient room to negotiate round corners. A ground floor room will be most suitable as the child will feel more included in family life. It has to be accepted that some homes will be unsuitable for this type of home care and the family's hopes should not be raised unrealistically.

Parents need to be aware of whom to call in an emergency. If the CCN is able to provide 24-hour cover, this is not a problem. If this facility is not available, it may be necessary to involve ward staff (Clayton 1997) or have a re-admission policy organised which would need to include the ambulance service. The family should have access to a telephone.

Liaison with the ambulance service will be necessary prior to discharge to prevent problems.

Parents should be aware of the dates of their outpatient appointments and transport should be arranged.

Equipment to be supplied by the hospital

- Traction frame either specially adapted (Clayton 1997) or a hospital bed
- Weights and pulleys
- Supply of traction extension kits, cord, bandages and securing tape
- Tincture benzoin compound
- Pressure-relieving device may be necessary (see Pressure Area Care, p. 235)

- Bedpan and urinal if required
- Incontinence aids if appropriate
- Hairwashing aids

Following discharge

Initially, there should be daily visits by the CCN to check traction and pressure areas and ensure that the family are coping.

Strategies for relieving boredom can be suggested to the family. Work can be sent from school for the school-aged child. A home tutor may be arranged via the school education department.

All children will benefit from the involvement of a community play specialist if available.

Before the child returns to hospital for removal of the traction, the family will need information and reassurance concerning the child's mobility following the removal. They may also require information concerning physiotherapy.

Children can be cared for with home traction most successfully, but there will need to be commitment from both family and professionals.

Do and do not

- Do check the condition of equipment before assembly.
- Do size the patient correctly for traction to ensure comfort and maximum therapeutic outcome.
- Do ensure that traction pull is maintained at all times.
- Do check visible skin daily for signs of irritation or blistering.
- Do ensure that traction cords run in a straight line to aid smooth running in the pulleys.
- Do not allow traction cord to become knotted and frayed.
- Do not allow weights to rest on the floor – they must be free hanging.
- Do not bandage over the knee when the leg is in traction – the knee should be visible.

References

Clayton M 1997 Traction at home: the Doncaster approach. Paediatric Nursing 9(2): 21–23

Davis P 1989 The principles of traction. Orthopaedic Nursing 3(34): 5–8

Department of Health 1996 Services for children and young people. HMSO, London

Heywood-Jones I 1990 Making sense of traction. Nursing Times 86(23): 39–41

Houston M S 1996 Care of the school-aged child in 90/90 traction. Orthopaedic Nursing 15(2): 57–64

Le Vieux-Anglin L, Sawyers E H 1993 Incorporating play interventions into nursing care. Paediatric Nursing 19(5): 459–463

Orr D J, Simpson H D, John P J, Bell D W 1994 Home traction in the management of femoral fractures in children. Journal of the Royal College of Surgeons of Edinburgh 39(5): 329–331

Pritchard A P, David J A 1990 The Royal Marsden manual of clinical procedures, 2nd edn. Harper and Row, London

Styrcula L 1994 Traction basics, Part II traction equipment. Orthopaedic Nursing 13(13): 55–59

Duckworth T 1984 Lecture notes on orthopaedics and fractures, 2nd edn. Blackwell Scientific Publications, Oxford

Jackson D W 1973 The adolescent and the hospital. Paediatric Clinics of North America 20: 903

Nicol D 1993 Preventing infection – orthopaedics, skeletal pins. Nursing Times 89(13): 78–80

Nicol D 1995 Understanding the principles of traction. Nursing Standard 9(46): 25–28

Smith C 1984 Nursing the patient in traction. Nursing Times 18(16): 36–39

Spansella P D, Stevens H M 1996 Handbook of paediatric orthopaedics. Little, Brown

Styrcula L 1994 Traction basics, Part II traction equipment. Orthopaedic Nursing 13(13): 55–59

Sutcliffe J R, Wilson-Storey D, Mackinley G A The Edinburgh experience. Journal of The Royal College of Surgeons 40(6): 411–415

Further reading

Department of Health 1991 The patient's charter. HMSO, London

40

Urine Testing and Urinary Catheterisation

Introduction

Development of the urinary and renal system starts around the third week of fetal development and continues until the fetus reaches a gestational age of 34 weeks (Hughes & Griffith 1984, Tortora & Grabowski 1996). At 34 weeks' gestation the urinary system is fully formed and the kidneys have their composite number of one million nephrons per kidney (Hughes & Griffith 1984, Tortora & Grabowski 1996). The glomerulus of the fetal kidney will filter approximately 0.5 ml/min of filtrate prior to 34 weeks' gestation, increasing thereafter in a linear fashion with age to approximately 120 ml/min achieved during adolescence (Hughes & Griffith 1984). In a healthy child, the volume and acidity of the urine and the concentration of solutes will vary according to the child's own metabolism. During pathological conditions, the composition of urine can change dramatically. An analysis of the chemical composition, the volume and the physical properties of the urine can tell us much about the metabolism of the child and the internal body environment (Lloyd 1993, Tortora & Grabowski 1996).

Learning outcomes

By the end of this section and following further reading and practice the nurse should be able to:

- identify the normal constituents of urine
- correctly use urine testing equipment
- recognise abnormal constituents in urine
- prepare a child and parents for urethral catheterisation
- select the appropriate size and type of urethral catheter
- safely insert an urethral catheter, minimising trauma and distress
- perform appropriate catheter care
- understand the need for suprapubic aspiration of urine
- provide comfort and support to child and parents during suprapubic aspiration
- understand the use of bladder irrigation

- recognise the need for bladder irrigation
- safely execute bladder irrigation.

Rationale

The observation of urine remains important in the diagnosis, monitoring and treatment of disease and also in helping to provide information on a child's health and well-being (Lloyd 1993, Thompson 1991).

Factors to note

- Daily urinary output will vary with oral fluid intake, environmental temperature and the child's activity (Marshall 1995).
- Urine volume can also be influenced by blood pressure, diet, temperature and general health (Tortora & Grabowski 1996).
- Urinalysis is frequently performed both within the hospital and in the community.
- Urine is normally transparent and amber in colour with a variable odour.
- Normally acidic in nature, urine has a pH range of 4.6–8.0 (Lloyd 1993).
- Specific gravity measurement of the urine gives an indication of the solute content. The normal range is 1.001–1.025 (Cook 1996).
- Traces of protein (less than 200 mg per day), normally albumin and globulin, can be present, but are not detectable using strip reagent tests. This is normal and is insignificant (Cook 1996, Marshall 1995).
- Minute traces of ketones and urobilinogen are normal in the urine; however, these are undetectable using strip reagent tests (Cook 1996, Lloyd 1993).

Urine testing

Urinalysis with reagent strips is a common routine examination seen both in the community and in hospital. It plays an important role in the diagnosis and screening of several diseases (Cook 1996). Urinalysis can also be used to monitor the progress of disease and in monitoring the efficiency of treatment. The reagent strips contain impregnated reagent areas and can test for one or more constituents when the reagent area comes into contact with the urine (Lloyd 1993). Urinalysis with reagent strips is overall a cheap, reliable and simple non-invasive method of detecting and monitoring disease (Thompson 1991).

The following practice guide refers to the testing of urine, using reagent strips, within the hospital or community setting.

Factors to note
- Urine examination can yield valuable information on the early signs of disease (Lloyd 1993).
- Careful and accurate use of reagent strips for urine testing can prove to be cost-effective as this may help to reduce the number of sterile specimens that are analysed within the laboratory (Lloyd 1993). Reagent strips are also used within the laboratory setting. The use of an automated urine chemistry analyser has been shown to improve accuracy of urine testing (Rowell 1998).
- If urine is not to be tested within 1 hour of being obtained, the specimen can be stored in a refrigerator until such time as it can be tested, when the specimen should be allowed to return to room temperature (Cook 1996).

Equipment
- Reagent strips
- Manufacturer's instruction for use
- Manufacturer's colour chart
- Urine container
- Stopwatch/watch with second hand
- Recording chart
- Non-sterile gloves
- Automated analyses (if available)

Method
- Explain to both the child and parent the reason for the test and how the specimen is to be collected.
- Obtain a sample of urine in a suitable container. A urine bag may be used in a young infant to obtain the sample. The container used to collect the sample should be clean, dry and free from contaminants, e.g. antiseptics or detergents (Lloyd 1993).
- Check the expiry date on the bottle of test strips; ensure that the test strips are not damp.
- Read the instructions carefully.

- Wearing non-sterile gloves, dip the reagent strip into the fresh urine specimen ensuring that all reagent areas are covered. Remove immediately and tap the edge of the strip on the side of the urine container to remove excess urine.
- Closely observe the reagent strip areas and compare with the manufacturer's colour charts at the stated times. If using automated analyser follow manufacturer's instructions.
- Record the findings on an appropriate recording chart and report any abnormalities.
- Replace the cap on the container tightly and store as per manufacturer's instructions.

Observations and complications
- Preferably use a fresh urine sample.
- Urine which has been stored in the refrigerator should be returned to room temperature before testing.
- Check that the reagent strips are dry and have not exceeded their expiry dates.
- Ensure accurate timing by using a stopwatch or a watch with a second hand. Inaccurate timing will give false results.
- Check the reagent area with the manufacturer's colour chart at the appropriate time.
- Always replace the lid of the bottle immediately after use, ensuring that it is tightly closed.

Do and do not
- Do ensure that the reagent areas are fully covered with urine.
- Do ensure accurate timing prior to comparing with the colour chart.
- Do record results on the appropriate chart.
- Do send a specimen of urine to the bacteriology laboratory for analysis should blood or protein be detected. This may indicate infection.
- Do send a specimen of urine to the bacteriology laboratory if the specimen is foul smelling, cloudy, dark red/brown in colour. This may indicate infection.
- Do not use damp reagent strips.
- Do not cut the strips as this may alter their effectiveness.
- Do not check more than one urine specimen at a time.

Urethral catheterisation

Urethral catheterisation is the insertion of a drainage device into the urinary bladder, using an aseptic technique. Catheterisation can be intermittent or continuous, when the catheter is referred to as being indwelling (Abernathy et al 1994, White & Oliver 1997).

The following practice guide is focused on the catheterisation of the acutely ill child or the child requiring investigation. Adaptations to the practice may be made for intermittent catheterisation of the chronically ill child or the child with long-term urinary problems, as indicated below.

Factors to note

- Urethral catheterisation may be performed for many reasons including the relief of urinary retention, following surgery to rest or help heal the bladder or urethra, to dilate an urethral stricture, for diagnostic testing such as voiding cystogram or urodynamics. In rare circumstances it may be performed to obtain a specimen of urine (Campbell & Glasper 1995, Gray 1996, Sugar et al 1993).
- Intermittent catheterisation may be performed on children. This can be the case for children with neurogenic bladder as a result of myelomeningocele. This is performed at home by the parents and/or the child and is a clean procedure rather than aseptic.
- For intermittent catheterisation the genital area may be cleansed with soap and water and thoroughly dried.
- Relaxation exercises may be taught to the child.
- The use of anaesthetic lubricant is indicated in both boys and girls (Gray 1996, MacKenzie & Webb 1995).
- Although research indicates that lubricants should not be used in intermittent catheterisation with a re-usable PVC catheter, as infection incidence is increased, they are often used until the child becomes accustomed to the catheterisation (Willis 1995a).
- Urinary catheters manufactured within the UK must conform to British Standard BS1695; thus they are tested to ensure a high level of safety (Willis 1995a). European Community Guidelines for medical equipment are also adhered to.

Equipment

- Sterile dressing pack
- Two pairs of sterile gloves
- Appropriate size of catheter
- Antiseptic solution, e.g. chlorhexidine in water
- Lignocaine gel
- Appropriate size of syringe for lignocaine gel (if required)
- Sterile water (for catheter balloon)
- Appropriate size of syringe for sterile water
- Urinary drainage bag

Method

- A careful explanation of the procedure and reasons for it being needed should be given to the child and the parent.
- The parent may be asked to comfort and support the child during the procedure.
- The child may be sedated prior to catheter insertion. Sedation is prescribed by the medical staff.
- Asepsis is important to prevent infection (see p. 39).
- Select an appropriate catheter size (see Table 40.1).
- Prepare sterile equipment.
- Wearing sterile gloves, cleanse the urethral meatus with the antiseptic solution.
- *For girls:* gently separate the labia and cleanse the meatus thoroughly, cleansing the full length of the labia from the front to back.
- *For boys:* gently retract the foreskin and cleanse the entire surface of the glans penis. Replace the foreskin once dry.
- Gently pat the genitalia dry with a clean sterile swab.
- Insert 2–3 ml (up to 10 ml for older children) of lignocaine local anaesthetic gel into the urethra, using the nozzle provided (Gray 1996).
- Allow 3–5 minutes for the gel to have full effect.
- Change gloves to ensure the utmost protection against infection.
- Cover the catheter with more lubricant and gently insert it into the urethra until urine is obtained. Allow the urine to flow into a sterile container. Obtain a specimen, if required, for bacteriology.
- Insufflate the catheter balloon (if used) with the appropriate amount of water as instructed by the manufacturer.
- If the catheter is to be indwelling and does not have a balloon, it should be secured to the child with surgical tape in such a fashion as to prevent undue tension.
- Attach the urine drainage bag.
- Reassure the child and parent.

Observations and complications

- An assistant to help with catheterisation is essential. Parents should not be used for this role.
- Assemble all equipment prior to going to the child and parent.
- Ensure that the anaesthetic gel has taken effect prior to inserting the catheter.
- Insert the catheter gently, using aseptic technique.
- Do not use excessive force to insert the catheter. Contact medical staff if any difficulty with insertion is experienced.

Table 40.1   **Selecting an appropriate size-for-age urethral catheter (Gray 1996)**

Age of child	Size of catheter	Rationale
Infants (0–1 year)	5 French feeding tube	Feeding tube secured with surgical tape. Sufficient for temporary use. Less expensive than other types of catheter
	6–8 French Foley catheter	Small French Foley catheters are preferred for long-term drainage or where urinary debris is present. Catheters are manufactured using inert material, which reduces urethral discomfort
13 months to 12 years	6–8 French Foley catheter with 3 ml retention balloon	Preferred to feeding tube for prolonged drainage. Standard balloon sizes preferred over larger sizes, which increase bladder neck irritation and bladder spasm
12–18 years	8–14 French Foley catheter with 5 ml retention balloon	Smaller sizes promote comfort and adequate drainage

- Ensure that urine is flowing freely before insufflating the catheter balloon (if applicable) or securing the catheter.
- Ensure that there are no kinks in tubing and that the drainage bag is properly positioned (see Catheter care, below).

Do and do not

- Do ensure that the catheter is secured in position.
- Do ensure that anaesthetic lubricant gel is used in both girls and boys.
- Do ensure that sterile gloves are changed prior to insertion of the catheter.
- Do record the type/size of catheter and the amount of water in the balloon in the child's nursing documentation.
- Do ensure that a trusted chaperone is present to support a child who has been, or is suspected of having been, sexually abused.
- Do not use excessive amounts of lubricant jelly. This may lead to infection (Willis 1995a).
- Do not use excessive force when advancing the catheter.
- Do not continue with the procedure if the child is extremely distressed.

Catheter care

Following urethral catheterisation, the care of the catheter is of the utmost importance. The primary aim of catheter care is to reduce infection, which accounts for some 30% of hospital-acquired infection in adult patients (Winn 1996). Although indwelling urethral catheters are uncommon in children, it is important to ensure that the risk of infection is reduced, as they are often used in children who are acutely unwell and at their most vulnerable and susceptible.

Factors to note

- There are two main routes of bacterial infection in the catheterised child. These are:
  - periurethral: bacteria travelling between the urethral wall and the outside of the catheter
  - intraluminal: bacteria travelling up the inside of the catheter lumen (Willis 1995b).
- Routine cleansing of the urethral meatus is a controversial issue. Studies have shown that there is no significant reduction in the incidence of bacteriuria when using antiseptic solution or soap and water (Winn 1996).

Equipment
- Catheter bag holder
- Alcohol wipes
- Urine container
- Gloves and apron

Method
- Catheter care commences with the selection and insertion of the urethral catheter (see Urethral catheterisation, above).
- Ensuring a closed system is important in reducing infection. However, all systems have points of entry for infection, normally at connection sites.
- Selection of drainage equipment is dictated by the reasons for catheterisation. Some drainage bags are designed for hourly or more frequent urinary volume measurement. Some are drainable, with others being totally closed.
- Always ensure that the catheter drainage bag is kept below the level of the bladder. This ensures good drainage and prevents backflow of urine. Some bags may be fitted with a non-reflux valve; however, it is good practice to position the bag below bladder level to ensure that there is minimal chance of backflow.
- Use an appropriate catheter bag hanger for suspending the bag.
- When emptying the catheter bag, wear gloves and apron. Clean the drainage tap with an alcohol wipe before and after emptying, and empty the urine into a clean container.
- Cleanse the urethral meatus with soap and water.
- Cleansing the urethra twice daily, morning and evening, is considered sufficient (Willis 1995b). The child may be bathed or showered at this time.
- *For boys:* cleanse around the glans penis by retracting the foreskin, then cleanse from the urethral meatus down the catheter for approximately 3 cm. Dry and replace the foreskin over the glans penis. In young boys it is not desirable to retract the foreskin, as this may cause discomfort.
- *For girls:* cleanse the labia majora, then the labia minora followed by the urethral meatus and down the catheter for approximately 3 cm. Dry the area.
- Always ensure that hands are washed before and after care.

Observations and complications
- Ensure that the catheter is secured with tape to the child's upper inner thigh. This will help prevent undue traction on the catheter.
- Observe the urethral meatus for signs of exudate and cleanse as necessary.

- Use a catheter bag holder to ensure that the bag does not come into contact with the floor.
- Ensure that hands are washed before and after emptying the catheter bag. Gloves should also be worn.

Do and do not
- Do involve parents.
- Do tape the catheter to the thigh to prevent undue traction.
- Do ensure that the urethral meatus is clear of debris.
- Do ensure that gloves are worn when cleaning the urethral meatus.
- Do keep the urine drainage bag below the level of the bladder.
- Do clean the drainage outlet before and after emptying.
- Do not allow the drainage bag to rest on floor.
- Do not use a variety of different cleansing agents for cleansing the meatus.

Suprapubic aspiration

Suprapubic aspiration of urine is performed by experienced medical staff to obtain a sterile specimen of urine for urinary investigation, in infants and children less than 2 years old. This technique is used when the specimen is required urgently, dictated by the child's condition, normally when the child is unable to produce a specimen by clean-catch technique. Suprapubic aspiration should be performed when the urinary bladder is known to contain urine, normally if the child has not passed urine for 1 hour or the bladder is palpable above the symphysis pubis (Campbell & Glasper 1995).

Factors to note
- Suprapubic aspiration of urine is normally performed in young children who are not toilet trained, normally less than 2 years of age and who are normally very unwell, a specimen of urine being required to rule out urinary tract infection (Carter & Dearmun 1995).
- It is important that the child's bladder contains urine; therefore this procedure should only be performed if the child has not passed urine for at least 1 hour.

Equipment
- Sterile dressing pack
- 70% alcohol

- Sterile gloves
- 5–10 ml syringe
- Size 20, 21 and 22 gauge needles
- Airstrip dressing
- Sterile urine container

Method
- Explain to the parent the need for the bladder aspiration.
- The parent may wish to comfort the child during the procedure. This should be encouraged; however, the parents should not be coerced as they may find the aspiration distressing.
- This is an aseptic procedure; therefore a sterile technique should be used.
- The child should be in a supine position with legs in the frog-leg position and securely restrained to prevent undue movement.
- The area above the child's symphysis pubis should be cleaned with 70% alcohol and allowed to dry.
- A member of the medical staff will insert the needle into the bladder approximately 1 cm above the pubic bone at a 90 degree angle.
- Urine is then aspirated from the bladder.
- The needle is then withdrawn. Pressure should be applied to the insertion site for 1–2 minutes. A dry dressing, e.g. Airstrip, should be applied.
- The urine should be put into an appropriate sterile urine container and sent for bacterial or biochemical analysis.

Observations and complications
- Ensure that the child is firmly held in the supine position during the procedure.
- Ensure that pressure is applied to the needle insertion site once the needle is removed. This helps to stem bleeding and leakage of urine.
- Advise parents that some fresh blood may be present in the urine for a short period following the procedure.
- Observe the child for signs of increasing abdominal pain, as bowel perforation during the procedure is possible.

Do and do not
- Do ensure that the child is held firmly.
- Do observe the insertion site for signs of bleeding.
- Do observe nappies for haematuria.
- Do not perform the procedure if the child has voided urine within the previous hour.
- Do not coerce parents or carers into holding the child firmly.

Bladder irrigation

Children with an indwelling urethral catheter may require bladder irrigation to relieve catheter blockage. The most common cause of catheter blockage is encrustation of the catheter surface caused by mineral constituents of the urine (Getliffe 1995, Winn 1996). In boys following hypospadias repair, where a urethral catheter has been inserted to aid urinary drainage and/or act as a stent, blockage of the catheter may occur which will result in the need for bladder irrigation (Campbell & Glasper 1995, Sugar et al 1993).

Factors to note
- Catheter blockage can be caused by bladder spasm, twisting of the tube or constipation (Getliffe 1995). Each of these should be considered if a child's urinary catheter drainage diminishes.
- Urine infection is known to increase the incidence of catheter blockage (Lowthian 1991).
- Urine infection produces an alkaline urine which encourages encrustations (Getliffe 1995).
- Increasing fluid intake to prevent catheter blockage, by reducing or preventing infection, is not indicated; however, maintaining a balanced diet will help to prevent susceptibility to infection (Getliffe 1995, Wilson 1996).

Equipment
- Sterile dressing pack
- Sterile gloves
- Sterile solution for irrigation
- Syringe (catheter-tipped if required)
- Drainage bag (if required)
- Sterile bowl for collecting returned fluid

Method
- Where possible, a closed system should be used, e.g. Urotainer system. Follow the manufacturer's instructions when using these systems.
- Explain to the child and parent the need for the bladder irrigation and what is to happen.
- This is an aseptic procedure and sterile equipment should be used.
- Wearing sterile gloves, draw 10 ml of irrigation solution into the barrel of a syringe.
- Clean the connection between the catheter and drainage bag (if used) with antiseptic solution, approximately 2.5 cm (1 inch) above and below the connection.

- Disconnect the drainage bag from the catheter and attach the syringe.
- Push the fluid into the catheter. This will flush out the inside of the catheter.
- Disconnect the syringe from the catheter and allow the fluid to drain into a sterile receptacle.
- Repeat the procedure until the returned fluid flows freely.
- Clean the insertion end of the catheter and attach a new drainage bag (if required).
- Record the total amount of fluid used and returned.

Observations and complications

- Prepare equipment prior to collecting the child.
- Ensure that the solution has been warmed to room temperature prior to insertion.
- Ensure accurate recording of all fluid instilled and drained.
- Observe the returned fluid for clarity, blood or any particles.

Do and do not

- Do ensure that the bladder irrigation fluid is at room temperature prior to insertion.
- Do use a closed system if available.
- Do record the volume of fluid instilled and returned.
- Do observe the returned fluid for clarity, blood and particles.
- Do not use excessive force to instil fluid.
- Do not apply negative pressure, using the syringe, to drain the bladder.

COMMUNITY PERSPECTIVE

There will be situations where parents are taught to test their child's urine, e.g. to monitor protein levels in Henoch–Schönlein purpura and nephrotic syndrome, glucose in diabetes. The families will be in direct contact with the hospital and are likely to have been taught the techniques prior to discharge. The role of the CCN will be to ensure that the parents are confident and to occasionally check techniques.

The CCN may be involved in teaching parents or children the technique of intermittent self-catheterisation, or this may be undertaken by the continence advisor.

References

Abernathy T L, Beck M L, Becuer S I et al 1994 Handbook of therapeutic interventions. Springhouse, Pennsylvania

Campbell S, Glasper E A (eds) 1995 Whaley and Wong's children's nursing. Mosby, London, ch 8

Carter B, Dearman A K 1995 Child health care nursing – concepts theory and practice. Blackwall Science, Oxford

Cook R 1996 Urinalysis: ensuring accurate urine testing. Nursing Standard 10(46): 49–52

Getliffe K 1995 Care of urinary catheters. Nursing Standard 10(1): 25–29

Gray M 1996 Atraumatic urethral catheterisation of children. Pediatric Nursing 22(4): 306–310

Hughes J G, Griffith J F 1984 Synopsis of pediatrics, 6th edn. Mosby, USA

Lloyd C 1993 Making sense of reagent strip urine testing. Nursing Times 89(48): 32–36

Lowthian P 1991 Using bladder syringes sparingly. Nursing Times 87(10): 61–63

MacKenzie J, Webb C 1995 Gynopia in nursing practice: the case of urethral catheterisation. Journal of Clinical Nursing 4: 221–226

Marshall W J 1995 Illustrated textbook of clinical chemistry, 3rd edn. Lippincott/Gower, London

Rowell D M 1998 Evaluation of a urine chemistry analyser. Professional Nurse 13(8): 533–534

Smith A B, Adams C C 1998 Insertion of indwelling urethral catheters in infants and children: a survey of current nursing practice. Pediatric Nursing 24(3): 229–234

Sugar E C et al 1993 Pediatric hypospadias surgery. Pediatric Nursing 19(6): 585–588

Thompson J 1991 The significance of urine testing. Nursing Standard 5(25): 39–40

Tortora G J, Grabowski S R 1996 Principles of anatomy and physiology, 8th edn. HarperCollins Publishers, New York

White M, Oliver H 1997 Developing guidelines on catheterisation in schools. Professional Nurse 12(12): 855–858

Willis J 1995a Intermittent catheters. Professional Nurse 10(8): 523–528

Willis J 1995b Catheters. Urinary tract infections. Nursing Times 91(35): 48–49

Wilson M 1996 Control of infection in catheterisation. Nurse Prescriber/Community Nurse 2(2): 31–32

Winn C 1996 Basing catheter care on research principles. Nursing Standard 10(18): 38–40

Further reading

Cook R 1996 Urinalysis: ensuring accurate urine testing. Nursing Standard 10(46): 49–52

Gray M 1996 Atraumatic urethral catheterisation of children. Pediatric Nursing 22(4): 306–310

Marshall W J 1995 Illustrated textbook of clinical chemistry, 3rd edn. Lippincott/Gower, London

41

Venepuncture and Cannulation

Introduction

Children may require blood sampling or the insertion of an intravenous cannula for many reasons, including the monitoring of the progress of a condition, the administration of medicine or the administration of fluids, blood or nutrition.

In the majority of circumstances the children's nurse will be assisting medical staff in this procedure by providing support to the child during the procedure.

However, more recently some nurses have been extending their scope of professional practice to include venepuncture and intravenous cannulation.

Learning outcomes

By the end of this section the nurse will be able to:

- demonstrate an awareness of the differences between arteries and veins
- identify the common sites for venepuncture and intravenous cannulation
- support the child during the procedure
- choose the appropriate size of intravenous cannula/needle for the individual child
- safely perform venepuncture/intravenous cannulation if extending the scope of practice under supervision and as per local policy
- apply the necessary precautions to prevent dislodgement of the needle/cannula
- safely dispose of equipment used during the procedure.

Rationale

Obtaining access to the blood vessel of a child is a relatively common occurrence within a children's hospital. Obtaining a blood sample or insertion of an intravenous cannula is a traumatic and distressing event. The children's nurse plays an important role during this procedure, not only in the provision of support and comfort to the child and/or parents but also in providing expert assistance to the health care professional obtaining the blood sample or inserting the intravenous cannula. Firm support of the child will help to reduce the distress that he may be experiencing.

Children's nurses, in a variety of settings, are extending their scope of professional practice to include such areas as venepuncture and intravenous cannulation.

Guidance from the UKCC emphasises knowledge and skills as prerequisites for taking the responsibility for practice (UKCC 1992, Davies 1998).

Factors to note

Intravenous access may be more difficult to obtain in young children owing to the size of their veins and the possibility of the veins being covered with subcutaneous fat, as well as their level of cooperation (Hazinski 1992).

Both arteries and veins are composed of three layers or tunics and have a hollow core called the lumen (Tortora & Grabowski 1996).

Arteries contain blood at higher pressure than within veins, with the blood moving within the artery in a pulsatile manner caused by the longitudinal arrangement of smooth muscle. Arterial blood is brighter in colour than venous blood.

When an artery is punctured, the blood will leave in a pulsatile fashion. Greater quantities of blood can be lost from an artery; however, constriction of the walls of the artery help to delay the escape of blood (Tortora & Grabowski 1996).

Veins have less elastic tissue and smooth muscle than arteries; however, they contain more white fibrous tissue.

Veins are distensible and adapt to changes in volume and pressure. Gentle squeezing of the area above a vein will cause the blood to pool within the vein and the vein to become palpable.

Veins tend to be more superficial than arteries.

The pressure of the blood within the vein is low and when the vein is punctured the blood will tend to flow out of the vein evenly.

The venous anatomy differs in each individual child; hence a thorough examination of all possible sites will help relieve distress by identifying the best site. Possible sites for intravenous cannulation and venepuncture are displayed in Figure 41.1.

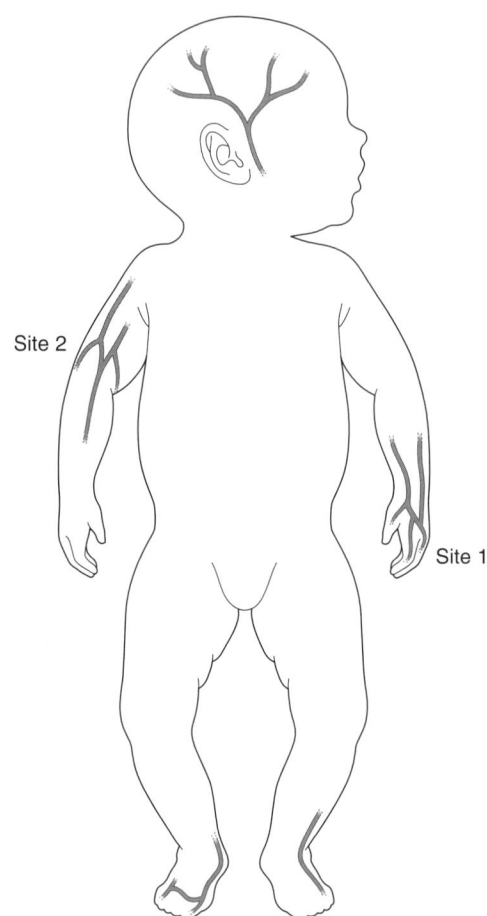

Figure 41.1

*Common sites for
venepuncture.*

Care must be taken to avoid adjacent structures, e.g. arteries, nerves.

Accidental puncture of an artery may cause painful spasm and will result in prolonged bleeding.

If the nerve is touched severe pain may result.

Venepuncture and intravenous cannulation are painful procedures. The use of local topical anaesthetic cream has been proven to reduce the pain of these procedures. EMLA (Eutectic Mixture of Local Anaesthetic) cream is one such cream that is universally used in children (Givens et al 1993, Lander et al 1996). In children less than 6 months the use of EMLA cream is contraindicated as the risk of methaemoglobinaemia is thought to be increased (Givens et al 1993). However, EMLA cream is only licensed in the UK for children aged 1 year and over. Ametop is another local anaesthetic and can be used in children/infants over 1 month old (Hewitt 1998). Local topical anaesthetics should be applied as prescribed by medical practitioners.

Methaemoglobinaemia is a condition wherein the haemoglobin of the blood has been altered to a form that cannot transport oxygen (Campbell & McIntosh 1992).

EMLA cream should be applied 1 hour prior to the needle puncture, Ametop can be applied 30 minutes prior to procedure. A thick layer of cream should be applied over the site and should be covered with an occlusive or semipermeable dressing, e.g. Tegaderm (Hewitt 1998).

It is important to have a thorough examination of all sites to ensure that the best site is chosen. Distal sites should be used to preserve the proximal sites in case the initial attempts are unsuccessful (Campbell & Jackson 1991).

Some hospitals/trusts employ phlebotomy technicians to perform venepuncture and cannulation. Health care assistants may also be trained to perform these tasks.

Registered nurses should be fully conversant with the Scope of Professional Practice guidelines produced by the UKCC (1992) if considering extending their scope of practice within this area.

Venepuncture

Venepuncture is the term used for the procedure of entering a vein with a needle, normally for the purposes of obtaining a blood sample for laboratory analysis.

Equipment
- Correct size of needle/butterfly needle
- Swabs soaked in 70% alcohol
- Non-sterile gloves
- Cotton wool balls
- Spot plasters

Method
- Explain the procedure to the child and parents prior to the venepuncture.
- Always examine all potential sites to ensure that the best vein is obtained. Ensure that this is explained to the child. Common sites used for venepuncture are the back of the hand and the antecubital fossa; however, the feet may be used (see Fig. 41.1, site numbers 1 and 2).
- Once sites have been identified, apply local topical anaesthetic cream, as prescribed, to the two most suitable sites for venepuncture and cover with a dressing.
- Firmly hold the child's limb and provide tourniquet by gently squeezing the limb. Parents can support and hold the child, to reassure him, but should not be used to provide tourniquet.
- Wipe off the local topical anaesthetic.
- Warming child's limb will help the vein to dilate.
- Palpate the vein to ascertain its calibre and direction.
- The area should be cleaned with an alcohol-impregnated swab, e.g. Mediswab, and allowed to dry.
- Wearing non-sterile gloves, insert the needle into the vein by about 0.5–1 cm at an approximately 30 degree angle.
- Because of the size and calibre of a child's veins, a flow-back of blood may not always be seen.
- Withdraw the appropriate amount of blood and instil into appropriate blood bottles. Paediatric

vacuum systems are available for obtaining blood samples and should be used wherever possible.
- Once all samples have been obtained, release the tourniquet, place a cotton wool ball or gauze swab over the insertion site and withdraw the needle. Then apply pressure over the site for approximately 2–3 minutes.
- Once bleeding has stopped, a dry dressing, e.g. airstrip dressing, may be applied if the child does not have an allergy to this type of dressing.
- Reassure the child and parents during the procedure and afterwards.
- Dispose of waste and sharps as per local policy.
- Most areas now give the child a bravery award following venepuncture. This may be a sticker, a badge or a certificate.

Intravenous cannulation

Peripheral intravenous cannulation is required when a child is to receive intravenous fluid therapy or intravenous medication. An intravenous cannula consists of a plastic catheter which is inserted with the aid of a stylet or needle placed in the lumen of the catheter with the sharp point protruding from the end.

Equipment
- Correct size of intravenous cannula
- Tape to secure cannula: this should be Steri-Strip or a sterile dressing for intravenous use, e.g. IV 3000
- Bandage
- Splint for limb/cover for cannula site (if sited in scalp)
- Swabs soaked in 70% alcohol
- Gloves

Method
- Examine potential cannulation sites thoroughly. Apply topical anaesthetic as prescribed.
- If the scalp vein is chosen, consent should be obtained from the parents for the shaving of the section of head. The parents may wish to keep the sample of hair.
- Select the appropriate size of intravenous cannula.
- Cut tape to desired length.
- Gently hold/support the child in a supine position if possible. Parents can assist in supporting their child and providing reassurance during the cannulation, if they feel able to.
- Wipe off anaesthetic cream and clean site with an alcohol-impregnated swab. Allow to dry.

- Insert the cannula at a 15–30 degree angle, advance the catheter and withdraw the stylet needle. A flashback of blood should be seen before advancing the catheter.
- Securely tape the cannula in place (see Fig. 41.2).
- Flush the cannula as per local policy to maintain patency.
- Immobilise the limb using a suitable splint, which immobilises the joint close to the site of insertion, hence preventing excessive movement (see Fig. 41.3).
- Protect a scalp cannula using a gallipot (see Fig. 41.4).
- Attach an intravenous fluid administration set to the cannula if it is to be used for intravenous therapy.
- Apply a sterile Luer lock cap if the cannula is to be used for intravenous medication.
- Dispose of waste and sharps as per local policy.

Observations and complications

- Ensure that blood flows freely and that there is no swelling at the insertion site.
- Blood spurting into the syringe may indicate puncture of an artery. If this occurs, remove the needle and apply firm pressure for 5 minutes.
- Extreme pain may indicate nerve involvement.
- If either of the two aforementioned complications arises, immediately remove the needle, allow the child to rest and then try again.
- Failure to ensure a free flow of blood may result in haemolysis and an inaccurate biochemical result.
- Using a needle that is too small may lead to haemolysis.

- Intravenous cannulae should be secured with sterile tape or dressings; however, approximately 1–2 cm above and below the insertion site should be clearly visible to allow for close observation.
- Splints should be used on limbs with an intravenous cannula sited, the aim being to immobilise the limb and prevent the cannula from becoming dislodged. These again should be secured in place by surgical tape and bandaged. Approximately 1–2 cm above and below the insertion site should be clearly visible to allow for close observation.
- Poor application of pressure following removal of the needle may result in bruising and swelling around the site.

COMMUNITY PERSPECTIVE

CCNs trained in the techniques of venepuncture and cannulation may be able to save families visits to hospital by undertaking these procedures in the home. This can save families many hours as outpatients and therefore the procedure becomes less of an issue for the child. However, in practice, the necessity for the procedure may arise so infrequently that the nurse may need to consider whether she is having sufficient practice to retain her skills.

Some areas may use Ametop, which is a quicker and cheaper alternative to EMLA and can be used on full-term babies from the age of 1 month. The CCN may carry sharps bins, although children having care requiring regular use of sharps may keep these in the home. Local collection for disposal can be arranged.

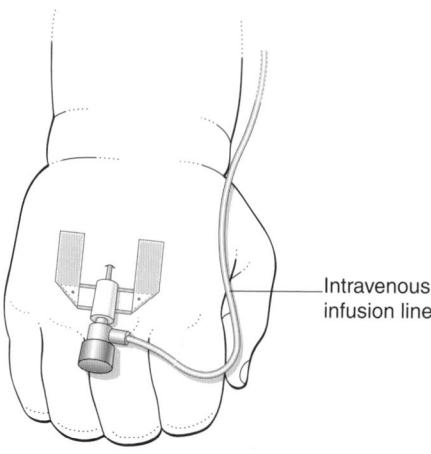

Intravenous infusion line

Figure 41.2

Taping of an intravenous cannula to secure its position.

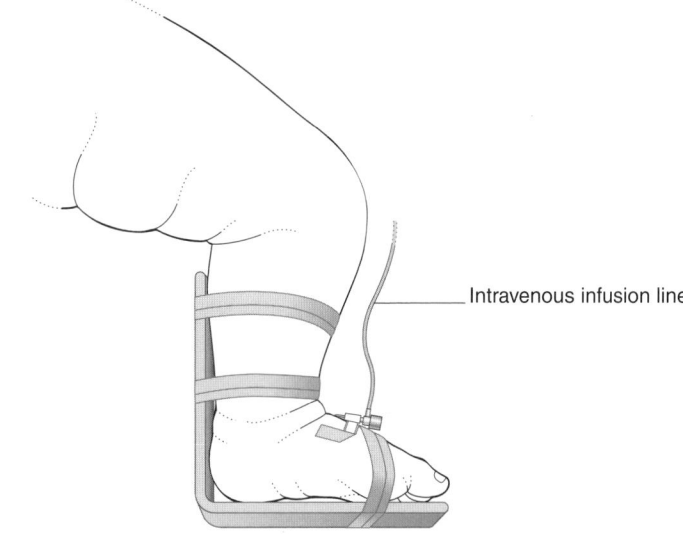

Figure 41.3
Immobilising the limb using a suitable splint.

Intravenous infusion line

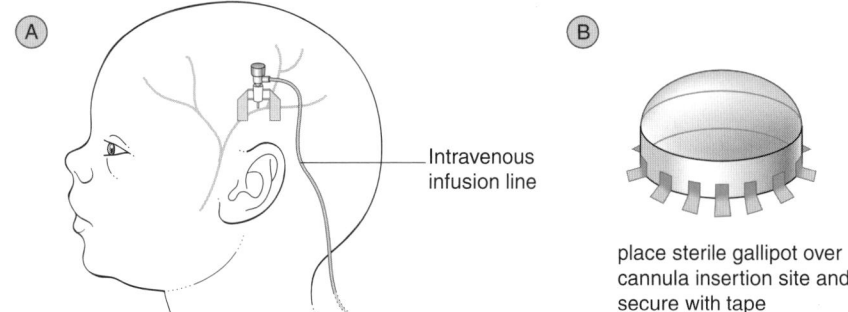

Figure 41.4
A, B Protecting the scalp cannula.

Intravenous infusion line

place sterile gallipot over cannula insertion site and secure with tape

Do and do not

- Do involve parents in the support of their child.
- Do ascertain the child's previous experience of venepuncture/cannulation.
- Do ensure that all possible sites for use are thoroughly examined.
- Do palpate the vessel to identify its position.
- Do ensure that topical anaesthetic (EMLA) is used, if the child wishes, to help prevent pain.
- Do ensure that the child has had an explanation of the procedure.
- Do use the play therapist/leader if available to help with explanation and assist with distraction.
- Do ensure that the child is firmly yet gently supported. An experienced assistant will help with a successful procedure.

- Do apply sterile tape or dressing to secure intravenous cannulae. The dressings should keep the site dry and prevent contamination. Dressings with a high water permeability should be used (Livesley 1996).
- Do not coerce parents into being present. Some parents may not wish to be present or may feel anxious and scared, which will heighten the child's anxiety.
- Do not ask the parents to restrain their child. They should be providing support and reassurance.
- Do not tell the child that it will not hurt.
- Do not use EMLA cream on children less than 1 year old.
- Do not use fragile, inflamed or fibrosed veins.
- Do not use sites that may interfere with a child's

normal activity, e.g. do not use the right hand of a right-handed child, avoid the feet of an active toddler if possible.

- Do not use wooden tongue depressors as splints.
- Do not use non-sterile tape to cover the insertion site of an intravenous cannula. This may contaminate the site (Oldham 1991).
- Do not use adult vacuum systems for venepuncture as these are often not suitable and may cause the vein to collapse.

References

Campbell A G M, McIntosh N 1992 Forfar and Arneil's textbook of paediatrics, 4th edn. Churchill Livingstone, Edinburgh

Campbell L S, Jackson K 1991 Pediatric update. Starting intravenous lines in children: tips for success. Journal of Emergency Nursing 17(3): 177–178

Davies S 1998 The role of nurses in intravenous cannulation. Nursing Standard 12(7): 43–46

Givens B, Oberle S, Lander J 1993 Taking the jab out of needles. Canadian Nurse 89(10): 37–40

Hewitt T 1998 Prolonged contact with topical anaesthetic cream: a case report. Paediatric Nursing 10(2): 22–23

Hazinski M F 1992 Nursing care of the critically ill child, 2nd edn. Mosby, St Louis

Lander J et al 1996 Evaluation of a new topical anesthetic agent: a pilot study. Nursing Research 45(1): 50–53

Livesley J 1996 Peripheral IV therapy in children. Paediatric Nursing 8(6): 29–33

Oldham P 1991 A sticky situation: microbiological study of adhesive tape used to secure IV cannulae. Professional Nurse 6(5): 265–266, 268–269

Tortora G J, Grabowski S R 1996 Principles of anatomy and physiology, 8th edn. HarperCollins College Publishers, New York

United Kingdom Central Council for Nursing, Midwifery and Health Visiting (UKCC) 1992 The scope of professional practice. UKCC, London

Further reading

Ashforth C D, Walker K R 1996 Education for practice: neonatal intravenous therapy. Journal of Neonatal Nursing 2(1): 6, 9, 10

Buckingham S, Bailey L 1995 Use of a phlebotomy service in a paediatric unit. British Journal of Nursing 4(7): 388–390

Dougherty L 1996 The benefits of an IV team in hospital practice. Professional Nurse 11(11): 761–763

O'Brien R 1991 Starting intravenous lines in children. Journal of Emergency Nursing 17(4): 225–230

42

Wound Care

Introduction

A wound can be defined as 'a loss of continuity of the skin or mucous membrane which may involve soft tissue, muscle, bone and other anatomical structures' (Collier 1996, p. 49). Wounds in children are produced in a number of different ways: resulting from elective and emergency surgery, accidental and non-accidental injuries, burns, pressure sores, extravasation injury, and animal bites.

A child's response to injury includes the inflammatory, destructive, proliferative and maturation phases. However, fetal wound healing is different as it occurs very rapidly and inflammation, fibrosis or scar formation does not take place (Longaker et al 1990). The mechanisms involved in fetal tissue repair are as yet unknown. In general, however, children other than premature infants and neonates have a vigorous healing reaction; increased metabolism and good circulation contribute to this increased rate of healing (Skale 1992).

The nurse's role in wound care begins with an understanding of the physiological processes involved in the healing process. This understanding is paramount in making an accurate assessment of any wound, and the subsequent treatment will depend on the outcome of that assessment. Following the assessment, the nurse, in collaboration with the multidisciplinary team, must be able to choose the appropriate cleansing technique, cleansing solution, and dressing. Nurses must understand the rationale for wound care and be accountable for their decision-making in relation to the management of a child's wound. Part of this process is recognising that each wound, child and family is individual and therefore care delivered must be on an individualised basis.

Learning outcomes

By the end of this section you will be able to:

- understand the physiological processes involved in healing
- describe the intrinsic and extrinsic factors that can delay wound healing

- use assessment skills to recognise and describe the tissue status of the wound, which may be epithelialising, granulating, sloughy, infected or necrotic
- use a wound assessment tool to assess and plan care effectively
- consider wound healing within the context of other childhood disorders
- have knowledge of the various cleansing agents, techniques and wound dressings available and how they are used to ensure safe and effective wound care
- recognise the role of the multidisciplinary team in the assessment and management of paediatric wounds.

Rationale

Children need expert and specialist care when skin integrity has been interrupted. Appropriate wound care should support the natural healing process and provide an environment conducive to the body's defence mechanisms so that healing takes place without complications or delay (Morison 1992). Many factors can delay and complicate healing: underlying medical condition, inappropriate wound cleansing and the incorrect use of a dressing/splintage may have adverse effects on a wound. The principal objectives of wound care are firstly to restore the function of injured tissue and secondly to do no damage during that process of restoration (Box 42.1).

What is healing?

Miller & Dyson (1996) state that healing refers to the body's replacement of destroyed tissue by living tissue. It is a complex integration of processes that results in regeneration of connective tissue, vasculature and epithelium (Wipke-Tevis et al 1996). Wounds heal in two different ways. Healing by primary intention indicates a process in which the wound edges are opposed as soon as possible (Morison 1992). There is no tissue loss; therefore healing is rapid and usually occurs within 24 hours. When wounds heal in this way, granulation

> Box 42.1 **Aims of wound care (Bale & Jones 1997, Dealey 1994, Morison 1992)**
>
> - Create the optimum environment for the natural healing processes to take place.
> - Promote moist wound healing.
> - Protect from trauma and cooling.
> - Prevent the build-up of devitalised tissue and excess exudate.
> - Prevent infection.
> - Promote dignity, comfort and well-being.
> - Restore the function of injured tissue.
> - Maintain the function of the skin.

tissue is not visible and scar formation is minimal. Surgical wounds without complications heal in this way. Healing by secondary intention is more commonly known as granulation. Granulation tissue is formed as part of the healing process in wounds where there is full thickness or deeper damage to the epithelium (Bale & Jones 1997), such as occurs as a result of accidental trauma or a burn.

Phases of wound healing

An understanding of the physiological process of wound healing is vital in making an accurate assessment of any wound; subsequent treatment will depend on the outcome of the assessment.

Inflammatory phase. When tissue is injured, blood vessels are also injured and a blood clot forms in the wound. Damaged cells release histamine causing vasodilatation and increased permeability of the blood vessels, delivering neutrophils and monocytes to the area (Collier 1996). As part of the inflammatory process, fluid leaks out of the surrounding tissues. This causes the swelling which leads to pain (Bale & Jones 1997). It is a normal and natural response and does not indicate infection. This fluid produced by the inflammatory response contains factors which actively promote healing. Its greatest importance is that it contains antibodies, leucocytes and macrophages. These collectively keep bacterial invasion and infection under control. Providing there is no infection or further injury or invasion, the inflammation gradually subsides and the exudate drains back into the circulation.

Destructive phase. During this stage, the leucocytes and macrophages clear the wound of devitalised and unwanted material. While leucocytes play a vital role, healing will continue in their absence (Morison 1992). However, the role of the macrophages is more important during this phase. As well as destroying unwanted material in preparation for cell renewal and wound repair, macrophages also stimulate the formation and multiplication of fibroblasts (Dealey 1994). Fibroblasts synthesise collagen, which is the main protein constituent of white fibrous tissue (Bale & Jones 1997). Collagen then produces a factor which stimulates angiogenesis, which is the growth of new blood vessels.

Proliferative phase. This is where collagen is synthesised by fibroblasts and the strength of the wound is increased (Davidson 1995). New blood vessels begin to infiltrate the wound through the process of angiogenesis. This new tissue formed is known as granulation tissue. The new capillary loops are numerous and very fragile and therefore are easily damaged.

Maturative phase. Collagen fibres that have been randomly laid down are reorganised during this phase. The scar appears large but as the collagen fibres reorganise into tighter positions, the scar is reduced. Owing to the disappearance of vascular granulation tissue during this stage, there is progressive decrease in the vascularity of the scar, thus changing its appearance from dusky red to white. Once the wound bed is filled with granulation tissue, re-epithelialisation begins. Epithelial cells divide and begin to migrate over newly granulating tissue. Epithelialisation occurs up to three times faster in a moist environment than in a dry environment (Morison 1992).

Factors to note

In order to manage a wound effectively, the paediatric nurse needs to be able to assess a wound accurately, because formal assessment of wound status is a prerequisite for good wound care (Gould 1984). Flanagan (1994) identifies that the purposes of wound assessment are:

- to monitor the progress of wound healing
- to evaluate the effectiveness of planned treatment/intervention
- to improve the morale of both patient (child and family) and staff

- to provide a valuable teaching tool for patients (child), staff and carers.

This supports the work of Dealey (1991) who states that wound assessment added to patient assessment has two main aims: to provide baseline information to enable progress to be monitored; and to enable the appropriate selection of dressing to be made. The second aim clearly helps nurses to use resources effectively. Documentation of the wound assessment should include 'the site, type and clinical appearance, incorporating colour and state of the surrounding skin. The amount or absence of exudate, the odour and how much pain the patient is experiencing should also be noted' (Milward 1995, p. 896). Wound appearance that denotes distinguishing differences between wounds expressing either epithelialisation, granulation, sloughy or necrotic areas should also be recorded. An effective wound assessment should include consideration of the components identified; an example of a wound-assessment tool is presented in Figure 42.1.

Figure 42.1
Wound assessment and treatment chart (front of chart).

Hospital No: _____ Ward: _____

Name: _____ Date: _____

Wound type: Surgical _____ Pressure sore _____

Burn/extravasation _____ Other_____

Overall Health Assessment:

Nutrition:

Related Pathology:

Medication:

Biochemistry Results

	Date	Date	Date			Date	Date	Date
ESR					Hb			
WCC					Diff			
Albumin					Glucose			

Additional information:

Signature: _____ Date:_____

Site of Wound:				
Date:				
Wound appearance Pink – epithelialisation Red – granulation Yellow/green – slough/infection Black/brown – necrotic Mixture of above				
Exudate Serous: straw-coloured Haemo serous: reddish Purulent: yellow green Volume: high/mod/low				
Signs of infection Redness, swelling, tender Pyrexia, slough, pain Wound swab sent Isolated organism				
Odour: Yes/No				
Surrounding skin Healthy, moist Oedema, e.g. erythema Dry, e.g. eczema				
Additional information				
Wound assessed by:				

Figure 42.1
*Wound assessment
and treatment chart
(back of chart).*

Before a wound can be assessed its history has to be ascertained, as there are potentially a number of factors that may affect wound healing.

Conditions or factors that may compromise wound healing should also be considered when undertaking wound assessment.

Nutrition

- All children require a diet which contains appropriate nutrients and vitamins. The value of nutrition in the healing process is paramount; there is evidence in the adult literature that wounds in malnourished patients are slow to heal (Shipperely 1997).
- Children who are deficient in nutrients as a result of illness or disease are susceptible to impaired healing:
  - vitamin C deficiency inhibits formation of collagen fibres and capillary development
  - protein deficiency reduces the supply of amino acids for tissue repair
  - zinc deficiency impairs epithelialisation.

- Children with special needs may have difficulty eating, drinking and swallowing; therefore skilled assistance is needed to ensure adequate intake of nutrition.

Disease or pathology

- Diabetes mellitus: hyperglycaemia impairs phagocytosis, which is the engulfing and destruction of bacteria, foreign bodies and necrotic tissue by phagocytes. It also inhibits collagen synthesis and impairs circulation and capillary growth.
- Anaemia: healing may be impaired through reducing oxygen transportation (McClaren 1992).
- Compromised immunological status, such as in children with a malignancy, HIV/AIDS or an immunodeficiency disorder: healing in these conditions is delayed because of reduced efficiency of the immune system. Secondary to this is a decreased resistance to infection, which in turn will delay healing (Morison 1992).
- Impaired circulation reduces the supply of nutrients to the wound area, and inhibits the inflammatory response and removal of debris from the wound.

Medication

- Cytotoxic drugs and radiotherapy interfere with cell proliferation during the process of healing (Morison 1992). Radiation inhibits fibroblastic activity and capillary formation; it may also cause necrosis.
- Prolonged steroid therapy delays healing during the inflammatory and proliferative phases (Bale & Jones 1997). It impairs phagocytosis, inhibits fibroblast proliferation, depresses formation of granulation tissue and inhibits wound contraction.

Other causes

- Pain and stress can affect the immune system and thus interfere with wound healing.
- Foreign bodies inhibit wound closure and increase the inflammatory response.
- Infection increases the inflammatory response and increases tissue destruction.
- Mechanical friction damages or destroys granulation tissue.

Guidelines when undertaking wound care

The approach to wound care encompasses consideration of wound assessment, wound cleansing techniques, wound cleansing solutions and wound dressings. The paediatric nurse, in consultation with other members of the multidisciplinary team, must make an informed decision on what approach is the most appropriate for a particular child and a particular wound. This will be based on ongoing assessment. It is essential for the nurse to have knowledge of the individual child prior to undertaking the practice. In addition, knowledge of the wound is required, noting cause, site, presence of sutures and drain. It is also important that nurses are aware of the future nursing and medical management of the wound. This information can be gained from the nursing and medical notes. Preparation includes collection and organisation of equipment, which includes cleansing solution, wound cleansing tools and dressing; informing the child and family; positioning the child; use of play and inclusion of a play therapist.

Wound cleansing techniques

Wounds are either swabbed or irrigated.

Swabbing.   Care must be taken in swabbing a wound when newly granulating or epithelialising tissue is present; healing may be interfered with as a result of swabbing, even when carried out in a gentle manner. In addition, there is some literature to suggest that fibres shed from cotton wool swabs can become entwined in granulating tissue and be the foci for infection (Briggs 1996). A clean granulating wound should be left untouched, leaving the exudate to nourish the natural healing process (Dealey 1994). However, a necrotic wound would require cleansing or debriding to remove dead tissue. Modern interactive dressings such as hydrocolloids and hydrogels can be used to soften and hydrate the wound before swabbing. This makes the process less traumatic when swabbing to remove dead tissue. This has implications for practice and suggests daily changes of dressing and cleaning of wounds should be discouraged where possible.

Irrigation.   Cleansing by irrigation with warmed solutions will prevent the shedding of fibres into the wound bed and avoid the complications already mentioned associated with swabbing. This technique is now being advocated. However, one of the difficulties of this method is in assessing the amount of pressure to be used when irrigating; it should be enough to dislodge debris without causing damage to the underlying tissues.

Cleansing by bathing and showering.   Bathing and showering are now recommended for wound cleansing (Briggs 1994, Oliver 1997). The use of bathing and showering in paediatrics is much less frightening and traumatic than other methods of wound cleansing and it can also be a playful experience. Many children prefer to remove their own dressings by soaking them off in the bath or shower (Bale 1996). In surgical wounds, once skin edges have sealed, bathing or showering is not likely to present any further risk (Briggs 1997). Gilchrist (1990, p. 66) suggests 'a shower may be preferable to a bath following surgery as there is less possibility of cross infection'. In hospitals the issue of cross-infection must be considered; therefore careful measures for disinfection must be taken between children.

Wound cleansing solutions

Paediatric nurses must be fully aware of the advantages and disadvantages of the different solutions available; research literature is often contradictory with no firm conclusions drawn. Critical analysis of the literature, applied to practice, has resulted in the development of guidelines (Table 42.1).

Wound dressings

Dressings have clear advantages and disadvantages and, if used incorrectly, adverse effects may occur. In addition, choosing an appropriate dressing is difficult, especially with the wide and confusing range that is available for use today. For children, the dressing must be easy to apply and remove and be able to withstand the rigors of children's activities (Teare 1997). It is also important that the dressing can be made secure enough to prevent the child from interfering with the wound. Therefore nurses have considerable responsibilities in choosing the most appropriate dressing for children. Critical analysis of the literature, applied to practice, has resulted in the development of guidelines (Table 42.2).

Table 42.1 **Guidelines for use of cleansing solutions**

Type	Advantages	Disadvantages
0.9% sodium chloride	Non-toxic to human tissues	No written documentation of disadvantages in literature
	Does not give rise to sensitivity reactions	
	Inexpensive	
	Most effective and appropriate solution and is least harmful (Trevelyn 1996)	
	Simple non-irritant solution	
	Isotonic solution – minimises the risk of cell damage during irrigation	
Betadine: povidone-iodine Aqueous solution and alcoholic solution	Has a wide spectrum of activity against most major pathogens	Action is reduced in contact with pus and exudate
	Used effectively to clean unbroken skin, e.g. preoperatively	Adverse reactions may be possible
	Cleans grossly infected wounds	Alcohol solutions should be avoided in wounds – may interfere with the healing process and can have toxic effect (Morison 1992)
	Active against methicillin-resistant *Staphylococcus aureus* (MRSA)	Need time to bring about the desired effect

Table 42.1 (Contd.)   **Guidelines for use of cleansing solutions**

Type	Advantages	Disadvantages
Chlorhexidine	Active against a wide range of Gram-positive and -negative organisms	Resistance in *Pseudomonas aeruginosa*, acid-fast bacilli, fungi and viruses
	Only 0.05% solutions recommended for use on wounds	Sensitivity and allergic reactions may occur
	Used effectively to clean unbroken skin	Toxic to fibroblasts even at high dilutions
		Ineffective against MRSA
		Activity reduced by blood, pus and soap
Hydrogen peroxide	Used to clean dirty, infected, necrotic, sloughy wounds	Caustic effect on wounds in concentrations above 6%
	Has an oxidising effect which destroys anaerobic bacteria	Hydrogen peroxide above 3% is toxic to fibroblasts, therefore delays healing (Miller & Dyson 1996)
		0.003% dilution is not effective against bacteria
		Loses its effect when it comes in contact with pus or cotton gauze

Factors to note:
Sodium chloride 0.9% is currently recommended as the solution of choice for wound cleansing (White 1997).
Povidone-iodine should only be used when the wound is infected and for not longer than 21 days.
Routine use of iodine-containing solutions should be avoided in very low birth weight infants.
Iodine absorption may cause hypothyroidism during a critical period of neurological development (Smerdely & Boyages 1989).

Equipment

- Dressing trolley or appropriate clean surface
- Sterile dressing pack containing plastic tray, non-woven swabs, pair of gloves, sterile towel
- Sterile gloves if not contained in dressing pack
- Hypoallergenic tape
- Plastic disposable apron
- Cleansing solution of choice
- Sterile additional non-woven swabs, if wound is large
- Large disposable plastic bag for soiled disposables
- Sterile syringe for irrigation
- Wound swab
- Appropriate dressing materials

Method

Preparation of the child

- Explain the procedure to the child in an age-appropriate manner and to the main caregivers. Ensure understanding and identify their role throughout the dressing change.
- Use play and involve the play specialist.
- Allow enough time between information giving and performing the practice – too much time may cause the child to become anxious, too little may not allow the play specialist time to prepare the child adequately.

Table 42.2 Guidelines for good practice in the selection of dressings (Dealey 1994)

Group	Type	Indications	Contraindications	Advantages	Disadvantages	Dressing changes
Absorbent	Cellulose wadding, cotton wool, Gamgee	Use only as secondary dressings when there is heavy exudate	As a primary dressing on open wounds / On the surface of a moist wound	Excellent secondary dressing for padding and protection	Adhere to the wound base / Dehydrate the wound 'Strike through' occurs / Shed fibres into the wound	Change using strict aseptic techniques / When exudate 'strikes through' / Up to 7 days
Hydrogels	Intrasite Gel, Vigilon, Geliperm (sheet hydrogel), Clearsite	Light to medium exuding, e.g. granulating wounds / To deslough necrotic or sloughy wounds / To remove black eschar	May cause allergic reactions / Contraindicated where anaerobic infection is suspected / Can support the growth of microorganisms	Provide ideal moist environment / Comfortable and soothing / Can be used with semipermeable films, thus allowing bathing (Bale & Jones 1997)	All hydrogels need a secondary dressing except Clearsite / Generally too expensive for routine use	Gel: applied at least 5 mm thick to the surface of the wound and covered with a moisture-retaining dressing / Sheet dressings are placed onto the surface and need a secondary dressing / On very dry wounds, Intrasite Gel needs daily changes / For sheet hydrogels, every 3–4 days is recommended
Alginates	Kaltostat, Sorbsan, Sorbsan Plus / Kaltostat Fortex / Sorbsan S.A.	Sloughy wounds, moderate to heavy exudate / Heavy exudate / Has a self-	On dry wounds with no or low exudate / On wounds covered with hard necrotic tissue	Provide ideal moist environment / Allow pain-free dressing changes / Fresh granulation tissue is not distributed	Kaltostat can cause maceration and excoriation of the surrounding area, dressings should be trimmed	Every effort should be made not to disturb the dressing. Even though manufacturers' instruction leaflets suggest daily dressing changes at first, this is not necessary if a thick

Dressing	Indications / use	Cautions	Advantages	Special considerations	Frequency of dressing change
			Sorbsan does not cause skin maceration and excoriations	adhesive (S.A.) border that attaches to the area surrounding the wound, thus preventing water penetration (can be worn while bathing)	absorbent pad is placed as a secondary dressing (Bux 1996)
			Have haemostatic properties		Change after 3–5 days at first, then after up to 7 days (Dealey 1994)
Kaltoclude		Worn for bathing			Change daily if infected; removal can be facilitated by irrigating with 0.9% sodium chloride solution
Ribbon and rope alginates		For packing cavity wounds			
Special consideration	Alginates can be used on infected wounds. Topical antibiotics or antimicrobial agents should not be used with alginates				
Foam dressing	Allevyn, Lyofoam, Spyrosorb, Tielle	To absorb exudate on exuding wounds	For dry eschar, non-exuding wounds	Encourages moist wound healing		Allevyn: allow 2–3 cm margin around wound. Tape white-patterned side to wound. Changing depends on the amount of exudate. Leave 3–5 days in situ for clean, non-infected wounds
		Allevyn and Lyofoam can be used with infected wounds	Known allergy to dressing	Makes for less painful dressing changes		Lyofoam: allow 2–3 cm overlap over wound edges. Change if exudate leaks along edge of dressing. Otherwise changing is not necessary for up to 7 days
		Spyrosorb and Tielle are not to be used on clinically infected wounds	May adhere if exudate becomes reduced	Easy to apply and to remove		Spyrosorb: change when exudate can be seen within 1 cm of the edge of the dressing. Up to 7 days
			Spyrosorb and Tielle will not absorb heavy exudate	Non-adherent		Tielle: frequency of change depends on amount of exudate. Up to 7 days

Table 42.2 Guidelines for good practice in the selection of dressings (Dealey 1994) (Contd.)

Group	Type	Indications	Contraindications	Advantages	Disadvantages	Dressing changes
Low-adherent dressings	Melolin	On dry or slightly exuding wounds	On heavily exuding wounds	Protect a wound Absorb a little exudate	Do not absorb excessive exudate	If very dry prior to changing, moisten before removal to protect viable tissue
	NA Dressing	As a secondary dressing			Some adherence to the wound	Up to 7 days
	Release				Secondary dressing are needed, i.e. adhesive tapes or bandages	
	Tricotex				Do not provide a moist environment	
Hydrocolloids	Granuflex	For granulating wounds which have low to medium amounts of exudate	Should not be used with children who have a known sensitivity to the type of hydrocolloid used	Can be used on infected wounds Create a moist wound environment	Some controversy in the past that the occlusive nature of hydrocolloid dressings may cause wound infection. Recent evidence suggests that this is unlikely (Dealey 1994)	Warm between hands Dressing should extend at least 2 cm beyond the edge of the wound. As it liquefies, there are characteristic odours and yellow appearance on reaction with exudate. Change when bubble reaches 1.5 cm from edge, then peel off from the edge
	Comfeel	Suitable for desloughing light to medium exuding wounds		Are absorbent or waterproof so patient can bathe Have barrier properties to bacteria. Control the spread of MRSA; no need to isolate	Non-transparent	Initially dressing may need changing daily. Once exudate decreases, dressing may be left in situ for up to 7 days. Infected wounds may need more regular dressing changes. If there is very heavy exudate demanding daily dressings, possibly change to alginate
	Tegasorb	For moderately exuding wounds		Break down devitalised tissue Stimulate the growth of new blood vessels Can be used as a secondary dressing Require no secondary dressing Provide pain relief by keeping nerve endings moist	Unpleasant odour from gel dressing Findings show gel becomes incorporated into granulating tissue (Rousseau & Niecestro 1991)	Frequency of changes will depend on amount of exudate. Change as needed for leakage

- Introduce the use of distraction, where appropriate.
- Assess the child for the need for analgesia, which should be given half an hour prior to cleansing the wound.
- Ensure that all the potential equipment required is on the dressing trolley.
- Positioning of the child will depend on the site or location of the wound; it will also depend on the chosen method for cleansing.
- Choose a position that is most comfortable and reasssuring for the child, ensuring that the wound is easily accessible.
- Infants or small children can lie or sit on an adult's lap, if the wound site permits.
- Ensure that the child is in a safe position throughout.
- Positioning children in the bath or shower may be another option, to soak off dressings (Bale & Jones 1997).
- Ensure that the child is kept warm and dressing time is kept to a minimum, thus decreasing heat loss and discomfort for the child.
- Ensure that a young child has her favourite cuddly toy or comforter with her throughout.

Wound care practice

- Ensure adequate time is available to undertake the wound dressing.
- Explain all the steps of the practice, in advance of them occurring, and throughout, to the child and parent.
- Perform the dressing using aseptic non-touch technique (see Aseptic Non-touch Technique, p. 39); ensure thorough handwashing.
- Moisten the dressing with warm, sterile solution such as normal saline. If appropriate, allow the child, in as far as is possible, to remove the dressing gently, avoiding damage to new granulation or epithelial tissue (this may be undertaken in the shower or bath).
- Warm the irrigation solution as this helps to maintain temperature at the wound site (Thomas 1994).
- Irrigate the wound using a syringe.
- Assess the surrounding skin together with categorising the tissue status of the wound (Milward 1995).
- The choice of dressing for the contact layer, which is the primary dressing, will depend on the type of tissue categorised (Harding & Jones 1996).
- The choice of secondary dressing used will often depend on the contact layer (Harding & Jones 1996).

- Assess pain at the wound site.
- Secure the dressing using an appropriate method.
- For children who have special needs, it may be difficult to carry out aseptic non-touch technique at dressing changes. With this group of children, it is even more important that their dressing is secured; to avoid the use of tape that can be easily removed may require some creative thinking.
- Document the assessment and management by completing the wound assessment and treatment chart, and record information in the child's nursing notes.

> ### COMMUNITY PERSPECTIVE
> The principles when undertaking wound care in the community are the same as in hospital; however, the CCN may need to be adaptable to maintain a safe practice in the home (see Aseptic Non-touch Technique, p. 39).
>
> Analgesia, if required, may be given prior to the CCN's visit, allowing time for the drug to work. Alternatively, Entonox may be self-administered by the child during the procedure.

Do and do not

- Do involve the child and family.
- Do ensure that the multidisciplinary team are involved.
- Do individualise the child's wound care.
- Do assess the wound systematically, using where possible an assessment tool, and categorise the tissue status.
- Do record wound assessment and wound care in the nursing notes.
- Do swab the wound if infection is suspected.
- Do minimise wound care problems by introducing evidence-based care.
- Do consider the factors that may influence wound healing.
- Do use play and distraction when undertaking wound care practice.
- Do assess the child for the need for analgesia.
- Do minimise the time taken to undertake the dressing change.
- Do not use cotton wool balls when swabbing.
- Do not use too much pressure when irrigating a wound.
- Do not use force to remove a dressing.
- Do not use forceps when cleaning a wound.
- Do not use high concentrations of Eusol and hydrogen peroxide on wounds.
- Do not use alcohol solution of Betadine on wounds.

References

Bale S 1996 Caring for children with wounds. Journal of Wound Care 5(4): 177–180

Bale S, Jones V 1997 Wound care nursing – a patient centred approach. Baillière Tindall, London

Briggs M 1994 Choosing wound care packs: a survey. Nursing Standard 8(23): 36–39

Briggs M 1996 The principles of aseptic technique in wound care. Professional Nurse 11(12): 805–810

Briggs M 1997 Principles of closed surgical wound care. Journal of Wound Care 6(6): 288–292

Bux M 1996 Selection and use of wound dressings. Wound Care for Pharmacists (Summer): 11–16

Collier M 1996 The principles of optimum wound management. Nursing Standard 10(43): 47–52

Davidson A 1995 Surgical infection. Nursing Times 91(39): 59–65

Dealey C 1991 Assessment of wounds. Nursing 4(27): 23–24

Dealey C 1994 The care of wounds. Blackwell Science, Cambridge

Flanagan M 1994 Assessment criteria. Nursing Times 90(35): 76–88

Gilchrist B 1990 Washing and dressing after surgery. Nursing Times 86(50 suppl): 71

Gould D 1984 Clinical forum. Nursing Mirror 159(16): 3–6

Harding K, Jones V 1996 Wound management: good practice guidelines. Macmillan Magazines, London

Higgins C 1996 Leucocytes and the value of the differential count test. Nursing Times 92(20): 34–35

Longaker M, Adzick N, Hall J et al 1990 Studies in fetal wound healing, VII. Fetal wound healing may be modulated by hyaluronic acid stimulating activity in amniotic fluid. Journal of Paediatric Surgery 25(4): 430–433

McClaren S 1992 Nutrition and wound healing. Journal of Wound Care 1(3): 45–55

Miller M, Dyson M 1996 Principles of wound care. Macmillan Magazines, London

Milward P 1995 Common problems associated with necrotic and sloughy wounds. British Journal of Nursing 4(15): 896–900

Morison M 1992 A colour guide to the nursing management of wounds. Wolfe, London

Oliver L 1997 Wound cleansing. Nursing Standard 11(20): 47–51

Rousseau P, Niecestro R M 1991 A review of the physiochemical properties of two gel and non-gel forming hydrocolloid dressings. Wounds 3(l): 43–48

Shipperely T 1997 The importance of assessing patients with leg ulceration. British Journal of Nursing 6(2): 71–80

Skale N 1992 Pediatric nursing procedures. Lippincott, Philadelphia

Smerdely P, Boyages S, We D 1989 Topical iodine containing antiseptics and neonatal hypothyroidism in very low birth weight babies. Lancet 2: 661–664

Teare J 1997 A home care team in paediatric wound care. Journal of Wound Care 6(6): 295–296

Thomas S 1994 Wound cleansing agents. Journal of Wound Care 3(7): 325–328

Trevelyn J 1996 Wound cleansing principles and practice. Nursing Times 92(16): 46–48

White C 1997 Wound cleansing: Guidelines for A&E staff. Nursing Times 93(2): 46–48

Wipke-Tevis D, Stotts N, Skov P, Carrieri-Kohlman V 1996 Frequency, manifestations and correlates of impaired healing of saphenous vein harvest incisions. Heart and Lung, Journal of Acute and Critical Care 25(2): 108–115

Further reading

Griffith G 1991 Choosing a dressing. Nursing Times 87(36): 84–90

Harding K 1992 The wound programme. Centre for Medical Education, University of Dundee

Jones I 1994 Removal of sutures and staples. Skills update, book 3. Macmillan Magazines, London

Lawrence J C 1997 Wound irrigation. Journal of Wound Care 6(l): 23–26

Morgan D 1994 Formulary of wound management products – a guide for health care staff, 6th edn. Euromed Communications, Haslemere

Morison M 1992 A colour guide to the nursing management of wounds. Wolfe, London

Roberts G 1988 Nutrition and wound healing. Nursing Standard 2(51 suppl): 8–12

Thomas S 1990 Wound management and dressings. Pharmaceutical Press, London

Thomas S 1991 Evidence fails to justify use of hypochlorite. Journal of Tissue Viability 1(1): 9–10

Thomlinson D 1987 To clean or not to clean. Nursing Times 92(16): 71–75

Appendix 1: Play

Introduction

Play forms an integral part of the care of the sick child. Most practical procedures involving the child will at some stage include some aspect of play. Play facilitates communication between the child and his carers, thereby providing a sense of control, trust and understanding. There are a variety of different types of play applicable to children according to their age and stage of development. These will be described, citing examples from practice of children who have successfully used play to help them understand and cope with their illness. Play programmes designed for the hospitalised child, taking into account the child's individual needs, age, cognitive understanding and illness, can provide a positive introduction to the ward environment, thus aiding the nurse in her holistic care of the child. The core of this text is designed to explore the importance of play in the life of the sick child. It is hoped that those who use this book will find this section a useful addition. Figures A1.1 and A1.2 show a visual interpretation of the nature and functions of play.

'Through play, a child will make sense of the world' (OMEP 1966, cited in Morris 1989). When children are provided with an environment where play occurs naturally, they are able to express feelings, indulge in fantasy and work through difficult situations if appropriate. This latter aspect is one where the intervention of skilled and trained adults may be needed. Hospital play specialists (HPS) are people who have undergone an appropriate training and have the in-depth knowledge and skills to work with children when they are sick, to help them cope with their illness through play. As play is a pleasurable activity, its normality helps to promote confidence in an unfamiliar environment, thus aiding the recovery process.

The use of play was initially introduced into paediatric wards in 1963, when Consultant Paediatrician, Dr Morris, noted how withdrawn and unnatural children appeared to be when admitted to hospital (Morris 1989). He believed that just because a child was in hospital, opportunities for play should not be taken away. Playschemes were set up by Save the Children Fund with the aim of reducing stress and anxiety and encouraging normal play.

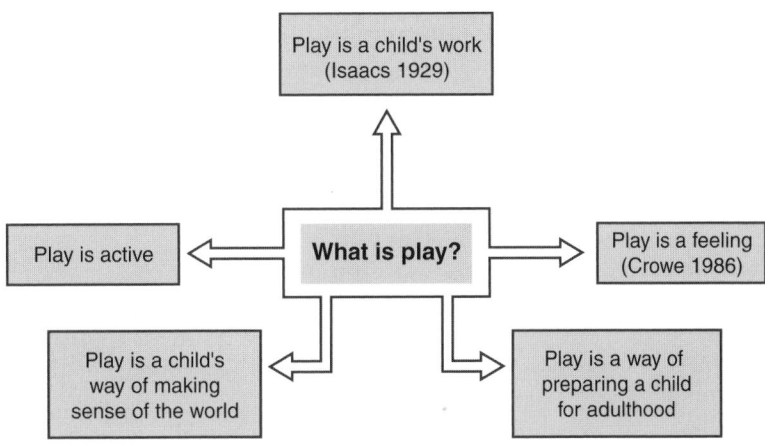

Figure A1.1
The nature of play.

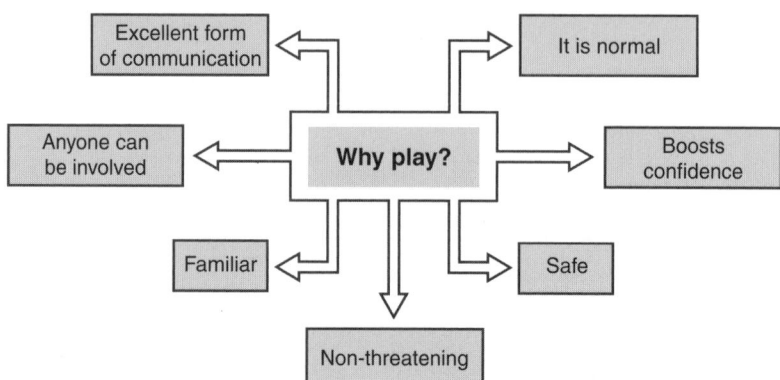

Figure A1.2
The functions of play.

Play is an activity that we are all involved in, often without realising it. From waving to a baby in a cot, which involves eye contact and communication, to a more involved imaginative play session with an older child, both are forms of play. The involvement and cooperation of the child with the adult has healing potential for the child. Some people may think that they have forgotten how to play, or have never experienced play themselves. To those of you in this situation, just relax and do what comes naturally, let the children take the lead, copy them, laugh with them, get down to their level physically as well as spiritually. The child's uncomplicated mind will easily show us how to enjoy play, but sometimes our expectations and inhibitions get in the way. Once the child's trust has been obtained, the ability to play becomes one of the greatest assets of a children's nurse.

Preparation

Play in hospital aims to inform children about the unusual situation in which they find themselves and thereby allay fears and increase confidence. It will also provide a much needed link with home and normality. Using play preoperatively, or prior to other frightening procedures (venepuncture, radiotherapy, nasogastric feeding), goes a long way in helping children to express their real feelings.

Before preparing a child for a procedure or operation, time should be taken to get to know the child. It is also important that whoever is leading the session is fully aware of the implications of the operation or procedure for the child. It is important to ascertain what the child already knows and to find out about any previous experiences. During preparation, the use of real hospital equipment is vital. The use of syringes, masks, EMLA cream patches, stethoscopes, etc. will allow children to familiarise themselves with and partially experience their future treatment or procedure. Picture books, photographs and videos may help a child by clarifying images and thoughts. Wolfer (1979) showed that by providing the child with accurate information about procedures in a safe, non-threatening environment the child was able to cope more effectively in a potentially stressful situation (see examples in Box A1.1).

During preparation sessions the child must be given physical and emotional space to express his feelings and fears. The session should not be rushed as this may add to the child's feeling of loss of control. The whole hospital experience tends to remove control from the child. If the child can be given space to think through and explore the forthcoming procedure through play, he can be given back some control over the situation, and this will help boost his confidence.

Note: The child should *always* be warned if the procedure is going to hurt as this will help build up a trusting relationship.

Preparation guidelines (see Table A1.1)
1. Always be honest with the child.
2. Information should be given to both child and family, ensuring that it is consistent and allowing time for questions.

> **Box A1.1   Examples of ways in which play can allay fear in children**
>
> 1. A 5-year-old with leukaemia, who was 18 months into his treatment, had a cannula inserted to administer antibiotics. During the procedure he displayed his anger by reacting violently. It was not until 2 days later, through a play session with the HPS, that the child realised it was only a piece of tubing in his arm and not a needle. He then became much more relaxed about the situation and cooperated well during follow-up procedures.
> 2. 'Jack', a doll with a Hickman line attached, allows children to work through their own personal medical experience (see Fig. A1.3).

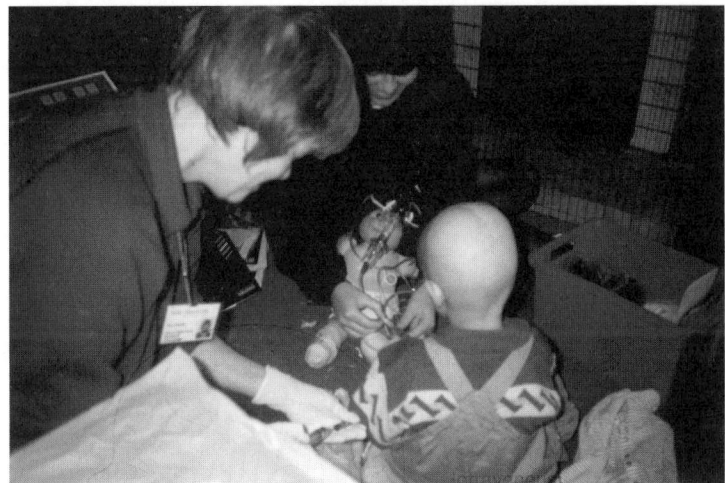

Figure A1.3
Child administering pretend drugs to 'Jack' whilst the nurse administers the child's drugs.

3. Use appropriate language, taking into account the child's age and understanding.
4. Avoid using phrases such as 'We will give you medicine to put you to sleep.' This can be confused with when a pet dies and is 'put to sleep'. 'Can I take your temperature?' may evoke anxiety as to where you are taking it: 'Will I get it back?'
5. Use breathing techniques. During venepuncture, some children will be helped by getting them to breathe in; then as the needle is inserted they can be asked to breathe out. This may help them feel that they have more control over the situation.
6. If the child is upset and screaming, in some situations it is possible to scream with him, thereby showing that this expression of pain and fear is understandable. This must be used with caution, as it can be most upsetting for other children and their parents.
7. It is important that everyone dealing with the child is as relaxed as possible, as this will give confidence to both child and family.
8. Children often regress whilst in hospital and may require repetitive explanations and information about their procedures.
9. Some parents may be anxious that telling their child about a procedure will cause him more anxiety. It is worth explaining that a child who is not given accurate information may fantasise and fear something worse.
10. All children and families are different, with a variety of previous experiences. The preparation must be tailored to fit the particular situation.

Emergency admissions and procedures often do not allow for effective preparation; it is worth ensuring that a preparation book (a book with a series of descriptive photographs about procedures) is always available.

Table A1.1 **Quick glance preparation guidelines**

Age	Developmental stage	Strategy
2–3 years	Short attention span Limited vocabulary Does not understand timescales	Prepare 1 day before at most Work with the parents Use real equipment, and a teddy/doll to demonstrate on
3–5 years	Attention span of approx. 5 minutes Questions: asks why and how? Eager to learn and absorb new experiences Believes all body parts are essential	Give short bursts of factual information, allowing time for questions Reassure and help to understand the operation/procedure Provide opportunities to play with real equipment.
6–11 years	Peer group important Good language skills Understands concept of time	Prepare child in privacy Provide specific information, using basic medical terminology Use body outlines and dolls to explain procedure Preparation can be given in advance
12 years to adolescent	Peer group very important Concern over body image May fear waking up during operation Values independence Capable of abstract thought	The involvement of another experienced adolescent may help Provide privacy and clear up any misconceptions Explain anaesthetist's role Offer preparation away from parents

Types of play

Play in hospital can be based around the work of Sylva (1993) who describes two main categories of play: normative and therapeutic.

The purpose of normative play is to establish norms and rules. This sort of play, which children use most often, engages others, including friends and siblings and uses the toys around the child. Normative play helps to bring familiarity to an unfamiliar situation such as an experience in hospital. Normative play is undertaken voluntarily and it is pleasurable. Very rarely does it have any

goals and the child is in control. In a safe, relaxed and inviting environment children can feel able to carry out their play.

Therapeutic play, the second category described by Sylva, is structured by adults and followed through by the child. Its purpose is to help the child to achieve 'emotional and physical well-being' by means of various activities, in order to achieve therapeutic ends. Through play, a child is given the opportunity to overcome fears and anxieties by bringing unconscious feelings to the surface. This play also incorporates desensitisation. A child who developed a needle phobia was able, with great pleasure, to work through his feelings of anxiety by handling and familiarising himself with the properties of a syringe, firstly without a needle, then progressed to using a needle and injecting into an orange. The mother was also present during this session and felt comfortable handling the syringe and working through her own anxieties relating to her son's treatment.

Puppets allow children to talk about their illness through the third person and are very simple and quick to create; for example, draw a face on your finger and bring the child into conversation. A 3-year-old with cancer was able to express her feelings of anger with ease when encouraged to do so with a finger puppet. She talked to the puppet about the horrible taste of the medicine in her mouth and about how cold it felt when it went into her tummy.

Another 4-year-old with arthritis expressed her anger at her consultant by using 'play-mobile' people. She positioned the characters in such a way that the one she had decided was to become the consultant was in a bed and she was the nurse inflicting pain on him; she squealed with delight when he cried. The most favourite activity postoperatively is 'gunging' the imaginary doctor or nurse with cornflour mixture. After an uncomfortable procedure has been carried out, silent play or simple discussion using any of the above examples can allow the child to be angry about the invasion of his or her body in a secure and non-threatening environment.

Messy play

Messy play is an activity which allows children to be as messy as they wish. This is very beneficial in the clinical environment of the hospital. It is a great kick against the system and an outlet for expression of emotion, be it frustration, anger, despair, loneliness or isolation. Playdough, cornflour and water, syringe painting, all provide therapeutic opportunities for expressive play. A young sibling showed great pleasure in thumping the playdough very hard when her sister was readmitted to the children's ward on her birthday, which was seen as a reflection of her inner feelings.

Use of paintings and drawings may also allow children to express how they are feeling about a situation.

Distraction

Distraction therapy during an unfamiliar procedure helps to limit the anxiety and stress that a child may feel.

Bubbles. Encourage the child to blow the bubbles high and low. Look at colours and shapes within them.

Counting. Use number games; count up and down.

Hangman. The game can be adapted to hang the person for whom the child feels anger.

Puppets. Encourage the child to talk about procedures, using the puppet.

Imagination. Talk with the child about his favourite activity or hobby.

Breathing. Encourage the child to control his breathing. Breathe in and hold for a few moments.

Relaxation tapes. Play the tape during a procedure. Gently talk the child through the forthcoming procedure.

Shouting. Allow the child to shout. Shout with him, if appropriate.

Squeezing. In stressful situations, give the child a ball to squeeze.

Design a distraction box full of bells, rattles, books, lights, musical tapes, party blowers and paper. Leave it in the treatment room for easy accessibility.

Visualisation

Visualisation exercises can be easily learned and can assist in the care offered to the anxious child (Ott 1996). Visualisation exercises are helpful when undertaken by those familiar with the procedure. They should be used with caution and not by inexperienced practitioners. There are possibilities for such exercises to be done pre- or postoperatively. Such exercises are a useful form of support which may be used to help children through other stressful times in their life (Ott 1996).

Play and the way forward

Siblings often experience feelings of abandonment, guilt, loss and uncertainty. Introducing play that includes the sibling will go a long way to encourage harmony within the family during an unfamiliar experience of hospitalisation.

Play specialists are now employed on most children's wards across the country. The introduction of a team member who works regular hours and is responsible for creating a safe, fun and non-threatening environment, gives the child some normality in an abnormal situation. The ability to create an environment where play occurs naturally is the best gift offered to sick children and their families.

The children's nurse who is able to understand the importance and value of play will add a vital component to her nursing skills, not only on the ward but also en route to theatre, in the anaesthetic room and in all other areas where children are nursed.

References

Crowe B 1986 Play is a feeling. Unwin Paperbacks, London

Isaacs S 1929 The nursery years. Routledge and Kegan Paul, London

Morris D 1989 Hospital – a deprived environment for children. A case for hospital playschemes. Save the Children Fund, London

Organisation Mondiale pour l'Education Prescolaire (OMEP) 1966 Play in hospital. Report by the World Organisation for Early Childhood Education.

Ott M 1996 Imagine the possibilities: guided imagery with toddlers and preschoolers. Pediatric Nursing 22(1): 34–38

Sylva, K 1993 Play in hospital – when and why it's effective. Current Paediatrics 3: 247–249

Wolfer J 1979 Psychological preparation for surgical patients: the effects on children's and parents' stress responses and adjustment. Paediatrics 56: 2

Further reading

Amylase R 1994 The excellence of play. Open University Press, Buckingham

Cohen D 1993 The development of play. Routledge, London

Davenport G 1991 An introduction to child development. HarperCollins, London

Hughes F 1991 Children, play and development. Allyn and Bacon, Massachusetts

Weller B 1980 Helping sick children play. Baillière Tindall, London

Appendix 2: Complementary Therapies

Introduction

Interest in complementary medicine has steadily increased over the past 10 years as witnessed by the numbers of people attending complementary practitioners. Barnes & Ernst (1997) suggest that one-third to a half of the population use some form of complementary therapy. There is a wide variety of books available on different therapies, which are targeted at both the lay person and the health care professional, as well as a range of courses available from certificate to higher degree level. With this interest and uptake comes the need for careful consideration when introducing the different therapies into nursing care.

The purpose of this appendix is to give a broad overview and definition of some of the more commonly used therapies; identify where and why they may be offered, particularly in relation to some of the procedures discussed in the main text; suggest aims for implementing complementary therapies; consider the question of consent; and provide some cautionary notes about specific therapies. At the end is a list of useful addresses and contacts where further information can be accessed by the reader. The therapies included are aromatherapy, reflexology, massage, therapeutic touch, hypnotherapy, visualisation and guided imagery, Bach flower remedies and craniosacral therapy.

The terms *complementary* and *alternative* therapies are often used synonymously and it is very difficult to define accurately what is meant by each – definitions may say more about the political stance of the authors than about exactly what is meant by the terms (Stone & Matthews 1996).

Complementary implies working alongside orthodox medical practice. It is used to imply cooperation with orthodox medicine as opposed to being in competition with it (Sharma 1992). Examples include aromatherapy and reflexology. There is not necessarily an expectation of cure attached and one has to be very careful with such terminology.

Alternative tends to mean outside of orthodox medicine and therapies may be associated with claims of their being curative. They are usually supported by a body of knowledge or theory about the causes of illness and health imbalance. The therapy may require some sort of technical intervention on the part of an expert practitioner. Examples include homeopathy, medical herbalism and osteopathy (Sharma 1992).

Complementary medicine is not new: some of the principal therapies used today have their roots in ancient times, with some such as aromatherapy going back 5000 years or more (Harrison 1995). But in spite of the relative antiquity of some therapies, it should not be assumed that they are automatically endowed with credibility and nurses must be rigorous in their understanding of each chosen therapy in order to ensure efficacy. They may also need to be able to answer their critics, for there is still considerable scepticism regarding the use of complementary medicine in health care today.

Smith (1995), writing in the *British Medical Journal*, suggested that commissioning health authorities should 're-think old prejudices' regarding complementary therapies, yet many nurses face difficulties in gaining acceptance for incorporating the therapies into practice. Some health care units in the UK, both hospital and community, offer complementary therapies to adults, when allopathic medicine may have nothing more to offer. This is particularly the case in the areas of chronic disease and palliative care. However, Barnes & Ernst (1997) suggest that the medical profession's level of interest in complementary medicine is increasing. It is not clear how many trusts and authorities offer therapies to children as a recognised part of care. The reasons for this scepticism are multifactorial and culturally and politically complex (Gabe et al 1994), in part based on historical prejudices (Lupton 1994). There is also some questioning over cost-effectiveness (Ernst 1997). Such discussion is certainly beyond the scope of this work, but nevertheless is an important part of the health care debate.

Nurses, who undertake courses should not be disheartened by challenges to their therapy, but should continue to develop their knowledge base and reflective skills. They should be rigorous and analytical of the quality of their work and also the literature they may use to argue the benefits of their chosen therapies. They should develop their communication and negotiation skills, in order to build a team around them of like-minded people for mutual support, whilst putting forward sound strategies for implementation of the therapies. Likewise they should value their role in furthering the dialogue within the health care arena to ensure that the interests and well-being of patients, practitioners and organisations are appropriately served. The RCN Complementary Therapies Forum is a useful means of networking with other practitioners around the country.

Once implemented, the benefits of the therapies should be evaluated and nurses in practice are in the best position to do this. A mechanism for evaluation and also for supervision and support for practitioners by specialists in the field of complementary medicine (Nicoll 1995) should be established.

Suggested aims of complementary therapies in child care

- To improve the quality of a child's experience, communications and continuity of care.
- To enhance the quality of a child's life, in terms of symptom management for acute, chronic and terminal conditions.
- To reduce anxiety and fear that may exacerbate the child's experience.
- To enhance the relationships between child and nurse, child and parent(s), nurse and family.
- To encourage fun and distraction.
- To improve motivation, alertness and healing potential.
- To provide different approaches to care to enable children to work towards realising their potential – to take some control.
- To provide an opportunity for nurses to observe and enhance their understanding of child development and behaviours and for the children to learn and understand more of themselves.

Complementary therapies have an important part to play in the care and well-being of children and, when offering a therapy, one should be cognisant of the individuality of children and the place each child holds in his family. Every child has his own story to tell and each visit or therapy session may bring different issues. Therefore, the therapist should be alert to the responses,

verbal and non-verbal, of children and their families and be skilled in the art of reflective practice.

Consent

The question of consent has been debated over the years and it is an important area for consideration, since any procedure carried out on a patient should be in that patient's best interests and decisions should be ethically based (Stone & Matthews 1996). Written consent is useful and, whilst not absolutely necessary other than as a record of what has been discussed, it may provide evidence of warnings given if there were to be a complaint about the practitioner afterwards.

Practitioners should not proceed with any therapy without at least verbal consent being given. Parental consent is required for children under 16 years of age, unless the therapist is absolutely sure that the child has sufficient maturity of understanding to be able to give informed consent. It is therefore important that the therapist offers information in a way that is unambiguous and comprehensible to the child so that the patient is 'informed'. Treatment should then include only what has been agreed. Children between 16 and 18 years have the statutory right to consent to medical and dental treatment as though they were adults; this may apply to complementary therapies, but has never been tested in a court of law.

'Consent should be viewed as an ongoing, dynamic process, which recognises the patient's ongoing co-operation and willingness to participate in treatment' (Stone & Matthews 1996).

A brief explanation of the therapies
Aromatherapy

Aromatherapy involves the use, for therapeutic effects, of concentrated aromatic or essential oils extracted from botanical sources, such as leaves, flowers, bark, berries, roots. René Gattefosse coined the term *aromatherapy* at the beginning of this century, but oils and herbs have been used for thousands of years for medicinal purposes (Rankin-Box 1995). The oils are used to treat the whole person. They can be applied in a variety of ways including massage, inhalation, compresses, creams, lotions, baths. They are very concentrated they should be diluted in a carrier oil or so cream/lotion before administration to the skin.

It is suggested that beneficial effects arise through activity in the limbic area of the brain, which is concerned with memory and emotion (Greer & Moorey 1992). The therapeutic properties of essential oils are thought to relate to responses to the chemical constituents (Price & Price 1995). There are possible harmful effects associated with some constituents and the use of oils that contain them may therefore be contraindicated in certain conditions, such as pregnancy or epilepsy.

Shenton (1996) identified the following conditions as benefiting from aromatherapy:

- stress-related conditions
- migraines
- sleeping problems
- skin problems
- pain
- anxiety
- constipation (Emly 1993)
- infections.

Some essential oils are toxic under certain conditions whilst others may cause skin sensitivities. It is important, therefore, that whoever uses the oils has a sound knowledge base and is accountable for their use. They are not the panacea for all ills and should be used with caution by appropriately qualified practitioners. It is important that the recipient likes the smell, because, by virtue of its links with the limbic system, it may evoke memories or emotional reactions or put in place memories for the future – either positive or negative. This is an important consideration in such areas as haematology/oncology where smells may be negatively associated with, for example, chemotherapy and may cause problems for the child and carers if they come into contact with the same smell at a later stage.

The dilutions need to be very much higher for children and even more so in newborn and preterm infants (Tisserand & Balacs 1995), who have fewer layers of epidermis than an older child or adult. The choice of oils is more limited in the younger age group because of the possibility of adverse reactions to some of the constituents of particular oils. This also has implications for the mode of administration. In-depth knowledge of oil derivation, constituents and actions is essential. Likewise, it is necessary to have a good knowledge of anatomy and physiology in order to understand the implications of application, e.g. the structure and development of infant skin, excretory capabilities of the immature kidney, the dynamics of dysfunctional systems, musculoskeletal splinting of an injured or unstable area.

Carrier oils are also of considerable importance, not least because of their varied therapeutic qualities and also their varying dermal uptake (Price & Price 1995). It would appear from anecdotal evidence that some hospitals will only allow the use of arachis (groundnut) oil as a carrier oil. If there is a risk of nut allergy it would seem sensible to use something like grapeseed oil instead.

Therapeutic massage

This healing art involves the use of touch in a formalised way using hands, elbows, feet, knees (Horrigan 1995) to bring about changes in soft tissues and circulation, and to promote a range of physiological and psychological effects, such as reduction in anxiety (Paterson 1990), relief of muscle tension, warmth, and pain relief (Fritz 1995). Massage is probably one of the oldest therapies known to man, but it is only in the last 150 years that it has become more formalised into the methodologies we know today. Massage offers a means of communicating through caring touch that is very different from the 'clinical' touch associated with much of nursing (Estabrooks 1992).

The beneficial effects of massage are well researched and recognised, but there are instances when caution needs to be exercised. For example, massage has been shown to improve the outcome for neonates in terms of weight gain, length of stay in hospital and subsequent development (Field et al 1986). It has also been shown to reduce cortisol (stress) levels (Acolet et al 1993). But it is also important that therapists recognise that preterm infants may be hypersensitive to touch and handling. Nerve pathways and pain modulation in the neonate need to be considered (Melzack & Wall 1994). It may be inappropriate for some neonates to receive massage.

Permission from a child may be acquired through nonverbal means and it is important to identify this (Russell 1993). For example, babies who have had a difficult delivery or received numerous heel pricks may reject or become distressed by specific contact, which may appear as a threat. Babies should always be approached with respect and openness and if a baby demonstrates, by means of facial expressions or other body language, that the contact is too close, that must be respected. It may be appropriate to make contact via another part of the body.

Careful assessment of need is required together with awareness of body language (Horgan et al 1996). A child who has a disordered perception of touch, as in abuse, is someone on whom massage must be used with extreme caution, if at all.

Reflexology/reflex zone therapy

Gentle pressure is applied to different parts of the body, particularly the hands and feet, to stimulate different systems and organs of the body. It is suggested that there are reflex zones, running in specific lines through the body, which are reflected on the surface of the hands and feet, and that by stimulating them through specific touch one can promote health and well-being (Griffiths 1995). It can be used very successfully in inducing a state of relaxation in an anxious person, in lowering blood pressure, in relieving distressing complaints such as constipation, or in improving sinus congestion, to name but a few benefits.

When working with children there is a general rule of thumb that they cannot tolerate the same length or depth of treatment as an adult (Bayly 1982). It is important to note that the therapy is not without its contraindications and a practitioner should be cognisant of these.

Therapeutic touch (TT)

This is defined as 'an energy field interaction between two or more people, aimed at re-balancing or re-patterning the energy field to promote relaxation and pain relief and activate self-healing' (Sayre-Adams & Wright 1995).

It is a therapy based on principles of quantum physics and the notion that we interact with our environment in an 'energetic' way. The view was promoted by Martha Rogers who suggested that human beings may be seen as dynamic energy fields, whole entities, not to be viewed in terms of their parts (Sayre-Adams & Wright 1995). Dr Dolores Krieger, formerly Professor of Nursing in New York University, studied and researched the particular method of 'laying on of hands' and coined the term 'therapeutic touch'. The therapist incorporates non-contact touch with a high degree of 'centredness' to promote balance and well-being. 'Intention' is at the core of the TT process and has been termed a 'healing meditation' (Sayre-Adams & Wright 1995). Studies have shown the healing potential of TT (Wirth et al 1993) and it has been a recognised part of nurse education in the USA for a number of years.

Bach flower remedies

During the early part of this century, Dr. Edward Bach, physician and bacteriologist, identified 38 flower remedies, one for each of the most common negative moods or states of mind. Bach flower remedies derive from non-poisonous wild flowers and act as a form of supportive therapy used to establish equilibrium and harmony through the personality, addressing such behaviours as fear, envy, jealousy, guilt, self-recrimination, rigidity of attitude, intolerance, impatience, procrastination, self-pity, and so on (Challoner 1990).

In order to store the essences, the remedies are preserved in brandy. They should be taken in non-carbonated spring water – although they can be taken neat. Dilution particularly applies to children who would probably find the effect of alcohol on the tongue too strong and unpleasant. Parents must be aware of the alcohol content of the remedies, but since only two to four drops are used at a time it should not be a problem for most parents to accept. Rescue remedy – a combination of five remedies – which offsets the effects of shock and severe anxiety and distress, calming the individual by 'quietening' the autonomic nervous system in response to shock, is probably one of the most useful of all the remedies.

Craniosacral therapy

This very gentle therapy involves the use of specific touch and holding techniques on different parts of the person's clothed body and 'listening' to the quality of that individual's expression of health in the tissues. It is based on the work of the osteopath Dr William Garner Sutherland, who believed that the body has within it a 'life force' which is considered to be the basic ordering and healing principle of the human body, and that the body has a way of expressing its health at all levels within the body. The therapy is the art of listening to the body's own story – its own intrinsic rhythms, movement patterns and patterns of congestion and resistance (Sills 1998). By forming a deep, intuitive 'relationship' with the child, the therapist can encourage release of resistances (tensions), whatever their origin, for example from birth trauma or accidents, in the tissues of the body.

Visualisation and guided imagery

Creative visualisation is the technique of using one's imagination to create pictures of a desired outcome (Grant 1993). One does this in daily life, but in this context it is done in a very focused way. Visualisation can be used as a means of handling a difficult situation more easily (Ryman 1995), such as prior to venepuncture. It is a form of relaxed, focused concentration and is a natural and powerful coping mechanism. It can be easily learned and used as an adjunct to the care of toddlers and preschool children, as well as older children, who are experiencing anxiety and pain (Bullock & Shaddy 1993, Ott 1996).

There are important steps that should be taken in preparation for the visualisation, which involves the therapist being very relaxed, 'centred' and focused on the child and his needs; the parents should be informed of goals and permission for the visualisation obtained; the therapist should have an open and honest relationship with the child about the visualisation, listen to any expressed concerns and then help the child to refocus his anxiety on the goals and images.

However, this is not a treatment to be used with those who are experiencing emotional instability. It can be harmful to those who are freely dissociating or acutely psychotic (Ott 1996). But it can be used to teach the child and parents relaxation techniques and to enable the child to cooperate with treatment, for example immunisations, venepuncture, bone marrow aspirations, biopsies or radiotherapy (Decker & Cline-Elsen 1992). It can improve self-esteem by enabling children to see themselves as having coped positively with a difficult situation.

Hypnotherapy

This is the conscious use of an altered level of consciousness or state of deep relaxation through suggestion to enhance the sense of health and well-being (Rankin-Box 1995). It may be used as a self-care technique in the management of difficult situations (Contach et al 1985), such as in pain management, reducing anxiety and phobias, and it has many potential benefits in child care. Whether it can be used effectively in the clinical setting depends largely on the clients' willingness to manage their own health care (Rankin-Box 1995).

The 'clinical' environment

Some therapies can, in part, be taught either to the child or the parent/carer and so encourage sharing, a sense of responsibility towards the child's own health, empowerment and positive coping mechanisms (Ott 1996). Consideration should be given to the environment in which therapies can be offered in terms of quiet, freedom from outside distraction where possible, privacy, lighting, warmth and so on.

They can be offered in a variety of settings:

- at home – by parents, dually qualified children's community nurses, play specialists, physiotherapists, occupational therapists, etc.
- in hospital wards
- in hospital departments, such as accident and emergency, or outpatient clinics
- general practice surgeries
- hospices
- schools and nurseries.

Conclusion

Complementary therapies have much to offer in health care settings and has the potential to encourage trust and coping behaviours in children and their carers (Pederson 1994). To apply them effectively requires sound education and skills acquisition through accredited organisations, together with access to supervision by experienced practitioners. The personal development that accompanies this learning can flourish with encouragement, experience and reflection. The health care arena is challenging to the complementary practitioner, but it offers an ideal setting for collaboration, evaluation and advanced patient care.

Useful addresses

Aromatherapy Organisations Council (AOC)
3 Latymer Close
Braybrooke
Market Harborough LE16 8LL
Tel: 01455 615 466

Association of Reflexologists
27 Old Gloucester Street
London WC1 3XX
Tel: 0171 237 5623

British Holistic Medical Association (BHMA)
179 Gloucester Place
London NW1 6DX
Tel: 0171 262 5299

British Hypnotherapy Association
1 Wythburn Place
London W1H 5W1
Tel: 0171 262 8852/0171 723 4443

Post graduate Medical Centre for Complementary
Medicine
University of Exeter
25 Victoria Road
Exeter EX2 4NT
Tel: 01932 264493

Craniosacral Therapy Education Trust
The Administrator
10 Normington Close
Leigham Court Road
London SW16 2QS
Tel/Fax: 07000 785778

Accredited courses for registered nurses, midwives and pharmacists

Council for Complementary and Alternative Medicine
(CCAM)
179 Gloucester Place
London NW1 6DX

Institute for Complementary Medicine (ICM)
PO Box 194
London SE16 1QZ

International Federation of Aromatherapists (IFA)
Department of Continuing Education
Royal Masonic Hospital
London W6 0TN
Tel: 0181 846 8066

Natural Medicines Society (NMS)
Edith Lewis House
Ilkeston
Derbyshire DE7 8EJ

Research Council for Complementary Medicine
(RCCM)
60 Great Ormond Street
London WCIN 3JF
Tel: 0171 833 8897

References

Acolet et al 1993 Changes in plasma cortisol and catecholamine concentrations in response to massage in preterm infants. Archives of Disease in Childhood 68(1 suppl): 29–31

Barnes J, Ernst E 1997 Complementary medicine. (Letter) British Journal of General Practice 47(418): 329

Bayly D 1982 Reflexology today – the stimulation of the body's healing forces through foot massage. Thorsons, England

Bullock E A, Shaddy R E 1993 Relaxation and imagery techniques without sedation during right ventricular endomyocardial biopsy in pediatric heart transplant patients. Journal of Heart and Lung Transplantation 39: 215–217

Challoner P M 1990 Illustrated handbook of the Bach flower remedies. C W Daniel, England

Contach P, Hockenbury M, Herman S 1985 Self-hypnosis as anti-emetic therapy in children receiving chemotherapy. Oncology Nurses Forum 12: 41–46

Decker T W, Cline-Elsen J 1992 Relaxation therapy as an adjunct in radiation oncology. Journal of Clinical Psychology 48: 388–393

Emly M 1993 Abdominal massage. Nursing Times 89(3): 34–36

Ernst E 1997 Complementary AIDS therapy: the good, the bad and the ugly. (Editorial) International Journal of STD and AIDS 8(5): 281–285

Estabrooks C A 1992 Toward a theory of touch: the touching process and acquiring a touching style. Journal of Advanced Nursing 17: 448–456

Field T, Schönberg S M, Scafidi M S et al 1986 Tactile/kinesthetic stimulation effects on pre-term neonate. Pediatrics 7(5): 654–658

Fritz S 1995 Fundamentals of therapeutic massage. Mosby Lifeline, USA

Gabe J, Kellerher D, Williams G 1994 Challenging medicine. Routledge, London

Grant B 1993 A–Z of natural healthcare. Optima Books, London

Greer S, Moorey S 1992 Adjuvant psychological therapy for patients with cancer: a prospective randomised trial. British Medical Journal 304: 675–679

Griffiths P 1995 Reflexology. In: Rankin-Box D (ed) The nurses' handbook of complementary therapies. Churchill Livingstone, Edinburgh, pp 133–140

Harrison J 1995 An introduction to aromatherapy for people with learning disabilities. British Journal of Learning Disabilities 23: 37–40

Horgan M, Choonara I et al 1996 Measuring pain in neonates: an objective score. Paediatric Nursing 8(10): 24–27

Horrigan C 1995 Massage. In: Rankin-Box D (ed) 1995 The nurses' handbook of complementary therapies. Churchill Livingstone, Edinburgh

Lupton D 1994 Medicine as culture – illness, disease and the body in western medicine. Sage Publications, London

Melzack R, Wall P 1994 Textbook of pain. Churchill Livingstone, Edinburgh

Nicoll L 1995 Complementary therapies and nurse education – the need for specialist teachers. Complementary Therapies in Nursing and Midwifery 1(3): 60–72

Ott M J 1996 Imagine the possibilities! Guided imaging with toddlers and preschoolers. Pediatric Nursing 22(1): 34–38

Paterson L 1990 Baby massage in the neonatal unit. Nursing 4(23): 19–21

Pederson C 1994 Ways to feel comfortable: teaching aids to promote children's comfort. Issues in Comprehensive Pediatric Nursing 17: 37–46

Price S, Price L 1995 Aromatherapy for health professionals. Churchill Livingstone, Edinburgh

Rankin-Box D (ed) 1995 The nurses' handbook of complementary therapies. Churchill Livingstone, Edinburgh

Russell J 1993 Touch and infant massage. Paediatric Nursing 5(3): 8–11

Ryman L 1995 Relaxation and visualisation In: Rankin-Box D (ed) The nurses' handbook of complementary therapies. Churchill Livingstone, Edinburgh, pp 141–149

Sayre-Adams J, Wright S 1995 The theory and practice of therapeutic touch. Churchill Livingstone, Edinburgh

Sharma U 1992 Complementary medicine today. Tavistock/Routledge, London

Shenton D 1996 Does aromatherapy provide an holistic approach to palliative care? International Journal of Palliative Nursing 2(4): 187–191

Sills F 1998 Biodynamic and biokinetic forces. Rhythm News Journal, Craniosacral therapy association, London

Smith I 1995 Commissioning complementary therapies. British Medical Journal 3(10): 1151–1152

Stone J, Matthews J 1996 Complementary medicine and the law. Oxford University Press, Oxford

Tisserand R, Balacs T 1995 Essential oil safety – a guide for health care professionals. Churchill Livingstone, Edinburgh

Wirth J T et al 1993 Full thickness dermal wounds treated with non-contact therapeutic touch: a replication and extension. Complementary Therapies in Medicine 1: 127–132

Index